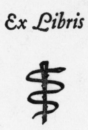

*The Pulmonary Circulation
in Health and Disease*

Academic Press Rapid Manuscript Reproduction

The Pulmonary Circulation in Health and Disease

Edited by

James A. Will
Department of Anesthesiology
Medical School and Department of Veterinary Science
College of Agricultural and Life Sciences
University of Wisconsin
Madison, Wisconsin

Christopher A. Dawson
Department of Physiology
Medical College of Wisconsin
Milwaukee, Wisconsin

E. Kenneth Weir
Cardiovascular Section
Veterans Administration Medical Center and Department of Medicine
University of Minnesota Medical School
Minneapolis, Minnesota

Carl K. Buckner
School of Pharmacy
Division of Pharmacology and Toxicology
University of Wisconsin
Madison, Wisconsin

1987

ACADEMIC PRESS, INC.
Harcourt Brace Jovanovich, Publishers

Orlando   San Diego   New York   Austin
Boston   London   Sydney   Tokyo   Toronto

ACADEMIC PRESS, INC.
Orlando, Florida 32887

United Kingdom Edition published by
ACADEMIC PRESS INC. (LONDON) LTD.
24–28 Oval Road, London NW1 7DX

LIBRARY OF CONGRESS CATALOG CARD NUMBER: 87-47723

ISBN 0–12–752085–6 (alk. paper)

PRINTED IN THE UNITED STATES OF AMERICA

87 88 89 90   9 8 7 6 5 4 3 2 1

Contents

Preface

Most previous symposia have addressed particular aspects of the pulmonary circulation, such as specific disease entities (primary pulmonary hypertension, hypoxic pulmonary vasoconstriction) or the role of a particular mediator or ion. It was the intent of this symposium to bring together an interdisciplinary group of acknowledged experts in order to create a more complete picture of the pulmonary circulation under normal and diseased conditions. We chose to include various aspects of the physiology (including hemodynamics and endothelial function), morphology, and pharmacology of the lung on which to base further presentations. Included are specific discussions on the relationship between gas exchange and blood flow through the lung, the mechanisms of pulmonary hypertension, and causes of clinical pulmonary hypertension (including epidemiology, management of pulmonary thromboembolism, and exogenous influences).

This book is primarily directed to basic scientists studying the lung, and clinicians such as cardiologists and pulmonologists. It should also be of interest to anyone confronted with the effects of alterations in lung function. It is clear that changes in the lung can affect virtually every other organ system whether directly or through complex interactions. Knowledge of the pulmonary circulation and these interactions is scattered and unfocused. We hope that this book will pull together and clarify the role of this secondary circulation.

JAMES A. WILL
CHRISTOPHER A. DAWSON
E. KENNETH WEIR
CARL K. BUCKNER

Acknowledgments

A symposium and a book like this cannot occur without the help and cooperation of the organizing committee and every speaker and chairman. The presentations by these participants were outstanding and I'm certain that you will find their chapters concise and informative. I am deeply indebted to all of these people who made this venture a success. My only regrets are that we had to disappoint some people and could not extend offers to them to present invited lectures. I apologize to those who feel left out; I am certain their contributions would have been valuable additions. I consider it a privilege to have been the director of this program. I hope that our time for programs focusing on the interdisciplinary aspects of the pulmonary circulation is not past and that we may bring together an equally dedicated group in the future.

I want to thank my family for being patient with me as I agonized over the difficulties in pulling together the financial support. It is relevant at this time to thank all of the contributors, who generously supported the symposium; the pharmaceutical companies; the Graduate and Medical Schools of the University of Wisconsin, who provided the seed funding; the Department of Anesthesiology of the Medical School, who understood my problems and cooperated to help whenever necessary; my secretaries, program assistant, and student employees, who helped whenever things got out of hand; and the Anesthesiology Department of the Medical College of Wisconsin, which stood by to help me financially if needed. Without these friends, we could not have reached our goals.

Finally, I want to thank my daughter, Lorna, whose expertise in editing and producing these chapters on a Macintosh computer contributed to the ultimate success of this volume.

J.A.WILL

The financial supporters of this symposium and book are listed below in alphabetical order:

Anaquest
Burroughs Wellcome Fund
The Council for Tobacco Research, Inc.-USA
Glaxo, Inc.
ICI Americas
Key Pharmaceuticals, Inc.
McNeil Pharmaceutical
Roerer Group, Inc.
Roerig
Smith, Kline and Beckman
The University of Wisconsin Graduate School
The University of Wisconsin Medical School
The Upjohn Company
Wyeth Laboratories, Inc.

EDITOR'S NOTE

The organizing committee and editors of this book wish to express special thanks to the Journal of Critical Care (Grune & Stratton, Inc., Harcourt Brace Jovanovich, Publisher) Editor-in-Chief David R. Dantzker, for the publication of the abstracts of posters presented at this symposium (Vol. 1, no. 2, June 1986). Many of the section summaries reflect information published in these abstracts and presented as posters.

Morphology

An Overview of the Microscopic Appearance of the Pulmonary Artery and the Problems of Its Quantitation

WILLIAM M. THURLBECK[1]
Department of Pathology
University of British Columbia
Vancouver, B.C., Canada

I. INTRODUCTION

This chapter will briefly discuss the microscopic anatomy of the human pulmonary arterial system. It will emphasise problems in quantitation and expression of data that exist at present, and how various authors have attempted to circumvent these. It is meant as an introduction to the paper by Dr. Wagenvoort, who, with his vast experience in the pathology of the pulmonary vascular system, will attempt to solve some of the problems that will be raised. I will also briefly outline some findings in the pulmonary arterial system in the National Institutes of Health (NIH) Nocturnal Oxygen Therapy Trial (NOTT), which illustrate well some of the problems.

Interest in the anatomy and pathology of the human pulmonary arteries became great in the 1950's when surgery for cardiac valvular disease lead to interest in arterial changes in mitral stenosis. Cardiac surgery for congenital heart disease further increased this interest, and special emphasis was placed on lesions that might indicate reversibility or otherwise of pulmonary hypertension. The classical grading system of Heath and Edwards was introduced (1). More contemporary

[1]*Supported by Grant # MT-7124, Medical Research Council of Canada, and a grant from the British Columbia Heart Association.*

The Pulmonary Circulation
in Health and Disease

3

interest has been aroused by the suggestion that intra-operative lung frozen sections may be important in guiding cardiac surgery (2). This topic will be amplified by Dr. Langston later in this chapter.

II.   PROBLEMS OF QUANTITATION AND DESCRIPTION

A.   The problem of vasoconstriction, and attempts at its solution

If vasoconstriction persists in the post-mortem interval, vessels may be falsely classified into vessels of a smaller order. The classic example is in the smallest arteries (less than 100 μm) that are generally non-muscular. If constriction of vessels of 100 μm and larger occurs, they will appear as the vessels of the smaller set. Since arteries more than 100 μm in diameter are usually muscular, their false inclusion may lead to the conclusion that there is abnormal development of muscle in the smallest arteries.

The reality, and the extent, of putative persistent vasoconstriction post-mortem is not known with certainty. One approach has been to distend the pulmonary arteries at high pressure so that all vessels dilate fully, and Reid's laboratory has been the chief proponent of this technique (3). Rabinovitch *et al.* (2), working in her laboratory, have indicated that medial thickness of the pulmonary arteries may be two and a half times as large in undistended arteries compared to distended arteries. Others have found a smaller change — an increase in thickness of media to wall ratio of 7.8% (4) and a decrease in lumen diameter of 0.34 to 0.30 mm and an increase in medial thickness of 0.09 to 0.095 mm in non-distended arteries compared to distended ones has been reported (5). These differences are not statistically significant. Another approach is to correct mathematically for the effect of vasoconstriction (6). This model assumes that the internal elastic lamina is circular in cross section when fully distended. The length of the crenated lamina is measured as seen in the undistended specimen and the circumference and diameter as a circle then calculated. The area of the media is measured and assumed to remain constant whether constricted or not. The thickness of the media when the artery is fully distended can then be easily calculated, from its area and the new diameter calculated from the internal elastica. This technique was modestly time consuming and difficult, but is now done much more quickly and easily with the use of computer-assisted digitizers. A third approach uses a similar assumption that medial area remains constant. It has been shown that the external adventitial diameter (from adventitial margin to adventitial margin) of the bronchovascular sheath is independent of vascular distension (5), although of course dependent on intrabronchial inflation. Under these circumstances, the ratio of medial or intimal area to total vessel area (marked at the edge of the adventitia and/or halfway betwen the arterial wall and bronchial wall) can be easily calculated (7). Whether the lumen area should be subtracted from total vessel area to give total tissue area is not clear. Theoretically, a smaller area is subtracted for total vascular area in the case of vasoconstriction, making the denominator larger and the ratio smaller.

Finally, vessel dimensions and thickness (or area) can be measured at marker structures, such as terminal bronchioles or respiratory bronchioles (8). This is particularly useful in infants and children where corresponding orders of vessel will normally be smaller than in adults.

The problems of morphometry of the pulmonary arterial system are further discussed by Langston and Holder in this chapter.

B.   Problems of counting

The number of arteries has been counted per unit area (2,9) and abnormalities found in disease states. The problem is that one is interested in the number per unit volume and the number per unit area is, in a sense, an optical illusion. This is because the number of structures per unit area (N_A) is related to the number per unit volume (N_V) as follows (10):

$$N_V = N_A^{3/2}/B \cdot V_{VS}$$

where B is the shape constant describing the ratio between the volume of the structure of interest and its average cross sectional area, and V_{VS} is the volume proportion that structure, s, forms of the whole organ.

When re-written:

$$N_{Aart}^{3/2} = N_{Vart} \cdot B \cdot V_{Vart}$$

Hence the number seen in two dimensions is dependent not only on N_{Vart} but also the shape constant and the volume proportion of the arteries. With constriction, the shape constant may change dramatically as the length:diameter ratio of the artery increases and will also change as the volume proportion of arteries decreases.

C.   Problem of different artery sizes

It is by no means certain that arteries of different sizes have the same thickness to diameter ratio, or muscle area to external elastic area or external adventitial area. It may be that, say, vessels 100-150 μm are different in medial or intimal thickness from vessels 150-200 μm in diameter. It may also be that vessels of different sizes respond differently to disease conditions. With modern computer processing, this problem may be easily and quickly solved, provided vasoconstriction is not a major problem. For example, we have a programme in which one touches the images of the lumen margin, internal elastica, external elastica and external adventitia. Calculations are made of appropriate thickness (intima, media, adventita) and placed in sets of 50 or 100 μm in diameter of either external elastic diameter or external adventitial diameter and the data, including statistics, processed automatically. The various areas can also be calculated by tracing the perimeter of the boundaries and dealt with in a similar fashion.

D.   The problem of normative data

It is generally taken for granted that control subjects should be without heart or lung disease. An important variable is smoking. It has long been known that smokers have increased intimal thickness (11), and more prominent bands of longitudinal muscle cells in the intima (12). These observations have been extended to show increased numbers of transected arteries less than 200 μm in diameter, increased medial muscle and intimal thickness in smokers (9). Others have shown that the proportion of intimal area was increased in smokers, and was more severe in patients with moderate compared to mild emphysema (7).

III.   THE NIH NOTT TRIAL

Lungs were available from 33 patients who entered this study. All had chronic airflow obstruction with a resting PO_2 of less than 60 mmHg and had no significant other disease. The average of death was 67 years. The first problem was the controls. Some 1400 autopsy cases were on file that had a detailed smoking history, autopsy report and paper-mounted whole lung sections. Only seven patients within this group met the criteria of having no chronic heart or lung disease (including chronic bronchitis) and had not smoked. Every measurement possible was made including intimal and medial thickness and area, and related to external elastica and external adventitial diameter and areas. The Yamaki correction was applied (6) and the internal diameter of the vessels measured. Vessels were placed in sets of 50 μm by external elastic diameter. All the measurements were closely inter-related. When the NOTT patients were compared to the controls, measurements of media were not significantly increased, whereas measurements of intima were. The changes were most marked in vessels 150-199 μm in diameter. The biggest difference between the groups was the intimal adventitia/total vascular area ratio (t = 8.01). The ratio of lumen diameter to external elastic diameter was as good as many of the other measurements (t = -7.49) in discriminating between the NOTT patients and the controls. A higher percentage of vessels less than 50 μm in diameter had well defined smooth muscle in the NOTT patients compared to the controls. Seven young controls (less than 50 years of age) were easier to find, and the difference between old and young controls was that the former had increased indices of medial enlargement, but no change in intimal variables. The value of lumen diameter to external elastic diameter was higher in the young controls. It may well be that this measurement, which is the easiest and quickest to make, is the most useful to study pulmonary arteries. In keeping with these observations, the mean lumen diameter to external elastic diameter ratio was significantly different between the groups, with values of 0.77 being found in the young controls, 0.67 in the old controls and 0.57 in the NOTT patients.

REFERENCES

1. Heath D and Edwards JE. (1958) *Circulation* **18**:533.
2. Rabinovitch M, Haworth SG, Castaneda AR, Nadas AS and Reid LM. (1978) *Circulation* **58**:1107.
3. Davies G and Reid L. (1970) *Thorax* **25**:669.
4. Wagenvoort CA. (1960) *Circulation* **22**:535.
5. Berend N, Woolcock AJ and Marlin GE. (1979) *Thorax* **34**:354.
6. Yamaki S and Tezuka F. (1976) *Circulation* **54**:805.
7. Wright JL, Lawson L, Pare PD, Hooper RO, Peretz DI, Nelems JM, Schulzer M and Hogg JC. (1983) *Am Rev Respir Dis* **128**:702.
8. Reid LM. (1979) *Am Rev Respir Dis* **119**:531.
9. Hale KA, Niewoehner DE and Cosio MG. (1980) *Am Rev Respir Dis* **122**:272.
10. Weibel ER. (1963) **Morphometry of the Human Lung.** Academic Press:New York.
11. Auerbach OA, Stout AP, Hammond EC and Garfinkel L. (1963) *N Engl J Med* **269**:1045.
12. Naeye RL and Dellinger WS. (1971) *Arch Pathol* **92**:284.
13. Nocturnal Oxygen Therapy Trial Group. (1980) *Ann Intern Med* **93**:391.

Innervation of the Pulmonary Circulation: An Overview

JOHN B. RICHARDSON
Montreal General Hospital
1650 Cedar Avenue
Montreal, Quebec Canada H3A 1A4

A description of the innervation to the pulmonary vessels was made three hundred years ago and at this time there was also speculation as to the function of these nerves (1). It was felt that the nerves had control over the calibre of both the vessels and the airways or, "those channels of inspired and expired blood and air" (1). It has since been assumed, more or less, that this general idea was true, but there exists a very incomplete understanding of the function of the pulmonary nerves, their anatomical distribution and their variation with different species. This is particularly true in the case of the human lung where little work has been done since the early detailed light microscopic studies (2-4). In the commonly used laboratory animals, the situation is also confused; this was clearly pointed out in a recent study on the rat lung which looked at the adrenergic system before and after the induction of pulmonary hypertension (5). The authors found the literature on the pulmonary innervation of the rat so contradictory that they had to clarify it themselves in the particular strain of rat they used before the experiments were started (5).

　　This review will attempt to briefly outline the autonomic pathways with their efferent components (the adrenergic, the cholinergic and the noncholinergic-nonadrenergic neural pathways) and then discuss the evidence for afferent reflex systems in the lung vasculature, which are probably similar in their complexity to those found in the airways and also as poorly understood. Studies on the human pulmonary vasculature have been hampered by the difficulty in obtaining the necessary vesssels in a viable state; this is similar to the situation in the human airways, where understanding of the innervation of the muscle, glands and

The Pulmonary Circulation
in Health and Disease

9

epithelium is not much ahead of that in the vasculature. The use of surgical and autopsy material, with suitable controls for the time interval from either removal or death, should remedy this situation. This is a very important point, as there are certainly species differences in the innervation and the pharmacology of the various parts of the pulmonary vasculature, and it is important that the human pattern be fully understood before extrapolations are made from animal models used to test various hypotheses.

The introduction of the fluorescent histochemical technique for the localization of catecholamines (6) led to numerous descriptions of the pulmonary innervation, and this technique combined with pharmacological methods for the depletion or augmentation of catecholamine stores has advanced our basic understanding of the roles of these nerves in the pulmonary vasculature (7-12). A detailed study of the dog lung showed adrenergic nerves in a dense pattern associated with the bronchial arteries (7), and in another study the pulmonary arteries and the larger veins were shown to have adrenergic nerves in their walls with the nerves localized to the adventitia and the outer aspect of the media of the arteries and the adventitia of the veins (8). Stimulation of the nerves, or infusion of norepinephrine led to an increased pressure in the vessels (8,13,14) and this response to stimulation was abolished by prior treatment with 6-OH-dopamine (8). Adrenergic nerves have also been described at the level of the capillaries, where their transmitter may act on pericytes (15). A comparative study of the adrenergic pulmonary vascular innervation of the rat and the monkey showed adrenergic innervation of all branches of the bronchial artery of the rat, but only in the small and medium bronchial arteries of the monkey. There was a difference in the distribution of the varicosities between the two, with varicosities ending on smooth muscle in the monkey, whereas in the rat the nerves passed through the smooth muscle without forming any varicosities (11). In the pulmonary artery there were adrenergic terminals in the adventio-medial junction only, while they were located in the media in the rat. In the pulmonary vein there were terminals in all pulmonary vein divisions in the monkey, whereas in the rat the veins lacked adrenergic nerves (8). In both the rat and the monkey there was a preponderance of adrenergic nerves in the vasa vasorum which has been suggested as a means of delivery of humoral agents to the vascular wall (11). In another study of the rat there was adrenergic innervation in the pulmonary vein, bronchial arteries and vasa vasorum of the larger pulmonary arteries and veins (5). No adrenergic innervation of the main pulmonary trunk was found, despite the rich innervation of the vasa vasorum (5). The axial pulmonary artery and its thick walled muscular branches were also devoid of adrenergic innervation although the vasa vasorum showed such innervation (5). When the pulmonary vasculature was examined after the production of pulmonary hypertension, the pattern of adrenergic innervation was found to be identical to the control animals; this was felt to be evidence that the changes in the smooth muscle which occur with hypoxia are independent of the presence of adrenergic nerves and not related to the innervation as had been suggested from studies on other vessels (15-18). The pulmonary vasculature of the cat has also been shown to have adrenergic innervation (9,19).

It is evident from the above discussion that controversy exists as to the innervation of the arteries and veins in the lung, and this is further complicated by the demonstration of a change in the innervation pattern with development from fetal to adult states, where adrenergic fibers present in the fetal tissue were no longer present in the adult bronchial tissue (20). This latter study points out the problematic area of the developing lung, which has been little studied, and the possible differences which could occur in its innervation as the lung matures, a fact which must be considered when comparing adult to fetal situations (20). The human lung has not been studied for the distribution of adrenergic nerves in either the adult or the fetal lung. Such studies are needed before meaningful extra-polations of animal experiments can be made to such conditions as muscular hypertrophy and adrenergic nerves (5,16-18) or cerebrally induced hemorrhagic edema (21).

Many of the earlier studies on the innervation were performed with nonspecific silver stains for acetylcholinesterase, and thus the cholinergic system is more defined than that of the adrenergic (2-4, 22). It is not clear, however, what the role of the efferent cholinergic fibers are, although vagal stimulation has been shown to dilate the vessels (13). A recent study in the cat, which has cholinergic innervation in small and medium sized intrapulmonary arteries (19), showed that stimulation of the vagus dilated the pulmonary vascular bed by a direct muscarinic action on the vessels which was blocked by muscarinic antagonists and by ganglionic blocking agents (23). This study also showed that the action of acetylcholine was not mediated by lipoxygenase metabolites via the endothelium, as had been demonstrated *in vitro* in strips of vessel without the endothelium (24), and was consistent with other *in vitro* work which showed a direct action for acetylcholine (25).

Although there are species differences, rather definite patterns of pulmonary innervation are assumed (26). Sympathetic and parasympathetic fibers are found in close association with pulmonary vessels, but these are sparse when compared to the bronchial innervation (26). The innervation is highest in the elastic arteries and diminishes toward the periphery, which has been interpreted as suggesting that it has a role in vessel stiffness rather than resistance (26). Finally, most studies indicate that the pulmonary veins are devoid of innervation, and thus unlikely to be under autonomic control (26).

Morphological studies have shown innervation of the vessels, but it is not known if these fibers are efferent or afferent. It is well known that the majority of fibers in the vagus are afferent (27,28), and a recent study on the innervation of the bronchi in the mouse showed that the majority of the nerves to the airways are afferent (29), but to date no such studies have been performed in the pulmonary vasculature in regard to the cholinergic fibers. Stimulation of the vagus nerve has shown an initial vasoconstriction and, after the adrenergic receptors are blocked, a vasodilation (particularly in the fetus), so there are definite efferent pathways to the vessels (23). In addition to the direct efferent pathways, there are numerous reflexes which are not completely understood. These reflexes involve hypoxia, stretch in the pulmonary vessels, and cerebral stimulation (26). An interesting reflex is that which occurs when a pulmonary artery is occluded and distended by a balloon (33-36). This distension leads to a rise in pulmonary artery pressure which can be maintained for weeks. This reflex can be abolished by local anesthetics (33,35), surgical denervation (33,35), or treatment with 6-OH-dopamine (33,35), and can be reduced or abolished by administration of arachidonic acid (36). Such a reflex exists in sheep (37), ponies (34), and human infants (38). The purpose of this reflex remains unclear, but it does point to our lack of understanding of the role of afferent nerves in the pulmonary vasculature. Another important reflex is edema seen with cerebral lesions, and this problem has recently been fully reviewed (21). There is some evidence that adrenergic vasoconstriction may play a role in the permeability and the hemorrhage, although the principal vascular activity seems to be with the systemic vessels which constrict and increase the resistance enough to strain the left heart (21).

Numerous peptides have been identified in the nerves of the lung (39-42), and some of these peptides have been implicated in the control of the vasculature (40,42,43). Bombesin and vasoactive intestinal peptide (VIP) in particular have been proposed as modulators of the vascular tone, and there is evidence that they may have some effect on the vessels (40,42,44,45). It is not clear, however, if this effect is direct or indirect through the mediation of another substance which is formed such as prostaglandins. There has been little work on the third autonomic nervous system in the pulmonary vasculature, the noncholinergic nonadrenergic system. There is some evidence that it affects other vascular beds, and some indication that there may be an action in the cat lung as well (46). Some of the above peptides have been localized to the neuroendocrine cells and the neuroepithelial bodies, and it has been recently shown that these bodies are sensory in nature (47) and therefore could release these peptides when stimulated. Studies to date, however, have not confirmed that the peptides have a direct role in the control of the smooth muscle of the vasculature, although an indirect or modulating effect is certainly possible.

REFERENCES

1. Willis T. (1965) Facsimile of the anatomy of the brain and the description and uses of the nerves in the remaining medical works of that famous and renowned physician.(W. Feindel ed., from manuscript published in 1683 by Samuel Pordage, Esq.) McGill University Press:Montreal, **2**:163.
2. Larsell G and Dow RS. (1933) *Am J Anat* **52**:125.
3. Spencer H and Leof D. (1964) *J Anat (Lond)* **98**:599.
4. Gaylor JB. (1934) *Brain* **57**:143.
5. McLean JR, Twaros BM and Bergofsky EH. (1985) *J Auton Nerv Syst* **14**:111.
6. Falck B and Owman C. (1965) *Acta Universitatis Ludensis, Section 2: Medica Mathematica, Scientiœ rerum Naturaliun* **7**:1.
7. Fillens M. (1970) *J Anat* **106**:449.
8. Kadowitz PJ, Knight DS, Hibbs RG, Ellison JP, Joiner PD, Brody JH and Hyman AL. (1976) *Circ Res* **39**:191.
9. Cech S and Dolexel S. (1967) *Experientia* **23**:114.
10. El-Bermani AW, McNary WF and Bradley DE. (1970) *Anat Rec* **167**:205.
11. El-Bermani AW. (1978) *Thorax* **33**:167.
12. O'Donnell SR, Saar N and Wood LJ. (1978) *Clin Exp Pharmacol Physiol* **5**:325.
13. Paulet G and Le Bars R. (1969) *J Physiol (Paris)* **1**:160.
14. Aarseth P, Nicolaysen G and Waaler BA. (1971) *Acta Physiol Scand* **81**:448.
15. Tranzer JP, Thoenen H, Snipes RL and Richards JG. (1969) *Prog Brain Res* **31**:33.
16. Bevan RD, Purdy RE, Su C and Bevan JA. (1975) *Circ Res* **37**:503.
17. Hart MN, Heistad DD and Brody JM. (1980) *Hypertension* **2**:419.
18. Scott TM and Pang SC. (1983) *J Auton Nerv Syst* **8**:25.
19. Knight DS, Ellison JP, Hibbs RG, Hyman AL and Kadowitz P. (1981) *Anat Rec* **201**:513.
20. Hung KS. (1980) *Am J Anat* **159**:73.
21. Malik AB. (1985)*Circ Res* **57**:1.
22. Larsell O. (1922) *J Comp Neurol* **35**:97.
23. Nandiwada PA, Hyman AL and Kadowitz PJ. (1983)*Circ Res* **53**:86.
24. Furchgott RF and Zawadski JV. (1980) *Nature* **288**:373.
25. Chand N and Altura BM. (1981) *Science* **213**:1376.
26. Dowing SE and Lee JC. (1980) *Ann Rev Physiol* **42**:199.

27. Agostoni E, Chinnock JE, de Burgh Daly M and Murray JG. (1957) *J Physiol (Lond)* **135**:182.

28. Bartlett D, Mortola JP and Sant'Ambrosio G. (1977) *J Physiol (Lond)* **268**:36P.

29. Pack RJ, Al-Ugaily LH and Widdicome JG. (1984) *Cell Tissue Res* **238**:61.

30. Colebatch HJ, Dawes GS, Goodwin JW and Nadeau RA. (1965) *J Physiol (Lond)* **178**:544.

31. Dawes GS. (1966) *Br Med Bull* **22**:61.

32. Nuwayhid C, Brinkman BR, Su C, Bevan JA and Assali NS. (1975) *Biol Neonate* **26**:301.

33. Juratsch CE, Jengo J and Laks M. (1977) *Chest* **71**:265.

34. Juratsch CE, Manohar M, Hockett D, Laks M and Will JA. (1978) *Physiologist* :21.

35. Juratsch CE, Jengo J, Castangna J and Laks MM. (1980) *Chest* **77**:525.

36. Juratsch CE, Grover RF, Rose CE, Reeves JT, Walby WF and Laks MM. (1985) *J Appl Physiol* **58**:1107.

37. Juratsch CE, Emmanouilides G, Thibeault DW, Baylen BG, Jengo JA and Laks MM. (1980) *Pediatr Res* **14**:1332.

38. Baylen BG, Emmanouilides GC, Juratsch CE, Yoshida Y, French WJ and Criley JM. (1980) *J Pediatr* **96**:540.

39. Dey DA, Shannon WA and Said SI. (1981) *Cell Tissue Res* **220**:231.

40. Said SI. (1982) *Ann NY Acad Sci* **384**:207.

41. Polak JM and Bloom SR. (1982) *Exp Lung Res* **3**:313.

42. Cutz E, Gillian JE and Track NS. (1984) *In* **Endocrine Lung in Health and Disease** (KL Becker and AF Gazdar, eds) Saunders:Philadelphia.

43. Lauweryns JM, Cokelaere M, Lerut T and Theunynck P. (1978) *Cell Tissue Res* **193**:373.

44. Kulik TJ, Johnson DE, Niemi T, Fuhrman BP and Lock JE. (1982) *Pediatr Res* **16**:102A.

45. Hakanson R, Sundler F, Moghimzadeh E and Leander S. (1983) *Eur J Respir Dis* **64**:115.

46. Hamasaki Y and Said SI. (1984) *Nippon Heikatsukin Gakkai Zasshi* **20**:59.

47. Lauweryns JM, Van Lommel AT and Dom RJ. (1985) *J Neuro Sci* **67**:81.

The Pathology of Human Pulmonary Hypertension Pattern Recognition and Specificity

C. A. WAGENVOORT
Department of Pathology,
Erasmus University
3000 DR Rotterdam, The Netherlands

I. INTRODUCTION

It would be a mistake to believe that hypertensive pulmonary vascular disease is an entity. Just as the etiology of pulmonary hypertension is extremely varied, so is its morphology. The lesions, particularly of media and intima of pulmonary arteries as well as of pulmonary veins, and sometimes even alterations of the lung tissue, form characteristic patterns. To recognize these in autopsy or lung biopsy material is essential for establishing the type of hypertensive pulmonary vascular disease and sometimes its etiology (1). There are some 15 morphologic patterns of the pulmonary vasculature, mostly associated with an elevated pressure in the pulmonary circulation. Many of these are either very rare or obvious when the lung vessels are studied. There is no opportunity nor necessity to discuss all of these. However, there are six patterns that will concern us now. These include the common ones and also those that often produce difficulties and confusion even though some of them are distinctly uncommon.

A. Plexogenic arteriopathy

Plexogenic arteriopathy occurs in a variety of conditions *e.g.*, as a primary form and secondary to congenital heart disease with a left-to-right shunt, hepatic disease, anti-appetite drug intake and schistosomiasis. The pulmonary arterial lesions of this pattern consist of medial hypertrophy and muscularization of arterioles followed by cellular proliferation and concentric-laminar fibrosis of the intima. In later stages dilatation lesions, fibrinoid necrosis and plexiform lesions may develop.

B.   Thromboembolic arteriopathy

Thromboembolic arteriopathy, in most instances without significant medial hypertrophy but with patchy eccentric non-laminar intimal fibrosis which is frequently obstructive, though over short distances. Particularly its "silent" form may clinically be confused with primary plexogenic arteriopathy.

C.   Hypoxic arteriopathy

Hypoxic arteriopathy may be due to chronic upper airway obstruction or chronic bronchitis and emphysema. Similar vascular changes occur also in high altitude residents. These consist of media hypertrophy of small pulmonary arteries with muscularization of arterioles, while medium-sized and larger arteries may be normal. The intima of arteries may contain longitudinal smooth muscle bundles in small veins.

D.   Congestive arteriopathy

Congestive arteriopathy occurs in any condition in which there is a chronic impediment to pulmonary venous outflow, whether resulting from stenoses of large pulmonary veins, mitral valve disease, congestive heart failure or pressure on the veins from mediastinal fibrosis. In the arteries medial hypertrophy and intimal fibrosis are pronounced. The latter is eccentric, non-laminar, not obliterating and present over considerable distance. The pulmonary veins are affected by medial hypertrophy and arterialization and sometimes by mild to moderate intimal fibrosis. Often there are hemosiderosis and interstitial fibrosis of the lung tissue.

E.   Pulmonary veno-occlusive disease

Pulmonary veno-occlusive disease is an uncommon disorder characterized by fibrotic obstruction of, particularly, small pulmonary veins, although in about half of the cases arteries are affected as well (2). The lesions are likely to be post-thrombotic. Patchy areas of congestion and interstitial fibrosis complete the picture.

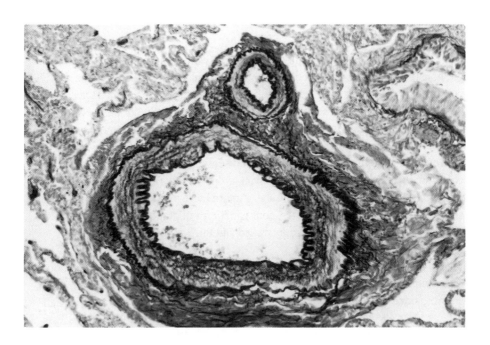

*Fig. 1. Medial hypertrophy of muscular pulmonary artery with
muscularization of a small branch, in a patient with ventricular septal defect.*

F.   Arteriopathy in lung fibrosis

Arteriopathy in lung fibrosisconsists of usually severe medial
hypertrophy and eccentric intimal fibrosis of pulmonary arteries as well as of
veins.

II.   PATTERN RECOGNITION

For the recognition of these patterns it is essential to know how specific
or characteristic the various vascular lesions are. Few vascular lesions are specific
on their own. However, combinations of lesions are either specific or at least
strongly suggestive of the type of pulmonary hypertension they are associated
with.

A.   Medial hypertrophy

Since medial hypertrophy of arteries as well as muscularization of previously non-muscular branches (Fig. 1) occurs in several forms of hypertensive pulmonary vascular disease, these changes are neither specific nor characteristic in themselves. Even so, the aspects of the arterial media should not be overlooked. If the medial thickness is normal in spite of proven significant pulmonary hypertension, it tends to exclude plexogenic and congestive arteriopathies. However, in patients with congenital heart disease and a left-to-right shunt, occasionally arteries with a normal or even atrophic media are found in the presence of a congenital stenosis of one or more large proximal pulmonary arteries. Also, as we will see later, confusion with dilatation lesions is possible, although then one would expect thin-walled and thick-walled arteries in combination.

In hypoxic pulmonary hypertension the arterial tree may be judged normal if attention is concentrated upon the easily detected medium-sized and larger arteries, since the lesions may well be confined to very small branches (Fig. 2).

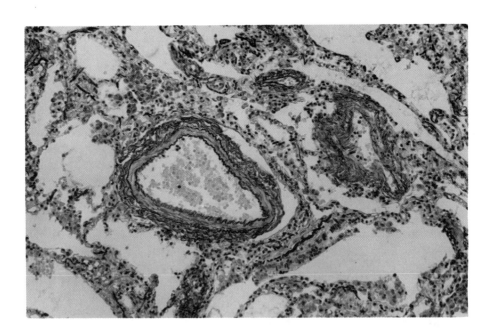

Fig. 2. Muscular pulmonary artery with normal media in a patient with Pickwickian syndrome and severe hypoxic pulmonary hypertension. Several small arterioles (arrows) are muscularized.

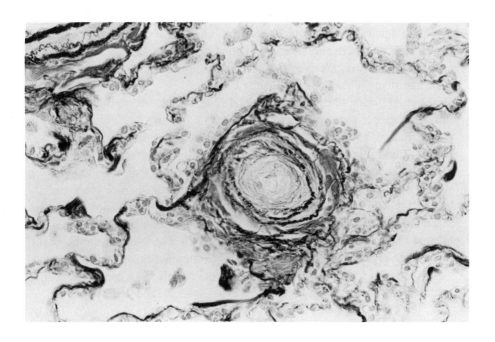

Fig. 3. Muscular pulmonary artery with concentric-laminar intimal fibrosis, in a patient with primary plexogenic arteriopathy.

It has often been maintained that no diagnosis is possible when increased arterial muscularity is the only alteration. Generally it is true that a diagnosis under these circumstances is hazardous. However, if medial hypertrophy is pronounced, if there are no other vascular lesions and if the pulmonary veins and the lung parenchyma are perfectly normal, plexogenic arteriopathy is the reasonable option.

B.   Intimal thickening

Intimal thickening of pulmonary arteries occurs in various types. Cellular intimal proliferation is suggestive of plexogenic arteriopathy while concentric-laminar intimal fibrosis (Fig. 3) is specific for this condition. The pathologist should not be led astray, however, by the occasional intimal lesions that mimic this type of intimal fibrosis such as the formation of a second muscular coat. Concentric-laminar intimal fibrosis should be distinct and preferably present, even in a biopsy specimen, in multiple arteries.

Eccentric intimal fibrosis, as we have seen, is found in several forms of hypertensive pulmonary vascular disease and is as such of little help. For a diagnosis of congestive arteriopathy it is good to keep in mind that in this condition it usually occurs over long stretches and particularly that it may cause severe narrowing of the lumen but hardly ever complete obliteration. Obviously, it is the combination of this type of intimal fibrosis with other lesions in pulmonary arteries and veins, that is decisive.

Eccentric intimal fibrosis resulting from organization of thrombi or thromboemboli (Fig. 4), though often obliterative, usually affects short stretches of the arterial wall. As a consequence, in any random histologic section it may be found in only few vessels, giving the impression that the resistance is not much elevated, while in fact numerous arteries are occluded, though at various levels. Recanalization, uncommon in other forms of intimal thickening, is regularly observed in post-thrombotic intimal fibrosis (Fig. 5). The intravascular fibrous septa may be regarded as pathognomonic for post-thrombotic lesions.

Bundles or layers of longitudinal smooth muscle fibers are common in eccentric intimal fibrosis but particularly in medium-sized and larger muscular

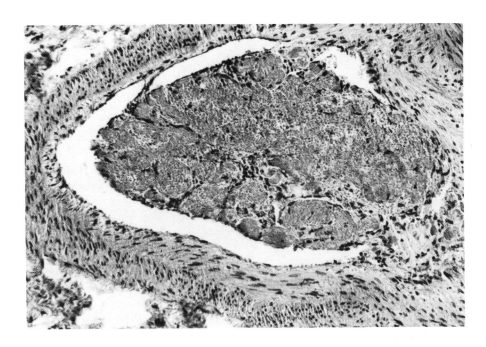

Fig. 4. Pulmonary artery with thromboembolus adherent to the wall and with early organization, in a patient with embolic pulmonary hypertension.

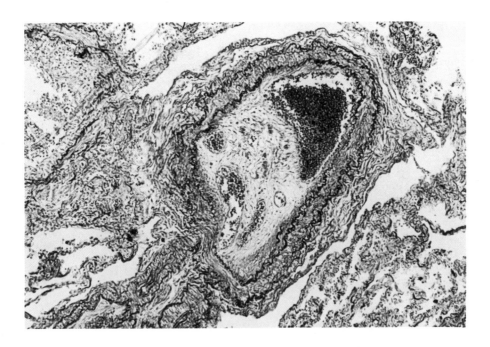

Fig. 5. Pulmonary artery with eccentric intimal fibrosis containing some
recanalization channels, in a patient with embolic pulmonary hypertension.

arteries. If they occur in muscularized arterioles it is suggestive that we are dealing
with chronic hypoxia (3). Occasionally such bundles are found in arterioles in
plexogenic arteriopathy (4).

C.   Combined changes

Severe alterations in the sense of medial hypertrophy and eccentric intimal
fibrosis in both arteries and veins occur in various forms of lung fibrosis or
granulomatosis. This means that confusion with congestive arteriopathy is easily
possible. Another problem is that such lesions, when found in a biopsy
specimen, may be taken as an indication of pulmonary hypertension, while in fact
the pressure may be normal. The reason is that the vascular changes are limited to
areas with fibrosis of lung tissue and therefore absent in normal lung fields. The
presence of pulmonary hypertension depends on the percentage of lung tissue
affected by fibrosis.

D.   Dilatation lesions

Dilatation lesions are characteristic of plexogenic arteriopathy but often difficult to identify unless they are numerous or form clusters of dilated vessels. Sometimes dilatation lesions can be taken for normal arteries. Fibrinoid necrosis is rarely found in conditions other than plexogenic arteriopathy but plexiform lesions (Fig. 6) are pathognomonic for this form of hypertensive pulmonary vascular disease. Of course, this is true for any lesion; the alteration must be typical enough for distinct identification.

E.   Venous changes

Changes in the pulmonary veins, particularly medial hypertrophy and arterialization (Fig. 7), generally indicate congestive arteriopathy. If intimal fibrosis in veins, including small veins, is severe and obliterative (Fig. 8) or when intravascular septa are formed by recanalization, pulmonary veno-occlusive disease should be considered (2).

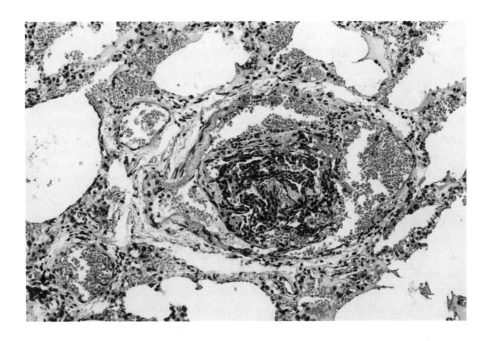

Fig. 6. Pulmonary arterial branch with a plexiform lesion, in a patient with ventricular septal defect.

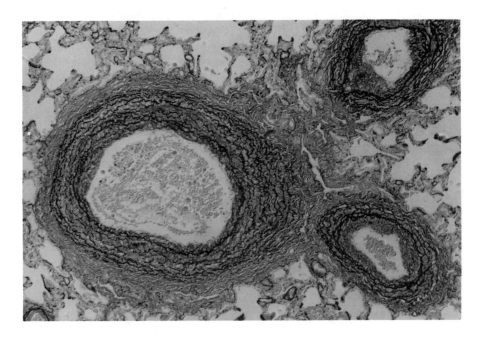

Fig. 7. Pulmonary veins with severe medial hypertrophy, arterialization and moderate intimal fibrosis, in a patient with mitral incompetence.

III.   DISCUSSION

Since few vascular changes in itself are pathognomonic for a certain form of hypertensive pulmonary vascular disease, it is clear that it is usually the combination of changes, including their eventual absence, which leads to the diagnosis. It should also be realized that it is not uncommon to find alterations belonging to different patterns at the same time. Sequelæ of occasional emboli may be found in hypoxic pulmonary hypertension and pulmonary venous changes may occur in plexogenic arteriopathy when cardiac failure develops in its late stages. Such combinations of patterns usually do not prevent an accurate diagnosis.

The significance of evaluation of the pulmonary vasculature in lung biopsy specimens is not limited to a classification. In cases of unexplained pulmonary hypertension it is often the only way to arrive at an exact diagnosis although unfortunately therapeutic measures are often unsatisfactory. An important point is whether the lesions in the lung vessels are reversible or not (5).

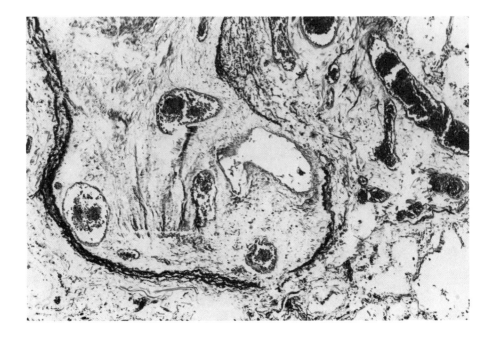

Fig. 8. Obliteration of pulmonary vein with some recanalization channels, in a patient with pulmonary veno-occlusive disease.

This applies particularly to plexogenic arteriopathy in patients with congenital cardiac disease, in whom the decision for corrective surgery may depend on the state of the pulmonary vasculature.

From a study (6) of such patients who underwent a banding procedure of the pulmonary artery and some years later a surgical correction of their cardiac defects, we now know something about the potential regression of the vascular changes. On both occasions a lung biopsy was carried out so that two specimens from each patient could be compared, one taken at the time that the lung vessels were exposed to a high pressure and one after the pressure had been considerably reduced.

It appeared that medial hypertrophy regressed distinctly, sometimes to normal. Cellular proliferation of the intima as well as the early stages of concentric-laminar intimal fibrosis also appeared to be reversible. However, when this type of intimal fibrosis was severe there was no regression but even progression of hypertensive vascular disease in spite of closure of a defect. The presence of fibrinoid necrosis and/or plexiform lesions had a similar ominous significance even though a fatal outcome was occasionally postponed for several years.

Regression of post-embolic lesions is limited in spite of recanalization. Complete obliteration of arteries apparently is not likely to be alleviated. In pulmonary veno-occlusive disease also it is unlikely that significant regression may be obtained. It is different with congestive arteriopathy. There are a few cases in which it was possible to compare the pulmonary vasculature in a biopsy specimen taken at the time of commissurotomy with that found at autopsy after the patient died of causes unrelated to his cardiac condition. From such cases it became clear that the often severe changes of congestive arteriopathy are largely reversible (7). Both medial and intimal thickness in these instances are influenced by interstitial edema and its removal may play a part in this regression. Little is known of morphologic regression of hypoxic pulmonary arteriopathy although experimental work suggests that the lesions are reversible to a large extent.

From this survey it may seem that there are few problems whenever an adequate open lung biopsy becomes available. To a certain extent this is true. The verdict "Pulmonary arteriopathy, unclassified" is fortunately unusual. But there is no rule without exceptions and sometimes the pathologist is confronted with a riddle that he is unable to solve. Even then a differential diagnosis, or the exclusion of certain possibilities, may be of some help to the clinician. If a decision for an open lung biopsy procedure has been made, the chance that the specimen will not provide useful information is indeed remote.

REFERENCES

1. Wagenvoort CA. (1980) *Chest* **77**:614.
2. Wagenvoort CA, Wagenvoort N and Takahashi T. (1985) *Human Path* **16**:1033.
3. Heath D. (1970) *Progr Resp Res* **5**:13.
4. Wagenvoort CA, Keutel J, Mooi WJ and Wagenvoort N. (1984) *Virchows Arch A* **404**:265.
5. Wagenvoort CA. (1985) *Histopathology* **9**:417.
6. Wagenvoort CA, Wagenvoort N and Draulans-Noë Y (1984) *J Thor Cardiovasc Surg* **87**:876.
7. Grimes ET and Abelman WH. (1968) *Amer J Med* **45**:975.

The Structure and Ultrastructure of the Pulmonary Microvasculature[1]

BARBARA MEYRICK
Vanderbilt University Medical Center
Pulmonary Circulation Center
Vanderbilt University Medical Center
Nashville, TN 37232

I. INTRODUCTION

There has been much discussion as to who first recognized that blood passed through the lungs during its circulation through the body — Servetus (1509-1553) or Columbus (1510-1599). Probably the first description to reach the West was that of Servetus in *Christianismi Restitutio* (1551) (1). He described how the blood passed from pulmonary artery to vein "by a lengthened passage through the lungs, in the course of which it becomes crimson in colour", and, "freed from fulginous vapours by the act of respiration." Harvey (1578-1657) is responsible for our modern understanding of circulation of the blood through the heart and lungs (2), although it was not until the advent of the light microscope that Malpighi (1628-1694) described the pulmonary capillary network (3).

Since these early descriptions of the pulmonary vascular bed our knowledge of the structure of the pulmonary circulation has vastly improved, through refinements in tissue preparation techniques and improved optics in the light microscopes. Additional insights were gained with the introduction of transmission and scanning electron microscopes.

[1]*Supported by Grants HL 19153 (SCOR in Pulmonary Vascular Research) and HL 340208.*

The following chapter falls into two parts. The first part is a description of the structure and ultrastructure of the pulmonary circulation with particular emphasis placed on the microvasculature. The description includes data collected from human, rat, sheep, dog, and cat (4-14). Such a description necessarily leads to the adoption of definitions for various levels of the pulmonary circulation. Many such definitions have evolved since Brenner's classic description of the pulmonary circulation (15). This chapter will utilize the definitions as described by Reid and colleagues over the last 20 years (4-10). These definitions rely on the structural characteristics of the vessel wall. The second part of the chapter deals with the pericyte, with its distribution and possible functions in the pulmonary vasculature.

II.   LIGHT MICROSCOPIC STRUCTURE
OF NORMAL PULMONARY ARTERIES

A.   Pre-Acinar Muscular Arteries

In man, the pulmonary artery can be divided into four structural regions as it passes from hilum to periphery : elastic, muscular, partially muscular and non-muscular. The wall of the larger arteries consists of a complete muscle coat, the media, as well as intimal and adventitial layers. The largest muscular arteries are called elastic arteries and by definition the medial coat of an elastic artery contains more than five elastic lamina, including the internal and external ones. In the distended pulmonary circulation elastic arteries are usually 2 mm or more in external diameter with a medial thickness expressed in relation to external diameter (2 x medial thickness divided by external diameter x 100) between 1 and 2% (6-8). These largest elastic arteries accompany the large preacinar airways and share the same connective sheath (16).

As one travels into the more distal regions of the lung, the number of elastic laminae in the media gradually decreases and an artery with between two and five elastic laminae in the media is usually referred to as a muscular artery. Medial thickness in the largest muscular arteries (< 2mm in external diameter) that run with the pre-acinar airways, is similar to that of the elastic arteries.

B.   Intra-Acinar Arteries

The arteries found at intra-acinar levels, that is, running with respiratory bronchioli, alveolar ducts or alveolar walls, generally have an external diameter of less than 150 µm. These smallest arteries may be muscular, partially muscular or non-muscular in structure (Figure 1). Muscular arteries may be found at alveolar

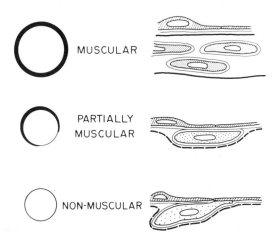

Fig. 1. Diagrammatic representation of the wall of muscular, partially muscular and non-muscular arteries. On the left is shown the complete muscle coat of the muscular artery, and the crescent of muscle in the wall of the partially muscular artery. On the right are the cell types that contribute to the various types of artery. Spindle-shaped smooth muscle cells containing myofilaments and surrounded by a basal lamina are found between elastic laminae in the media of the muscular regions of both muscular and partially muscular arteries. A spindle-shaped cell containing fewer filaments than the smooth muscle cell is sometimes found in the non-muscular regions of the partially muscular arteries. This cell is surrounded by a basal lamina that fuses with the adjacent endothelial cell and lies within a single fragmented elastic lamina. The pericyte is found in the walls of the non-muscular arteries. This cell is stellate, contains occasional filaments, shares the same basal lamina as the adjacent endothelial cell and lies internal to a single fragmentary basal lamina.

wall level with an external diameter as small as 30 μm and non-muscular arteries may be found running with respiratory bronchioli with an external diameter as large as 120 μm (7). In general, the intra-acinar muscular arteries are similar in structure to the larger ones described above, save that as their external diameter decreases so does the thickness of the intima, media and adventitia. Additionally, as they extend more distally into the lung the elastic laminæ become thinner and their number is reduced to two. Finally, the internal of these two laminæ disappears. For external diameter the smaller muscular arteries have a thicker medial coat than the larger arteries, *i.e.*, in the smallest muscular arteries (30 to 100 μm external diameter) percent medial thickness may be a high as 5% (6). It has been suggested that these small muscular arteries at intra-acinar level are perhaps responsible for, or at least contribute to, maintenance and alterations of pulmonary vascular resistance.

1.   Partially muscular arteries

As the name suggests, the partially muscular artery has a muscle coat in only part of its wall (Figure 1). This appearance is caused by the spiral arrangement of muscle in the wall as the complete muscle coat of the larger arteries disappears (6). This oblique arrangement of muscle in small pulmonary vessels is well documented in a number of species including man, rat, sheep, cat and dog (6,8,11-14). Arteries with an external diameter between 50 and 100 μm are predominanty partially muscular in structure (6). In the muscular region of the partially muscular arteries, the smooth muscle cells lie between both an internal and external elastic lamina while in the non-muscular region of wall only a single fragmented elastic lamina separates the intima from the adventitia.

2.   Non-muscular arteries

By light microscopy, the wall of the non-muscular arteries is similar in structure to the non-muscular region of the partially muscular arteries, and also to the thick portion of the blood/gas barrier (10). Non-muscular arteries are distinguished from alveolar capillaries by their external diameter—generally a capillary is defined as being less than 15 μm in diameter. Additionally, non-muscular arteries are often surrounded by a thin layer of connective tissue.

While it is known that many of the arteries run and branch with the airways of the lung—the conventional arteries—there is a group of thin-walled arteries whose pathway is short and that do not accompany the airway system. These are called supernumerary arteries (6). In the preacinar regions, the supernumeraries contribute about 25 % of the cross sectional area of the arterial side branches and within the acinus, they contribute about 33% (7). It is likely that in the normal lung these arteries carry blood for oxygenation to the alveoli adjacent to large arteries, veins and airways and represent a short cut for the blood supply to reach these relatively remote alveoli. In diseased states the supernumerary arteries could have important functions such as carrying blood distal to an occluded conventional artery.

III. LIGHT MICROSCOPIC APPEARANCE OF PULMONARY VEINS

In general, all the descriptions outlined above can be applied to the venous circulation. There are, however, several features that enable distinction between arteries and veins. The veins usually lie in interlobular septa, while arteries often run in close association with airways. For each structural type of vein the external diameter is larger than that of an artery. The walls of the veins contain more connective tissue and less muscle than the walls of arteries of a similar size. The veins do not have an internal elastic lamina separating the intima from the media (5,12). The supernumerary veins are more numerous than the arteries (5). A more precise method for distinguishing arteries from veins is to inject and distend either side of the pulmonary circulation with a medium that does not cross the pulmonary capillary bed. This technique has been used to great effect in many normal and pathologic studies (4-8,12) and also has the great advantage of allowing more precise measurements of vessel size and wall thickness (6,7).

IV. ULTRASTRUCTURE OF PULMONARY CIRCULATION

The majority of cell types and connective tissue components found in the walls of the entire pulmonary circulation are similar and have been described in detail elsewhere (10,12,13,17,18). The following therefore includes only a brief description of the cell types found in the walls and mentions specific differences in cell types or organelles at the various levels of the pulmonary circulation where they are known to occur. Again, the descriptions allude to the pulmonary arterial circulation but the same cell types are found in the walls of the veins.

A. Intima

The intima of the muscular arteries is composed of endothelial cells, basal lamina, collagen, microfibrils and elastin, all of which lie, in the case of muscular arteries, inside an internal elastic lamina (Figure 2), and in the case of non-muscular arteries, internal to a single fragmentary elastic lamina (Figure 1; 10). In the alveolar capillaries the intima is comprised of endothelial cells resting on a basal lamina. The endothelial cell of the larger pulmonary arteries exhibits several differences when compared to those of the small arteries. The endothelial cells are larger in diameter than those in the smaller arteries (19,20), endothelial turnover time is faster in the smaller arteries than in the large (21), the frequency of rod-shaped organelles decreases from hilum to periphery (19), the basal lamina of the peripheral arteries is more complete than that of the large arteries, and the overall thickness of the intima is greater in the larger versus the smaller vessels (19). In

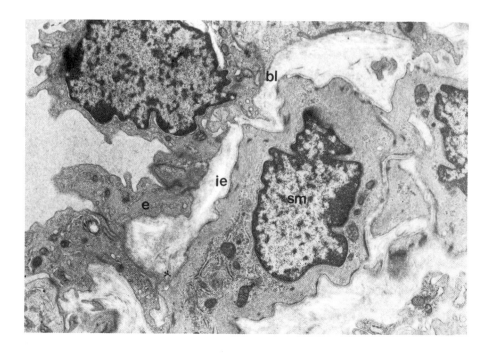

Fig. 2. Electron micrograph of part of the intima of a muscular artery showing endothelial cells (e), basal lamina (bl) and the internal elastic lamina (ie). A myoendothelial junction is seen at *. Smooth muscle cells (sm) X 13,700.

addition, myoendothelial junctions (Figure 2) are less frequent per unit length of wall in the larger than in the small pulmonary arteries and also than in pulmonary veins (12). This might suggest that the veins as well as the smaller arteries have greater control over the pulmonary circulation than the larger arteries. Additional differences exist between the endothelial cells of the arteries and veins. For example, using freeze-fracture techniques it has been shown that the tight junctions of the intra-acinar veins are less complex than those of the arteries, indicating that the veins are leakier than the arteries (22).

B.   Media

The media of the muscular arteries consists of smooth muscle cells, elastic laminæ, elastin, collagen and microfilaments. The smooth muscle cells on the arterial side of the pulmonary circulation lie between an internal and external elastic lamina and on the venous side they lie internal to the external lamina. The

smooth muscle cell is spindle shaped (Figures 1 and 2), has a centrally placed
nucleus and is surrounded by a basal lamina. The characteristic features of the
smooth muscle cytoplasm are the myofilaments with their associated dense bodies.
As the caliber of the vessel decreases, the number of myofilaments and dense
bodies in the cell declines. Pinocytic vesicles and attachment devices are found
along the cell membrane (10).

C.   Adventitia

The adventitial layer of the pulmonary circulation is composed of
fibroblasts, elastin and larga bundles of collagen. The thickness of the adventitia,
like the media, decreases with caliber of the vessel and the demarcation between the
two coats becomes less distinct. Nerve fibers are sometimes seen at the junction
between the media and adventitia (23).

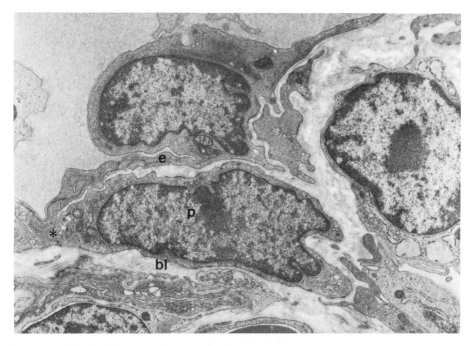

*Fig. 3. Electron micrograph of a pericyte (p) in the wall of a non-
muscular artery. The main body of the cell is surrounded by a basal lamina (bl)
but to the left (*) the pericyte is immediately adjacent to the endothelial cell (e) X
13,700.*

D.   Pericyte and Intermediate Cell

Pericytes and their processes are often encountered in the intimal layer of the non-muscular arteries, *i.e.* internal to the single fragmented elastic lamina. This cell is stellate in shape and shares the same basal lamina as adjacent endothelial cells (24,25). Pericyte processes often lie immediately adjacent to and abut onto the neighboring endothelial cell (Figures 1 and 3). Processes from a single pericyte may be shared by several capillaries. Occasional bundles of filaments that stain for actin and myosin are seen in the pericyte (26-28); these filament bundles are often at the tips of pericyte processes. As described for the smooth muscle cell, pinocytic vesicles and attachment devices are seen along the cell membrane of the pericyte.

A cell with structural features intermediate between a pericyte and smooth muscle cell lies internal to the fragmentary elastic lamina of the non-muscular region of the partially muscular artery. This cell is spindle-shaped, surrounded by a basal lamina which in regions fuses with that of the adjacent endothelial cell and contains myosin filaments (Figure 1). It seems that this cell type both by its position and structure warrants the name intermediate cell (10). Since both the pericyte and intermediate cell have been shown to contain contractile filaments, it may be that these cells can contribute to vascular tone in the peripheral arteries. Additionally, it has been shown that these cells can undergo hypertrophy and division in certain clinical and experimental conditions where pulmonary vascular resistance is increased (7).

V.   ULTRASTRUCTURE OF ALVEOLAR CAPILLARY WALL

As has been noted above, the structure of the alveolar capillary wall, especially the thick side, is similar in structure of the wall of non-muscular arteries. On its thin side the alveolar capillary wall is composed of a thin cytoplasmic process of a Type I pneumonocyte, an endothelial cell and a fused basal lamina between (24). In its thinnest portions the blood/gas barrier is probably about 0.4 μm in thickness. The thicker regions of the alveolar capillary wall often contains collagen, elastin and processes of fibroblasts. Pericyte processes are sometimes visualized internal to the basal lamina of the capillary endothelial cell. Thus all the vascular cell types seen in the walls of the non-muscular regions of vessels are present at capillary level.

VI.   FUNCTION OF THE PERICYTE

In recent years there has been renewed interest in the pericytes in the lung and other organs and their function (for review see ref 29). Pericytes were first described in the late 18th century (30,31) and they were thought at this time to be a contractile cell (Rouget cell) found in most mammalian capillary beds. Later studies in capillary beds of omenta and salamander larvæ failed to demonstrate a relationship between these cells and capillary contraction (32,33), but more recent studies with sophisticated histochemical techniques have documented the presence of contractile proteins within these cells, again indicating a contractile role for these cells (26-28). This finding together with the morphologic description that a pericyte can be shared by more than one capillary segment are of particular importance in the pulmonary microvasculature and suggest that such cells could contribute to control of pulmonary vascular tone. Additional data indicating a contractile role for these cells comes from models of chronic pulmonary hypertension (7,34-36). For example, in rats exposed to hypobaric hypoxia, it has been shown that the pericyte and intermediate cell are responsible for appearance of muscle into smaller and more peripheral arteries than normal. During the first three to four days of hypoxia when pulmonary artery pressure and pulmonary vascular resistance are increasing, these precursor smooth muscle cells (see above) hypertrophy (21,35). By five days, increased uptake of ^{3}H-thymidine is apparent in the cells, indicating their division (21) and finally, by ten days of hypoxic exposure, when pulmonary artery pressure has reached a plateau (37), these cells have differentiated to a cell which by electron microscopy has the characteristics of a mature smooth muscle cell (10,34).

Scanning electron microscopy shows that pericytes form a series of ridges around microvessels (29). These ridges may be arranged obliquely; in the smallest vessels where the pericyte is not as numerous, they may be seen as a rather erratically placed network. Some workers have noted that in bovine lung, pericyte processes are often located close to interendothelial junctions and in the thicker portions of the blood/gas barrier (38). Such findings may suggest that the pericyte has a protective function in the lung acting as a barrier, additional to the barrier formed by the endothelial cells and basal lamina, to escape of proteins and cells from the capillary lumen into interstitium.

Along this same line, the pericyte has also been suggested to have a phagocytic role, especially in the central nervous system, and rat cremaster muscle and skin (29,39). But thus far such a function has not been noted for the lung.

Perhaps more importantly with regard to the lung, especially lung growth, the pericyte has been suggested to play a role in regulation of capillary growth and maturation (40,41). Additionally, because of its position in small arteries and in alveolar capillaries, the pericyte may be involved in maintenance of alveolar architecture. *In vitro* studies suggest that the pericyte contributes to production of the basal lamina that enfolds both it and the endothelial cell (42).

Finally, in large vessels a "pseudo-endothelium" has been reported to migrate from the subendothelial layer to replace large areas of damaged endothelial cells (43). These cells are thought to be smooth muscle in origin (43-48), are non-thrombogenic (49,50) and when in their luminal position, the morphology of these cells is similar to that of normal endothelium (50). The position of the pericyte in the microcirculation, immediately beneath and often in contact with the adjacent endothelial cell, might suggest that the pericyte represents a "pseudo-endothelial cell", that under certain conditions, could migrate to the surface and replace a single damaged endothelial cell. In recent studies with the endothelial layer of intimal explants from bovine main pulmonary artery (51,52), we have

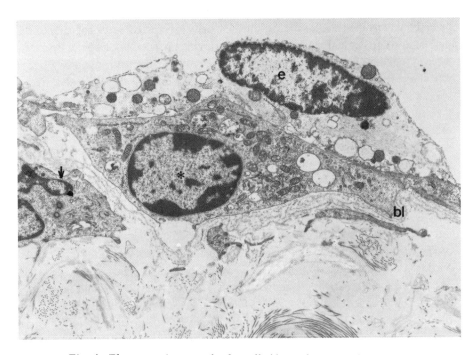

Fig. 4. Electron micrograph of a cell (*) in a bovine pulmonary artery intimal explant with pericyte-like features which seems to have replaced a damaged endothelial cell (e). This cell is within the endothelial basal lamina (bl). Another pericyte-like cell is seen at arrow and lies external to the endothelial basal lamina. X 9,100.

noticed a cell in the subendothelial layer with features reminiscent of a pericyte (Meyrick B.; unpublished observations). This cell is stellate, surrounded by a basal lamina, contains filaments and has been seen to make contact with endothelium. This cell is most obvious when the endothelial layer of the explants is damaged. Micrographs suggest that this cell can form junctions with the endothelial cells on both sides of the damaged cell and eventually replace it (Figure 4), thereby maintaining the integrity of the endothelial layer without division of adjacent endothelial cells or endothelial spreading. Endothelial replacement in the absence of cell proliferations been described previously in the aorta (43,53,54). Such data imply that pericyte-like cells may be found in pulmonary vessels much larger than the microvasculature and that pericytes may be responsible for replacement of single damaged cells, even at capillary level. Further work is needed to examine these ideas.

VII.   SUMMARY

The structure of the pulmonary circulation from hilum to periphery has been described as has the ultrastructure of the various cell types found in the wall of the pulmonary vessels. The descriptions of the cell types include a more detailed look at the pericyte, a cell that is found in the walls of most mammalian capillary beds. This cell type as yet has no identified function, but its position and frequency in the wall of pulmonary vessels, both large and small, warrant further study.

REFERENCES

1.   Coppola ED. (1957) *Bull Hist Med* **31**:44.
2.   Harvey W. (1628) **De Mortu Cordis. Movement of the Heart and Blood in Animals** (translated from the original Latin by KJ Franklin, 1957). Blackwell:Oxford.
3.   Young J. (1929) *In* Malpighi's **De Pulmonabis** [direct translation of letters to Borlius (Pisa) from Marcellus Malpighius Bologna, 1661]. *Proc Roy Soc Med* **23**:1.
4.   Elliott FJ and Reid L. (1965) *Clin Radiol* **16**:193.
5.   Hislop A and Reid L. (1973) *Thorax* **28**:313.
6.   Reid L. (1979) *Amer Rev Resp Dis* **119**:531.
7.   Meyrick B and Reid L. (1983) *Clin Chest Med* **4**:199.
8.   Hislop A and Reid L. (1978) *J Anat* **125**:71.
9.   Meyrick B, Hislop A and Reid L. (1978) *J Anat* **125**:209.

10. Meyrick B and Reid L. (1979) *Anat Rec* **193**:71.

11. Meyrick B and Brigham KL. (1983) *Lab Invest* **48**:458.

12. Michel RP. (1982) *Am J Anat* **164**:227.

13. Rhodin JAG. (1978) *Microvasc Res* **15**:169.

14. Kay JM. (1983) *Amer Rev Resp Dis* **128**:S53.

15. Brenner O. (1935) *Arch Int Med* **56**:211.

16. Murray JF. (1976) **The Normal Lung**. Saunders:Philadelphia.

17. Rhodin JAG. (1968) *J Ultrastruct Res* **25**:452.

18. Simionescu M, Simionescu N and Palade GE. (1975) *J Cell Biol* **67**: 863.

19. Meyrick B and Reid L. (1980) *Lab Invest* **42**:603.

20. Reid L and Meyrick B. (1980)*In* **Metabolic Activities of the Lung**. Ciba Foundation Symp 78. Excerpta Medica: Amsterdam, pp 37-60.

21. Meyrick B and Reid L. (1979) *Am J Pathol* **96**:51.

22. Schneeberger EE. (1981) *Circ Res* **49**:1102.

23. Meyrick B and Reid L. (1980)*Am J Pathol* **101**:527.

24. Meyrick B and Reid L. (1970) *Brit J Dis Chest* **64**:121.

25. Schulz H. (1959) **The Submicroscopic Anatomy and Pathology of the Lung**. Springer-Verlag: Berlin.

26. Meyrick B, Fujiwara K and Reid L. (1981) *Exp Lung Res* **4**:303.

27. Herman IM and D'Amore PA. (1985) *J Cell Biol* **101**:43.

28. Davies P, Smith B, Maddalo F, Fujiwara K and Reid L. (1984) *Amer Rev Resp Dis* **129**:A309.

29. Sims DE. (1986) *Tiss Cell* **18**:153.

30. Rouget C. (1873) *Arch Physiol Norm Pathol (Paris)* **5**:101.

31. Eberth CJ. *In* **Handbuch der Lehre von den Gewebwn des Menschen und der Tiere**. (S Stricker ed), Bd l: Liepzig.

32. Florey HW and Carleton HM. (1926) *Proc Roy Soc* **100**:23.

33. Clark ER and Clark EL. (1925)*Am J Anat* **35**:265.

34. Reid L and Meyrick B. (1975) *INSERM* **51**:145.

35. Meyrick B and Reid L. (1978) *Lab Invest* **38**:188.

36. Meyrick B and Reid L. (1982) *Am J Pathol* **106**:84.

37. Rabinovitch M, Gamble W, Nadas AS, Mietinen O and Reid L. (1979) *Am J Physiol* **236**:H818.

38. Sims DE and Westfall JA. (1983) *Microvasc Res* **25**:333.

39. Majno G. (1965) *In* **Handbook of Physiology**. Am Physiol Soc (WF Hamilton and P Dowie, eds) **3**:2293.

40. Crocker DJ, Murad TM and Geer JC. (1970) *Exp Molec Pathol* **13**:51.

41. Orlidge A and D'Amore PA. (in press) *Microvasc Res.*

42. Cohen MP, Frank RN and Khalifa AA. (1980) *Invest Ophthal Vis Sci* **19**:90.

43. Reidy MA. (1985) *Lab Invest* **53**:513.
44. Stemerman M, Spaet TH, Pitlick F, Clinton J, Lejnick S and Tiell M. (1977) *Am J Pathol* **87**:125.
45. Schwartz SM, Stemerman MB and Benditt EP. (1975) *Am J Pathol* **81**:1.
46. Clowes AW, Collazzo RE and Karnovsky MJ. (1978) *Lab Invest* **39**:141.
47. Moore S. (1981) *Lab Invest* **44**:301.
48. Clowes AW, Reidy MA and Clowes M. (1983) *Lab Invest* **49**:327.
49. Groves HM, Kinlough-Rathbone RL, Richardson M, Moore S and Mustard JF. (1979) *Lab Invest* **40**:194.
50. Reidy MA, Clowes AW and Schwartz SM. (1983) *Lab Invest* **49**:569.
51. Meyrick B, Hoffman LH and Brigham KL. (1984) *Tiss Cell* **16**:1.
52. Meyrick B and Brigham KL. (1984) *Exp Lung Res* **6**:11.
53. Reidy MA and Schwartz SM. (1981) *Lab Invest* **44**:301.
54. Ross R. (1986) *New Engl J Med* **314**:488.

The Pulmonary Vasculature and Experimental Pulmonary Hypertension in Animals

J. MICHAEL KAY
Department of Laboratory Medicine
St. Joseph's Hospital
Hamilton Ontario
Canada L8P 2C1

I.   SPECIES VARIATION IN STRUCTURE AND MICROANATOMY
       OF PULMONARY VASCULATURE

There are species differences in the course and structure of the pulmonary blood vessels that need to be considered when planning investigations of the pulmonary circulation using animals (1). These differences in structure and their physiological implications must also be considered when interpreting morphological data derived from animals and extrapolating the results to human subjects. Table I includes data about the structure of muscular pulmonary arteries and pulmonary veins in mammals (1). In the following paragraphs comparative aspects of the structure and function of the elastic pulmonary arteries, muscular pulmonary arteries, pulmonary arterioles and pulmonary veins are reviewed.

A.   Elastic Pulmonary Arteries

The elastic pulmonary arteries are the capacitance vessels of the lung, in contrast to the muscular pulmonary arteries and arterioles, which are the resistance vessels. In humans the elastic pulmonary arteries measure more than 1000 μm in external diameter and have a medial coat composed of concentric regular elastic

41

TABLE I. Pulmonary vascular morphologic characteristics in mammals.

| Animal Species | Muscular pulmonary arteries | | | Pulmonary veins |
	Diameter range (μm)	Medial thickness	Distinctive features	
Human	100-1000	2.0-6.9		Thin,mainly fibrous wall
Cat	20-500	8.0-25.0	Pulmonary artery medial hyperplasia occurs spontaneously	Thin,mainly fibrous wall
Cow	20-150	6.2-16.4		Follow bronchial tree. Thick spiral bundles of smooth muscle in intima
Beagle dog	30-120	3.9-11.7		Thin,mainly fibrous wall
Ferret	20-225	2.3-9.0		Thin,mainly fibrous wall
Goat	100-300	2.2-4.0		Thin,mainly fibrous wall
Guinea pig		4.3±0.2 SEM	Discontinuous segments of medial smooth muscle	Thin, fibromuscular wall
Horse	40-300	5.1-10.3		Follow bronchial tree. Thin, mainly fibrous wall
Monkey (*Erythrocebus patas patas*)	50-160	2.1-5.2		Thin,mainly fibrous wall
Mouse	20-300	4.4-11.7		Follow bronchial tree. Cardiac muscle in media
Pig	25-70	7.4-17.6		Follow bronchial tree. Thick intimal pads of smooth muscle
Rabbit	40-150	3.8-10.6		Thin,mainly fibrous wall
Rat	20-350	2.6-26.0	Thick walled oblique muscular segment. Discoid bodies in endothelium	Intimal pads of smooth muscle. Cardiac muscle in media.
Sheep	30-200	5.2-11.8		Follow bronchial tree. Thin muscular wall

laminæ interspersed with circular smooth muscle. In other animals, the basic structure of this class of vessel is similar to that in humans, but there is considerable variation in the medial thickness expressed as a percentage of the external diameter. The pulmonary arterial tree in humans, deer, monkey, dog, cat and mouse is smoothly tapering so that elastic pulmonary arteries blend imperceptibly and without irregularity of wall thickness into muscular pulmonary arteries. This contrasts with the rabbit, rat and guinea pig where the elastic segment is thin-walled, and branching is associated with abrupt changes in lumen diameter and wall thickness (2). In all species, the length of the arterial segment distal to a point where the external diameter is 1000 μm is similar. The difference in total length of the pulmonary arterial tree is accounted for by a variation in the length of the elastic pulmonary arterial segment. The increase in the length of the pulmonary arterial tree which occurs during postnatal growth is mainly due to an increase in the length of the elastic pulmonary arteries.

B.   Muscular Pulmonary Arteries

The basic structure of this class of vessel is an intima of endothelium, an internal elastic lamina, a media of circular smooth muscle, an external elastic lamina and an adventitia of fibrous tissue. In humans, the muscular pulmonary arteries range in external diameter from 100-1000 μm and the thickness of the tunica media ranges from 3-7% of the external diameter with a mean value of 5% (Figure 1). In the baboon, ferret, goat, llama and monkey the medial thickness of muscular pulmonary arteries is similar to that in humans. However, in most other animals the muscular pulmonary arteries are more muscular than those in humans. Accordingly, it is important that, when histological material from laboratory animals is examined, that normal thick-walled muscular pulmonary arteries, such as those that occur in the cow (Figure 2), are not mistakenly diagnosed as being affected by medial hypertrophy associated with pulmonary hypertension.

The amount of pulmonary artery smooth muscle inherent within each species may be a major determinant of the pulmonary hypertensive response to chronic alveolar hypoxia and may contribute to the interspecies variation in this response. Tucker *et al.* exposed seven animal species to hypobaric hypoxia for 19-48 days (3). The pulmonary hypertension that developed in the hypoxic animals varied in the following order of decreasing severity: calf and pig (severe); rat and rabbit (moderate); sheep, guinea pig and dog (mild). Right ventricular hypertrophy developed in proportion to the severity of the pulmonary hypertension. These interspecies variations in response did not correlate with the degree of systemic arterial hypoxemia, polycythemia, tachycardia or postnatal age. However, there

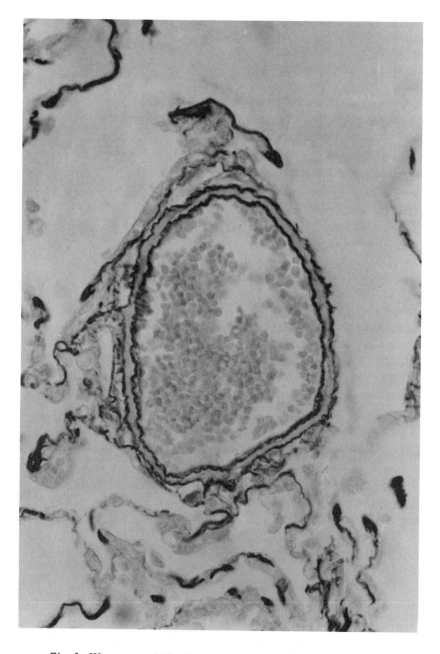

Fig. 1. Woman aged 37. Normal muscular pulmonary artery. The
tunica media is thin and bounded by internal and external elastic laminæ.
Elastic-van Gieson stain, x500.

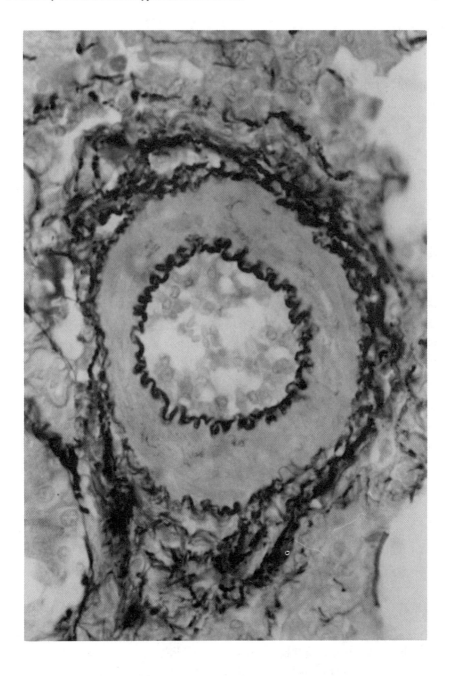

Figure 2. Cow. Normal muscular pulmonary atery with thick tunica media. Elastic-van Gieson stain, x 800.

was a significant relation between the medial thickness of small pulmonary arteries in control animals on the one hand, and the severity of pulmonary hypertension and right ventricular hypertrophy in hypoxic animals, on the other hand. The susceptibility or resistance to high altitude pulmonary hypertension in cattle may be determined genetically (4). Lung biopsy specimens from calves susceptible to high altitude pulmonary hypertension showed thicker muscular pulmonary arteries than lung biopsy specimens obtained from calves resistant to high altitude pulmonary hypertension (5). It is interesting that the llama (6) and the mountain-viscacha (7), which are genetically adapted to life at high altitude, have thin muscular pulmonary arteries. While the amount of pulmonary vascular smooth muscle may be a significant determinant of chronic hypoxic pulmonary hypertension, it does not seem to be the determinant of the pulmonary vasoconstrictor response to acute alveolar hypoxia. Peake *et al.* measured steady-state stimulus response relationships of the pulmonary circulation to graded hypoxia in the isolated lungs of pigs, dogs, rabbits, cats and ferrets (8). Marked species differences were apparent in both the level of PO_2 required to elicit responses and the amplitude of the responses. The ferret and the pig had the largest vasoconstrictor responses to hypoxia, the cat and the rabbit were intermediate responders, and no significant response was obained in the dog. The pig has relatively thick muscular pulmonary arteries with the medial thickness ranging from 7.4-17.6% while the ferret has thin pulmonary arteries resembling those found in humans with a medial thickness ranging from 2.3-9% (1).

The cat is not an ideal subject for experiments on the pulmonary circulation because it may suffer from a spontaneously arising condition known as pulmonary artery medial hyperplasia (PAMH). The incidence of PAMH has been reported to range from 1.3-68.8%. Hamilton (9) concluded that the condition was a result of infestation with the lung worm *Aelurostrongulus abstrusus*. However, Rogers and co-workers (10) observed PAMH with the same frequency in both specific-pathogen-free and conventional cats. In the guinea pig, the tunica media of muscular pulmonary arteries is irregular. It is composed of crescentic masses of circular smooth muscle disposed in discontinuous segments resembling sphincters (Fig 3). In the areas between the sphincter-like masses of smooth muscle, the wall consists only of an elastic lamina. The functional significance of this unusual arrangement of pulmonary vascular smooth muscle is unknown. Along the course of many of the muscular pulmonary arteries of the rat is a short segment where the tunica media is thickened and composed largely of obliquely orientated, closely packed smooth muscle cells with no external elastic lamina (11). In this so-called "thick walled oblique muscle segment", the medial thickness may be as much as 33% of the external diameter. The physiological significance of the thick walled oblique muscle segment is unknown but it is

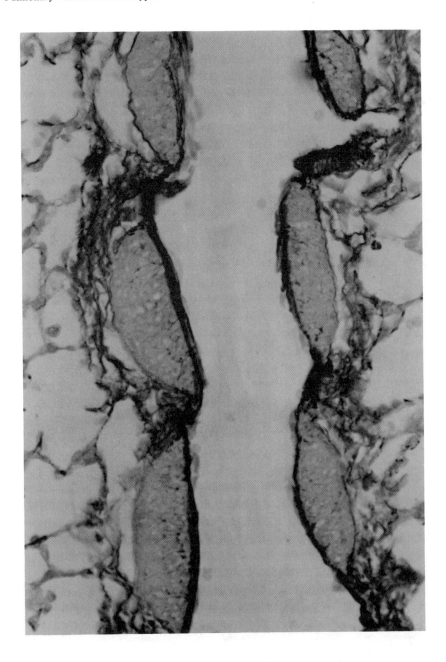

Figure 3. Guinea pig. Muscular pulmonary artery in longitudinal section. The tunica media is composed of crescentic masses of circular smooth muscle disposed in discontinuous segments. Elastic-van Gieson stain, x500.

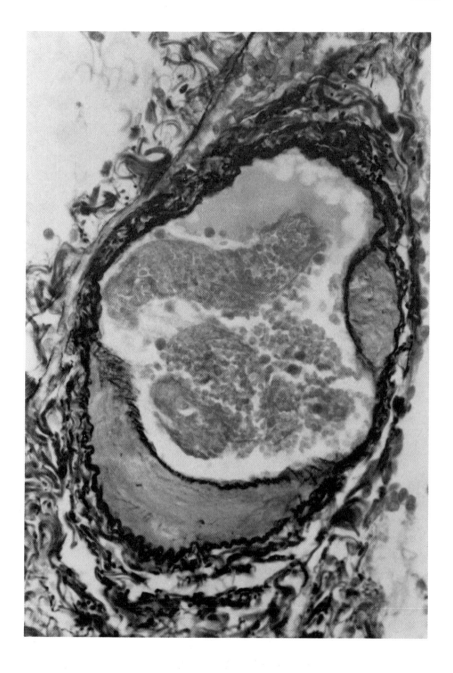

Figure 4. Cow. Normal pulmonary vein. Thick, spiral bundles of muscle are present in the intima. Elastic-van Gieson stain, x500.

important to realize that it is a nomal anatomical feature of the pulmonary arteries of rats. It should not be misinterpreted as medial hypertrophy associated with pulmonary arterial hypertension.

C.   Pulmonary Arterioles

In humans the transition from muscular to non-muscular pulmonary arterial vessels is seen over a diameter range of 100-70 μm. Accordingly, pulmonary arterioles that arise as terminations or lateral branches of muscular pulmonary arteries are normally devoid of histologically discernible smooth muscle, except near their site of origin. The smaller pulmonary arterioles consist of a single elastic lamina lined by endothelium. The goat is similar to humans in that the muscular pulmonary arteries terminate at an external diameter of about 100 μm. However, in most other animals smooth muscle is present in pulmonary arterial vessels of much smaller external diameter (1). Specifically, the pulmonary arterial vessels in the cat, cow, ferret, mouse and rat are muscularized down to an external diameter of 20 μm. The earliest morphological evidence of pulmonary arterial hypertension is muscularization of pulmonary arterioles. Accordingly, in the human lung the finding of large numbers of small muscular arterial vessels measuring less than 70 μm in diameter is pathognomonic of hypertensive pulmonary vascular disease. Clearly, this criterion cannot be applied to the lungs of many laboratory and domesticated animals where such small muscular vessels with a diameter of as little as 20 μm are merely the smallest muscular pulmonary arteries and have no pathological significance.

D.   Pulmonary Veins

There is pronounced variation between the species in the course and structure of the pulmonary veins. In humans, the pulmonary arteries and arterioles follow the bronchial tree and are thus located in the central regions of the pulmonary lobules. In contrast, the pulmonary veins are located at the periphery of the lobules in the interlobular fibrous septa. Thus the pulmonary veins are situated away from the pulmonary arteries and pursue an independent course towards the hilum of the lung. This anatomical relationship is not present in the cow, horse, mouse, pig or sheep where the pulmonary veins accompany the bronchial tree. In humans, the pulmonary veins measuring more than 100 μm in external diameter have walls that are thinner than those of an artery of comparable size. The intima is composed of an internal elastic lamina lined by endothelium. The tunica media is composed of a haphazard arrangement of elastic fibrils, smooth muscle and collagen. There is no clear demarcation between the media and adventitia. Pulmonary veins with thin fibrous walls are also present in the cat, civet, dog, ferret, fox, goat, horse, monkey and rabbit. However, the pulmonary veins are muscular in the cow, guinea pig, llama, pig and rat. In the cow the pulmonary veins present a beaded appearance in longitudinal section due to the presence of thick spiral bundles of smooth muscle in the intima (Figure 4). It is important not to misinterpret these thick muscular pulmonary veins adjacent to bronchi as pulmonary arteries. In humans, the left atrial cardiac muscle extends for a short distance along the course of the large extrapulmonary veins. Most large animals are similar to humans in that the intrapulmonary veins are devoid of cardiac muscle. However, the intrapulmonary veins of the mouse, rat, squirrel and mountain-viscacha are characterized by a thick medial coat of striated cardiac muscle continuous with the left atrium. In the rat, pulmonary veins down to an external diameter of 80 μm have a medial coat of cardiac muscle. In the larger intrapulmonary veins, the cardiac muscle is arranged into an external longitudinal layer and an internal circular layer. The ultrastructure of these medial cardiac muscle cells is similar to that of rat myocardium. Electrophysiological studies show that the action potential shape and propagation velocity along the myocardial coat of the rat pulmonary veins are similar to those observed in the left atrium and so is their sensitivity to locally applied acetylcholine. The physiological direction of propagation in rat pulmonary veins is towards the lung. This finding lends support to the hypothesis of a rhythmic valve-like action of the striated musculature of the pulmonary venous wall during systole, and a possible role in the capacitance of the pulmonary circulation (12).

II.   EXPERIMENTAL MODELS OF CHRONIC PULMONARY HYPERTENSION

Chronic pulmonary hypertension may arise as a result of increased pulmonary blood flow (hyperkinetic pulmonary hypertension), prolonged left atrial hypertension (passive pulmonary hypertension), pulmonary vasoconstriction (vasoconstrictive pulmonary hypertension) and organic vascular obstruction (obstructive pulmonary hypertension). Experimental models have been described for hyperkinetic, passive and vasoconstrictive pulmonary hypertension but it has been surprisingly difficult to establish a satisfactory model for obstructive pulmonary hypertension (13,14). Pulmonary hypertension has also been reported in experimental models of parenchymal lung disease such as emphysema (15). Severe pulmonary hypertension and pulmonary vascular disease may be produced in some animals by the administration of pyrrolizidine alkaloids (16,17).

A. Hyperkinetic Pulmonary Hypertension

Pneumonectomy, or simple ligation of the pulmonary artery to one lung, which approximately doubles the pulmonary blood flow through the contralateral lung, causes slight elevation of the pulmonary artery pressure. However, ligation of a pulmonary artery combined with chronic hypoxia does result in pulmonary hypertension (13,14). Pulmonary hypertension and severe hypertensive pulmonary vascular disease such as occur in human left to right shunts have been produced by creating shunts between the systemic and pulmonary circulations in dogs. A problem in these experimental models is the development of left ventricular failure and pulmonary edema after opening the shunt. However, in successful preparations the most severe grades of hypertensive pulmonary vascular disease have been reported including plexiform lesions and necrotizing arteritis (18,19).

B. Chronic Pulmonary Venous Hypertension

Most of the experiments designed to cause chronic pulmonary venous hypertension have been carried out in dogs with limited success (13,14). The methods used have included the production of mitral stenosis and invagination of the left atrium by implantation of a silastic ball. The most successful model for chronic pulmonary venous hypertension was developed in the calf, in which constriction of the pulmonary veins resulted in progressive pulmonary hypertension over a period of 3-4 months (20). The animals developed medial hypertrophy of the small pulmonary arteries and there was a relation between the pulmonary arterial pressure and the histological grade of hypertensive pulmonary vascular disease. The calf is particularly suited to this experimental procedure because the veins from all segments of the right diaphragmatic lobe join the left diaphragmatic lobe vein before entering the left atrium. This common pulmonary vein is easily dissected out and constricted.

C. Chronic Hypoxic Pulmonary Hypertension

Alveolar hypoxia is one of the most significant factors regulating the hemodynamics of the pulmonary circulation. An important aspect of hypoxic pulmonary vasoconstriction is that it is widespread throughout the animal kingdom, although there are considerable differences between the species in the pulmonary vascular reactivity to hypoxia (3,8). The most commonly used method of inducing chronic hypoxia is to place the experimental animal in a hypobaric chamber. The most extensively studied animal is the rat (21-25) but calves, pigs, rabbits, sheep, guinea pigs and dogs have also been studied in hypobaric chambers (3,13,14).

When rats are placed in a hypobaric chamber (380 mmHg) for about three weeks they develop polycythemia, pulmonary hypertension, right ventricular hypertrophy and musuclarization of the pulmonary arterioles (21-23). Ultrastructural studies to determine the origin of the new muscle which develops in the pulmonary arterioles have yielded conflicting results. Meyrick and Reid stated that the pulmonary arterioles became muscularized as a result of proliferation and differentiation of smooth muscle cells derived from pericytes and intermediate cells (24). Sobin *et al.*, on the other hand, considered that new smooth muscle cells were derived as a result of proliferation, migration and transformation of fibroblasts derived from the interstitial areas where the alveolar septa were adjacent to the arterioles (26). Pulmonary hypertension, right ventricular hypertrophy and muscularization of pulmonary arterioles develop rapidly in rats exposed to chronic hypoxia and are detectable after four days. These lesions regress slowly and at different rates if the rats are allowed to recover under conditions of continuous normoxia. Intermittent normoxia is ineffective (22,23). In a recent experiment rats were placed in a hypobaric chamber (380 mmHg) for 24 days then allowed to recover in room air (27). The times taken for right ventricular hypertrophy, pulmonary hypertension and muscularization of pulmonary arterioles to regress were 34 days, 56 days and 132 days, respectively. Ultrastructural studies of the pulmonary arterioles during the recovery period have shown de-differentiation of vascular smooth muscle cells with loss of contractile apparatus and reduction in cytoplasm (26).

D.   Pyrrolizidine Alkaloids and Pulmonary Hypertension

Monocrotaline is a pyrrolizidine alkaloid which occurs in the seeds of the leguminous plant *Crotalaria spectabilis*. When young rats are given a diet containing 0.1% of powdered *Crotalaria spectabilis* seeds they develop severe pulmonary hypertension and eventually die within 36-60 days (28). The pathological findings include right ventricular hypertrophy, an increase in the medial thickness of the pulmonary trunk, medial hypertrophy of muscular pulmonary arteries and muscularizatin of the pulmonary arterioles. About one-third of treated animals show an acute or healing pulmonary arteritis. Similar changes occur in rats given the pure alkaloids monocrotaline or fulvine by subcutaneous or intraperitoneal injection (29,30). Younger rats are more susceptible to monocrotaline than older rats (31). Monocrotaline pulmonary hypertension has also been described in monkeys (32) but mice, rabbits, hamsters and dogs are relatively resistant to the pulmonary hypertensive effects of this alkaloid (14). The mechanism which by the pyrrolizidine alkaloids produce pulmonary hypertension is not clear (33). One of the most intriguing problems is the latent period which elapses between the administration of the alkaloid and the development of pulmonary hypertension and hypertensive pulmonary vascular disease. In a recent experiment a group of rats was given a single subcutaneous injection of monocrotaline (60 mg/kg body weight). The sequence of changes was as follows: muscularization of pulmonary arterioles and medial hypertrophy of muscular pulmonary arteries occurred after 7 days; pulmonary hypertension occurred after 10 days; right ventricular hypertrophy was detected after 12 days (34). There is evidence that the pyrrolizidine alkaloids themselves are not toxic substances, but that they are dehydrogenated in the liver to produce highly reactive pyrrole derivatives which may then be transported to the lungs (35,36). The metabolism and excretion of a single toxic dose of a pyrrolizidine alkaloid take place rapidly and are virtually complete within 24 hours. Thus the delayed onset of the pulmonary vascular disease cannot result from a prolonged exposure to a toxic metabolite circulating in the blood but must follow a short exposure during the metabolism of the alkaloid. In addition to the pulmonary vascular disease, the lungs of rats treated with monocrotaline show proliferation and desquamation of alveolar cells, pulmonary edema, intra-alveolar hemorrhage, interstitial fibrosis, osseous nodules and mast cell hyperplasia (16). Since all of these changes may be the direct or indirect result of leakage of fluid from lung vessels, it has been suggested that endothelial injury may be an early or possibly the earliest event after monocrotaline administration (37). Recently it has been shown that inflammatory changes in the lung precede the development of right ventricular hypertrophy and hypertensive pulmonary vascular disease in rats given monocrotaline (38). Furthermore, the administration of dexamethasone supresses these inflammatory changes and completely prevents the development of right ventricular hypertrophy and hypertensive pulmonary vascular disease (39).

E.   Reduction in Number of Arteries in Pulmonary Hypertension

The technique of postmortem angiography followed by histology in the assessment of pulmonary vascular disease has recently been subjected to detailed criticism. In this technique, a pressure of 100 cmH$_2$O or 75 mmHg is used to force a barium-gelatin mixture into the pulmonary arteries. Vessels containing barium are then counted in histological sections. This technique has resulted in the concept that monocrotaline pulmonary hypertension (40) and chronic hypoxic pulmonary hypertension (41,42) in rats are characterized by a reduction in the number of pulmonary arteries. The same technique has purported to show a reduction in the number of pulmonary arteries in primary pulmonary hypertension (43) and congenital heart disease (44). In contrast, direct counts of pulmonary blood vessels have failed to demonstrate any reduction in the number of pulmonary arteries in rats with monocrotaline pulmonary hypertension (45) and chronic hypoxic pulmonary hypertension (45-47) and humans with pulmonary hypertension due to congenital heart disease (48,49). Mooi and Wagenvoort (50) have recently compared the effect of various fixation techniques on the number of recognizable pulmonary arteries in histological sections of lung. There was a marked difference between specimens fixed by high pressure vascular perfusion on the one hand and those fixed by intratracheal instillation on the other hand. In the perfused lungs there was a varying degree of mechanical destruction to the lung tissue apparently resulting from high presssure gradients across the vessel walls. The larger blood vessels were very thin-walled so that many pulmonary arteries showed a media only partly discernible between internal and external elastic laminae. Many small arteries in the perfused lungs showed a media so stretched as to be hardly recognizable. These workers concluded that much of what has been reported about decreased numbers of pulmonary blood vessels in pulmonary hypertension may well be due to artefactual changes in the lung tissue caused by unsatisfactory fixation techniques and the fact that the areas of lung tissue subjected to quantitative analysis were too small. Barium-gelatin mixture is erratic in its penetration of the pulmonary vasculature (51). The use of pulmonary angiography cannot distinguish between absence of blood vessels on the one hand, and total or subtotal destruction by severe constriction or intimal thickening on the other hand.

REFERENCES

1. Kay JM. (1983) *Am Rev Resp Dis* **128**:S53.
2. Ferencz C. (1969) *Johns Hopkins Med J* **125**:207.
3. Tucker A, McMurtry IF, Reeves J, Alexander AF, Will DH and Grover RF. (1975) *Am J Physiol* **228**:762.
4. Weir EK, Tucker A, Reeves JT, Will DH and Grover RF. (1974) *Cardiovasc Res* **8**:745.
5. Weir EK, Will DH, Alexander AF, McMurtry IF, Looga R, ReevesJT and Grover RF. (1979) *J Appl Physiol* **46**:517.
6. Harris P, Heath D, Smith P, Williams DR, Ramirez A, Kruger H and Jones DM. (1982) *Thorax* **37**:38.
7. Heath D, Williams D, Harris P, Smith P, Kruger H and Ramirez A. (1981) *J Comp Pathol* **91**:293.

8. Peake MD, Harabin AL, Brennan NJ and Sylvester JT. (1981) *J Appl Physiol* **51**:1214.

9. Hamilton JM. (1970) *Br Vet J* **126**:202.

10. Rogers WA, Bishop SP and Rohovsky MW. (1971) *Am J Vet Res* **32**:767.

11. Meyrick B, Hislop A and Reid L. (1978) *J Anat* **125**:209.

12. Almeida OP, Bohm GM, Carvalho M de P and Carvalho AP. (1975) *J Morphol* **145**:409.

13. Herget J and Palecek F. (1978) *Int Rev Exp Pathol* **18**:347.

14. Reeves JT and Herget J. (1984) *In* **Pulmonary Hypertension.** (EK Weir and JT Reeves, eds) Futura:Mount Kisco, New York.

15. Will JA and Kay JM. (1974) *Respiration* **31**:208.

16. Kay JM and Heath D. (1969) *Crotalaria spectabilis:* **The Pulmonary Hypertension Plant.** Charles C. Thomas:Springfield.

17. Heath D and Kay JM. (1978) *In* **Progress in Cardiology.** (PN Yu and JF Goodwin, eds) Lea and Febiger:Philadelphia.

18. Heath D, Donald DE and Edwards JE. (1959) *Br Heart J* **21**:187.

19. Esterly JA, Glagov S and Ferguson DJ. (1968) *Am J Pathol* **52**:325.

20. Silove ED, Tavernor WD and Berry CL. (1972)*Cardiovasc Res* **6**:36.

21. Abraham AS, Kay JM, Cole RB and Pincock AC. (1971) *Cardiovasc Res* **5**:95.

22. Kay JM. (1980) *Am Rev Respir Dis* **121**:993.

23. Kay JM, Suyama KL and Keane PM. (1981) *Am Rev Respir Dis* **123**:454.

24. Meyrick B and Reid L. (1978) *Lab Invest* **38**:188.

25. Rabinovitch M, Gamble W, Nadas AS, Miettinen OS and Reid L. (1979) *Am J Physiol* **236**:H818.

26. Sobin SS, Tremer HM, Hardy JD and Chiodi HP. (1983) *J Appl Physiol* **55**:1445.

27. Kay JM, Suyama KL and Keane PM. (1985) *Thorax* **40**:587.

28. Kay JM and Heath D. (1966) *J Pathol and Bacteriol* **92**:385.

29. Kay JM, Smith P, Heath D and Will JA. (1976) *Cardiovasc Res* **X**:200.

30. Kay JM, Heath D, Smith P, Bras G and Summerell J. (1971) *Thorax* **26**:249.

31. Sugita T, Stenmark KR, Wagner WW, Henson PM, Henson JE, Hyers TM and Reeves JT. (1983) *Exp Lung Res* **5**:201.

32. Allen JR and Chesney CF. (1972) *Exp Mol Pathol* **17**:220.

33. Lafranconi M and Huxtable RJ. (1981) *Rev Drugs Metab Drug Interact* **3**:271.

34. Kay JM, Keane PM, Suyama KL and Gauthier D. (1982) *Thorax* **37**:88.

35. Mattocks AR. (1968) *Nature* **217**:723.

36. Boyd MR. (1980) *CRC Crit Rev Toxicol* **7**:103.

37. Meyrick B, Gamble W and Reid L. (1980) *Am J Physiol* **239**:H692.

38. Kay JM, Suyama KL and Keane PM. (1986) *Am Rev Respir Dis* **133**:A159.

39. Keane PM and Kay JM. (1984) *Clin Invest Med* **7**(Suppl 2):82.

40. Hislop A and Reid L. (1974) *Br J Exp Pathol* **55**:153.

41. Hislop A and Reid L. (1976) *Br J Exp Pathol* **57**:542.

42. Rabinovitch M, Gamble W, Nadas AS, Miettinen OS and Reid L. (1979) *Am J Physiol* **236**:H818.

43. Anderson EG, Simon G and Reid L. (1973) *J Pathol* **110**:273.

44. Rabinovitch M, Haworth SG, Castaneda AR, Nadas AS and Reid LM. (1978) *Circulation* **58**:1107.

45. Kay JM, Suyama KL and Keane PM. (1982) *Thorax* **37**:927.

46. Emery CJ, Bee D and Barer GR. (1981) *Clin Sci* **61**:569.

47. Hunter C, Barer GR, Shaw JW and Clegg EJ. (1974) *Clin Sci Mol Med* **46**:375.

48. Takahashi T and Wagenvoort CA. (1983) *Arch Pathol Lab Med* **107**:23.

49. Wagenvoort CA. (1985) *Histopathology* **9**:417.

50. Mooi W and Wagenvoort CA. (1983) *J Pathol* **141**:441.

51. Barer GR, Finlay M, Bee D and Wach RA. (1982) *Bull Europ Physiopathol Resp* **18**(supp 4):69.

Pulmonary Vascular Changes in Infants and Children

CLAIRE LANGSTON
PAMELA HOLDER
Department of Pathology
Texas Children's Hospital and
Baylor College of Medicine
Houston, Texas   77030

I.   INTRODUCTION

Little is known of the embryogenesis and early development of the pulmonary vasculature which would account for the congenital abnormalities of this system. Alternately, a great deal of attention has been paid to the mechanism of adaptive changes necessary for transition from the fetal or intrauterine state of the pulmonary vasculature to extrauterine existence. These studies have established that there is marked instability of the pulmonary vasculature during this transition period, and that a host of factors may influence the ease and completeness of the transition phase. Investigation of the status of the pulmonary vasculature in utero has led to the observation that certain infants begin extrauterine life with an already altered pulmonary vascular bed. Consequently, the concept that alterations of the pulmonary vascular bed are caused exclusively by post-natal alterations of vascular flow and pressure has now changed. The importance of the prenatal state of the vascular bed is now recognized and the influence of prenatal events on morphologic and functional changes in the pulmonary vasculature is becoming more widely appreciated.

This chapter will briefly review the normal development of the pulmonary vasculature including both pre-natal and post-natal changes, selected abnormalities both congenital and acquired, and will critique the techniques employed to study the pulmonary vasculature in infants and children.

II.   NORMAL DEVELOPMENT

Embryogenesis of the pulmonary vasculature begins with the appearance at 32 days of the 6th branchial arches. These form connections to the developing vascular plexus within the primitive lung buds. The basic pattern of the pulmonary vasculature is established by about 50 days, at which time the lung buds have developed through the stage of formation of bronchopulmonary segments (1).

The pulmonary arterial supply initially follows the branching pattern of the airways. Arteries that branch with the airways throughout their course have been termed "conventional" arteries. There are additional arteries called "supernumerary" arteries which arise as branches from the conventional arteries and directly supply the acinus (2). These arteries may arise from either pre- or intraacinar conventional arteries. The basic pattern of the arterial supply is established shortly after bronchial branching is complete at 16 weeks gestation (3). Supernumerary arteries which arise from preacinar branches are also established early, however, those which arise from intraacinar branches are added as the acinus continues to develop in late gestation and throughout early childhood.

The pulmonary veins lag slightly behind the arteries in their development. In the human, the pulmonary veins, unlike most other visceral veins, do not course with the arteries but rather are located at the periphery of lobules and follow an independent course to the pulmonary hilum.

Bronchial arteries arise from the thoracic aorta and from intercostal arteries and supply the non-respiratory structures of the lung. These arteries also course with the airways. Bronchial veins may connect with both the azygos or hemiazygous venous system and the pulmonary veins themselves.

In the fetus the main pulmonary trunk structurally resembles the aorta, being both thick walled and having many elastic lamina. After birth it gradually decreases in thickness relative to the aorta; while it contains more elastic tissue than the aorta, that elastic tissue is more fragmented (4). The pulmonary arteries form a continuum from elastic to muscular to non-muscularized vessels, with a gradual transition between morphologic types and with a gradual rather than an abrupt diameter change (5). The elastic vessels are the capacitance vessels in the lungs and the muscular vessels are the resistance vessels. It is primarily the elastic vessels which increase in length with increasing somatic growth, while the resistance vessels remain relatively constant in their length (5).

Beyond the main pulmonary trunk, progressive generations of pulmonary arteries show decreasing numbers of elastic lamina between the internal and external elastic layers until the vessels are about 1000 µ in diameter. At that size the vessels become muscular arteries with poorly developed elastic lamina and gradually taper to about 100 µ in diameter. These small muscular arteries lie adjacent to terminal bronchioles and represent the major resistance sites within the pulmonary vasculature. The small arteries decrease in diameter peripherally, but the amount of muscle decreases less than the diameter, so there is a relative increase in muscle thickness in smaller artery walls (2,6). The intact muscle layer is gradually lost as the muscle invests the peripheral arteries in a spiral fashion and finally disappears. The non-muscularized arteries or precapillary arterioles which follow, connect with the capillary network of the alveoli. It appears that the amount of muscle in the small pulmonary arteries of fetal lungs is relatively constant over the last half of gestation, although the numbers of such vessels per unit lung volume increases markedly (7).

The limited studies of pulmonary pulmonary vascular development in utero have focused largely on understanding the basis for the vascular changes that accompany the transition from intrauterine to extrauterine life. These developmental and adaptive changes in the pulmonary vascular bed must be understood in order to appreciate early changes associated with pulmonary vascular disease. They can be divided into two phases: the first phase includes those adaptive changes that lead to an abrupt and marked decrease in pulmonary vascular resistance at birth while the second phase involves remodeling of the vasculature. In fact, these changes merge as a continuum.

From birth to approximately 10 days of age arterial wall thickness decreases. This decrease is most prominent in vessels less than 200 µ in diameter (1,2). The rapidity of this change is such that it is generally agreed to be due primarily to dilatation (2,8,9). Following this change, a further, more gradual decrease in muscle thickness in the small arteries occurs such that adult values for arterial medial thickness are achieved by about 2 months of age (9). The decrease in muscle thickness in larger arteries (greater than 200 µ) is slower and adult levels are not reached until several years of age. With lung growth, arterial muscle also extends gradually into more peripheral vessels so that by about 10 years of age muscle can be seen throughout the intraacinar course of the arteries.
Concommitant with these changes in medial thickness are changes in the sizes of the various arterial segments. After birth there is an initial increase in the size of the smallest muscular and largest non-muscular arteries which continues to about age 10. Later there is a decrease in size. This sequence of events suggests that there is initial dilatation of these arterial segments and then muscle growth

proceeds at a slightly slower pace than vessel growth, although regression and regrowth of medial muscle is also a possibility.

Because the branching of the small arteries parallels alveolar proliferation, the alveolar/arterial ratio and arteries/unit area remain almost constant through early childhood. Once alveolar proliferation has slowed and ceased, alveoli increase gradually in size leading to a slight decrease in the arterial/unit area ratio as the lungs approach adult size (9).

III.   CONGENITAL ABNORMALITIES OF THE
        PULMONARY VASCULATURE

A.   Aberrant arterial supply to the lung — "Intralobar" sequestration

Intralobar sequestration is defined as a portion of lung tissue within the normal pleural investment which is supplied by a systemic artery and also has no bronchial connection (10). Its existence as a developmental anomaly is debated (11,12). While it is three times more common than extralobar sequestration, it is not described in stillborn infants or neonates. In our series of 15 cases (13) with aberrant systemic arterial supply to lung in children, we found 9 cases of aberrant systemical arterial supply to normal lung. In those children less than one year of age peripheral extension of pulmonary arterial smooth muscle was often seen. In those over one year there were more advanced vascular changes and occasionally fibrinoid necrosis and plexiform lesions could be found. There were also 5 cases of aberrant arterial supply to cyctic adenomatoid malformation and one case that could not be accurately categorized. No intralobar sequestrations were found. We believe that most cases of intralobar sequestration represent acquired changes in an initially normal portion of lung supplied by a systemic artery.

B.   With lung developmental abnormalities

1.   The vasculature in pulmonary hypoplasia.

Pulmonary hypoplasia of various etiologies is regularly associated with abnormalities of the pulmonary vasculature (14). The basis of these changes is a relative increase in pulmonary vascular flow in utero because of the decreased cross-sectional area of the vasculature in hypoplastic lungs. These changes are acquired during intrauterine development and relate to the degree of under-development of the pulmonary vascular bed. Although these have been most extensively studied in the lungs of infants with congenital diaphragmatic hernia

(15-18), similar changes occur in pulmonary hypoplasia arising in other settings. When the lung is hypoplastic, there is regularly peripheral extension of pulmonary vascular smooth muscle. This finding is generally more marked with more severe degrees of hypoplasia. In infants with congenital diaphragmatic hernia, treated early surgically, post-operative survival appears to correlate with the degree of pulmonary hypoplasia present (18). Those with the smallest lungs have persistent hypoxemia following surgery and have smaller arteries with more prominent muscularization. Those with somewhat larger lungs often have a transient period of stability following surgery and then develop hypoxemia probably on a vasoconstrictive basis. These infants also have increased medial muscle in their small arteries, but the structural abnormalities are not as severe. Another group of infants with presumably less reduction in pulmonary volume and less abnormality of the pulmonary vasculature successfully weathers the post-surgical period.

2.   The vasculature in Trisomy 21

Earlier onset and severity of pulmonary hypertension in congenital heart disease associated with Trisomy 21 is a recognized clinical entity (19-21). A morphologic basis for the pulmonary hypertension has been identified in the developmental deficiency of the lung described in Trisomy 21 (22). A small group of patients with Trisomy 21, both with and without associated cardiovascular abnormalities, were found to have inadequate alveolarization of terminal lung units with accompanying alveolar enlargement. This suggests an accordingly reduced pulmonary vascular bed. Many of these lungs also showed retention of the fetal double capillary pattern in their alveolar septa. Infants with Trisomy 21 often demonstrate prominent peripheral extension of pulmonary arterial smooth muscle, again likely related to a modest reduction in pulmonary vascular cross-sectional area.

C.   Abnormal intrapulmonary vascular development — Malposition
        of intrapulmonary veins

As discussed above in section II, pulmonary veins in man do not accompany the pulmonary arteries and bronchial tree as they do in some species (5). Rather, venous drainage is to the periphery of the lobule and then by an independent course from the arteries to the pulmonary hilum.

There are, however, rare instances in which this pattern is not observed, and venous drainage is via aberrant veins which accompany the pulmonary artery and bronchus. This condition has been associated with respiratory distress and a clinical course resembling persistent pulmonary hypertension of the newborn; that is, a full term infant with cyanosis, hypoxemia, acidosis, and evidence of right-to-left shunt without anatomic heart disease (23). These lungs show the same peripheral extension of pulmonary arterial smooth muscle seen in the lungs of infants with persistent pulmonary hypertension of the newborn but their venous drainage and alveolar capillary development are also abnormal. Alveolar septa are thickened and hypovascular. The number of blood-air interfaces is reduced. With time, the septa become fibrotic and the number of capillaries decreases even further, while muscularization of small pulmonary arteries becomes more pronounced. Survival of these infants is limited. Those who present beyond the neonatal period do so with failure to thrive, cardiomegaly, and pulmonary hypertension (personal observation).

IV.   PULMONARY VASCULAR CHANGES IN CONGENITAL HEART DISEASE

A.   Associated with abnormal premature development

It is clear that the pulmonary vascular changes associated with certain forms of congenital heart disease have their genesis in abnormal intrauterine development of the pulmonary vasculature and/or the lungs themselves on the basis of abnormalities of intrauterine pulmonary blood flow. In other instances blood flow may be normal in utero and the pulmonary vascular changes which proceed post-natally are imposed on essentially normally developed lungs and pulmonary vascular systems.

In a variety of conditions best exemplified by pulmonary atresia, critical pulmonary stenosis, and tricuspid atresia without intraventricular septal defect, pulmonary blood flow in utero is entirely ductus dependent as it is post-natally. In pulmonary atresia without significant systemic collateral circulation, prenatal development of the pulmonary vasculature is abnormal (24). These infants have decreased number, size and muscularization of both pre- and intraacinar arteries. When there is significant systemic collateral circulation, advanced vascular disease may develop rapidly; whether this occurs in the setting of abnormal intrauterine pulmonary vascular development in these cases is not understood (25).

In contrast, when cardiac lesions which significantly obstruct left ventricular outflow (critical aortic stenosis, aortic atresia, hypoplastic left heart syndrome) exist in utero, systemic flow is entirely ductus dependent and cardiac output is exclusively from the right ventricle. In these instances there is also abnormal intrauterine development of the pulmonary vasculature, here related to increased pulmonary flow and/or increased pulmonary artery pressure in utero (26). The pulmonary vascular changes in these instances are quite different. These lungs show an increased number of intraacinar arteries, increased muscularity of pre- and intraacinar arteries and veins and peripheral extension of pulmonary arterial smooth muscle. In these cases the small arteries also do not dilate normally after birth.

B.   Morphologic grading systems

In their definitive study, Heath and Edwards (27) classified the changes of "plexogenic pulmonary arteriopathy" into six grades of increasing severity. Although defined as distinct groups, these changes represent a gradually changing spectrum of involvement. While the Heath and Edwards system was primarily formulated using patients with post-tricuspid shunts (*i.e.*, VSD), the descriptions also apply generally in idiopathic pulmonary hypertension and pre-tricuspid shunts (*i.e.*, ASD). Notable exceptions are that grade I change in atrial septal defects usually consists of intimal proliferation rather than medial hypertrophy, and that Grade IV to VI changes are unusual in pretricuspid shunts (28,29). In truncus arteriosus, plexogenic pulmonary arteriopathy tends to occur earlier at a given pressure than it does in VSD, in which muscular hypertrophy is generally more marked. This increased medial muscle mass may protect against more advanced lesions (30,31). Other causes of pulmonary artery hypertension such as pulmonary venous congestion, mechanical arterial obstruction, alveolar hypoxia, and destruction of the distal capillary bed, can also give rise to the changes described by Heath and Edwards; however, in these instances the changes are generally not as severe as those seen with intracardiac shunts (28).

There are two drawbacks to the use of the Heath and Edwards grading system in predicting clinical outcome. In the first two years of life, grades IV to VI changes are seldom seen, even in the face of markedly elevated pulmonary vascular resistance. Secondly, it has been noted that advanced changes of grades IV to VI are often irregularly distributed, making interpretation of small biopsies difficult (32). It should be noted, however, that some studies have not found irregular distribution, and lung biopsies may be representative of the status of the entire lung (33,34). Because of the lack of correlation between physiologic and morphologic parameters in the young child with pulmonary vascular disease a different grading system using morphometric analysis has been proposed to assess pulmonary vascular disease in those less than two years of age (35). In this sytem the diameter and thickness of artery walls are evaluated, as well as the peripheral extension of vascular smooth muscle and the alveolar/arterial ratio. Using these features, three grades of disease, A,B and C, are proposed. In grade A, there is peripheral extension of vascular smooth muscle into intraacinar arteries. This change, the earliest seen, is usually associated with an increase in pulmonary blood flow and not in pulmonary artery pressure. Grade B is marked by an increase in the thickness of the medial muscular coat (this is equivalent to grade I of Heath and Edwards) and is always associated with peripheral extension of vascular smooth muscle. More severe degrees of this grade are usually associated with an increase in pulmonary artery pressure, and in prolonged cases can be associated with a decrease in the size of small intraacinar arteries. Grade C shows in addition to the changes of grades A and B, a reduction in number of small peripheral arteries. This grade is almost always associated with a marked increase in pulmonary artery pressure, and is usually accompanied by the changes of Heath and Edwards grade III. The changes in the A,B,C grading system have a uniform distribution throughout the lung with the exception of the lingula (33).

In order for this grading system to achieve widespread application, both normal and abnormal must be readily definable and consistent, and the system must also predict reversibility. The described increase in alveolar/arterial ratio (grade C) has been the most controversial finding. Others have not been able to confirm this finding except when accompanied by changes of severe pulmonary artery hypertension (grade IV to VI) and usually only in children older than 2 and adults (36-38). Moreover, it appears that grade C changes, when not accompanied by advanced changes of the Heath and Edwards system, have little predictive value and may be reversible (39,40). Some of the discrepancies in various studies may be attributable to the different techniques employed. The grading system for infants and young children was devised using necropsy specimens in which the pulmonary arteries were injected. Others have generally studied uninjected specimens, as lung biopsy specimens do not lend themselves to vascular injection. The application of this grading system also may be hazardous in association with cardiac lesions in which some of these changes may occur during development. For example, patients with Tetralogy of Fallot who have a very low pulmonary blood flow have a decrease in the alveolar/arterial ratio, whereas those with a higher than normal flow may have an increase in this ratio (41). A quantitative decrease in lung volume in these patients has also been demonstrated (42).

V.   FAILURE OF TRANSITION — PERSISTENT PULMONARY
        HYPERTENSION OF THE NEWBORN

Failure of the pulmonary circulation to adapt normally to extrauterine life is often seen as a secondary phenomenon in which the pulmonary vasculature does not undergo the dilatation and decrease in smooth muscle which usually occurs rapidly after birth. This failure is most often associated with asphyxia and may be seen in premature infants with respiratory distress syndrome. It is also seen in term infants with meconium aspiration, is associated with early onset neonatal infection, and occasionally occurs in term infants without any recognized etiologic factors. In those infants with respiratory disease associated with prematurity or infection, this failure is likely an acquired problem secondary to the pre-existing pulmonary disease. However, in patients with no recognized antecedent event and in many of those term infants with meconium aspiration and persistent pulmonary hypertension, studies suggest that the failure of the circulation to adapt normally is the result of abnormal muscularization of the small pulmonary arteries occurring in utero (43-45).

Another group of infants with persistent pulmonary hypertension associated with occlusion of small pulmonary arteries by fibrin-platelet thromboemboli has been described (46-48). The thromboembolic phenomenon may be a complication of the altered hemodynamics of persistent pulmonary hypertension or may be an important etiologic factor (46). These infants are characterized by thrombocytopenia and failure to respond to therapeutic measures aimed at pulmonary vasodilatation (47).

VI.   ACQUIRED ABNORMALITIES AND PULMONARY VASCULAR CHANGES

A.   Bronchopulmonary dysplasia

Pulmonary vascular changes have been recognized pathologically as part of the spectrum of pathologic changes in bronchopulmonary dysplasia. The pathologic correlates of pulmonary hypertension, increased medial muscle mass of small pulmonary arteries, elastin plates in large pulmonary arteries, and right ventricular hypertrophy, have been seen in infants dying with bronchopulmonary dysplasia (49-53). These are not, however, uniform morphologic findings (54), and physiologic studies of these infants have also been variable with some studies showing elevated pulmonary vascular resistance (55) and others not (56). Despite this heterogeneity, it is clear that there is at least a group of patients with bronchopulmonary dysplasia who have elevated vascular resistance and high pulmonary arterial pressure. Many of these infants also show a poor response to oxygen, suggesting that they will not respond to drug therapy and implying a reduced cross-sectional area of their pulmonary vascular bed.

B.   Iatrogenic lesions of the pulmonary vasculature

1.   Long term prostaglandin administration and the pulmonary vasculature

When either systemic or pulmonary blood flow is ductus dependent, maintenance of ductal patency is critical to post-natal blood flow. In pulmonary and aortic atresia syndromes, PGE_1 infusion has been employed to maintain ductal patency prior to surgical intervention. The effects of PGE_1 therapy on the pulmonary vasculature in pulmonary atresia have been studied (57). In treated cases arterial muscularity is further reduced over that seen in untreated cases and normal controls, and muscle does not extend as peripherally in the circulation. This reduction in arterial muscle mass increases with duration of PGE_1 infusion. A concomitant of this decreased muscle mass, dilatation, occasionally aneurysmal, is largely effected in pre-acinar arteries while intraacinar arteries remain abnormally small but show an increase in number over untreated cases. This increase in intraacinar arteries is likely due to recruitment of vessels in these relatively short-term therapeutic intervals rather than to development of new vessels.

PGE_1 is now being used on a longer term basis to support infants with hypoplastic left heart syndrome prior to surgical intervention either with Norwood's procedure or cardiac transplantation. The effects of this therapy on the altered pulmonary vascular system of infants with hypoplastic left heart syndrome have not been reported. We have studied a single infant with hypoplastic left heart syndrome who received PGE_1 for 39 days prior to attempted surgical repair (unpublished observations). At postmortem the lungs showed severe chronic congestive changes with evidence of old and recent hemorrhage, interlobular septal edema and fibrosis, and alveolar wall thickening and fibrosis. The small pulmonary arteries had thickened media and there was marked peripheral extension of smooth muscle into intraacinar vessels. In addition to these well-recognized lesions reflecting increased pressure and flow within the pulmonary circulation, there was also a severe necrotizing vasculitis affecting widely scattered small pulmonary arteries. In several areas these necrotic vessels were seen within areas of pulmonary infarction. A similar necrotizing vasculitis was also seen in small resistance arteries in the small intestine, pancreas, kidney, and brain. We have since administered PGE_1 chronically to newborn beagle puppies and have reproduced the necrotizing pulmonary vascular lesions (Goddard-Finegold J, Hawkins EP, Langston C, unpublished observations).

2.   Intravenous lipid infusions and the pulmonary vasculature

There is another recently described lesion of the pulmonary arteries associated with therapeutic intervention in sick neonates. Lipid deposition has been reported in the pulmonary arteries in infants treated with intravenous lipid infusions as part of parenteral nutrition (58-60). In rare instances this deposition has been associated with morphologic changes of pulmonary hypertension (58) and some infants have also shown increased pulmonary vascular resistance related to lipid infusion (61). The more usual situation is a few lipid microemboli of no apparent clinical significance (59,60).

VII. PULMONARY VEINS

The pulmonary veins are a frequently overlooked site of pathologic change. Pulmonary venous obstruction may occur at several levels. In infants and children, anomalous pulmonary venous connection, pulmonary vein atresia or stenosis, and pulmonary veno-occlusive disease are causes of pulmonary venous obstruction. The obstruction, although it occurs at different levels in the pulmonary venous system, produces a similar picture with medial hypertrophy of arteries and thickening of vein walls, engorgement of the microcirculation, edema of intralobular septa and dilatation of lymphatics, peripheral extension of pulmonary arterial smooth muscle, and hemosiderin-laden macrophages (62-64). Occasionally with anomalous pulmonary venous connection, high grade lesions of pulmonary hypertensive vascular disease have been seen, but this is not the usual case (64-66). The increase in pulmonary arterial and venous muscle is observed in the newborn (67).

Stenosis or atresia of individual pulmonary veins, a rare congenital defect, may produce a similar histologic picture (68). One, all, or any combination of veins may be involved. The most frequent finding is stenosis of two veins unilaterally. Atresia usually involves only a single vein. The site of stenosis is at or near the venoatrial junction and histologically is usually an intimal fibrous proliferative lesion. These abnormalities appear to be acquired late in development, long after the veins are formed and connected (69-71). The vascular changes of venous obstruction are said to occur bilaterally even when vein stenosis is unilateral (62). Untreated cases are fatal within a year or two even when unilateral.

Pulmonary veno-occlusive disease, while it affects all ages, is predominantly a disease of children and young adults. This condition is a rare cause of pulmonary hypertension in which there is acquired intimal fibrous obstruction of intrapulmonary veins and venules without developmental cardiovascular defects (73). Presentation in infancy is uncommon, and when it occurs is non-specific with feeding difficulties, failure to thrive, and respiratory symptoms predominating. The course is usually brief, and some of these infants die suddenly and unexpectedly (73-75). We have seen two infants who presented as sudden infant death who subsequently were shown to have pulmonary veno-occlusive disease pathologically (75 and unpublished personal observation). The clinical histories and gross findings of these infants resembled those of cases of sudden infant death syndrome. As the lesions involving the pulmonary veins and venules may be easily overlooked or misinterpreted, it is possible that this condition is a more common cause of sudden infant death than has been recognized.

VIII.   MORPHOMETRIC ANALYSIS

In reviewing both pulmonary vascular development and the vascular changes occuring in various abnormal conditions, major discrepancies between the conclusions of studies become evident. While there is general agreement concerning what parameters should be assessed (a measure of arterial density, a measure of arterial size, and a measure of muscularity), there is little agreement on the techniques used either to assess these parameters or to prepare lung samples for evaluation. Because of this the normal ranges of these parameters have been difficult to establish. Part of the problem lies in the different techniques used by various investigators. Lung tissue employed for the evaluation of the pulmonary vasculature has been variously inflated or uninflated, injected or uninjected, and different materials, time courses and pressures have been used. For example, Haworth and Hislop (9) examined uninjected lung specimens and found that intraacinar arteries were more muscular than previously had been suggested when the pulmonary arteries were injected at high pressure prior to fixation (2,6,7). Injection of the pulmonary arteries at the pressure used in these studies results in marked vascular dilatation and an apparent decrease in smooth muscle thickness when related to the external vessel diameter. The potential artifactual changes produced by high pressure injection likely account for the discrepancy between the two studies.

The main advantages of vascular perfusion with a marker material are the ability to visualize the vascular tree radiographically, and the degree of confidence with which non-muscularized arteries can then be differentiated from venules histologically. Vascular perfusion, however, is not a simple procedure. It is technically difficult and time-consuming. It is not clear what pressure choice is appropriate and whatever choice is made the pressures are difficult to maintain. Distention of arteries is not uniform; some dilate excessively and others not at all (10). Intimal changes may also affect distensibility.

Inflation-fixation of the lung is useful for the histologic evaluation of pulmonary tissue. It permits evaluation of the density of vessels and a more accurate recognition of the location of structures within the acinus. It is well known that comparisons of inflated and uninflated lung preparations do not produce comparable data in terms of pulmonary parenchymal evaluations (77).

Despite the differing methods of preparation of the lungs for study of the pulmonary vasculature, there have been very few assessments of the effect of vascular perfusion or inflation-fixation on the parameters generally measured in the evaluation of the pulmonary vasculature. Those studies which have been carried out suggest that measurements of vessel size are altered by high pressure vascular perfusion, but not by inflation-fixation (78). It has been suggested that this does not occur when physiologic pressures are used for vascular perfusion (79,80). Others have tried to compensate for the differences produced by vascular perfusion by the application of "correction factors" to normal values derived from the literature to provide controls for uninjected biopsy specimens. These sorts of manipulation can produce widely varying conclusions. It is important to remember that investigations done using injected and or perfused whole lungs may not apply directly to the diagnostic study of smaller biopsy specimens. In the biopsy specimens it is inevitable that the degree of inflation is variable and that vascular perfusion is not possible. Extrapolation from cases studied using inflation and/or perfusion to lung biopsies cannot be made without extensive mathematical manipulations based on tenuous assumptions.

Many studies have been poorly controlled and this further complicates review in this area. Although control values are difficult to obtain, because suitable cases are unusual, it is possible with foresight to overcome this problem. The use of small numbers of historical controls casts doubt on the validity of conclusions in these studies where both biologic variability and interobserver differences must be considered.

Normal values available in the literature (Table I) reflect these problems. The deviations from "normal" described in various studies most likely reflect genuine trends; however, it is unlikely that they have great clinical utility. The better controlled studies have shown differences in morphometric parameters in the extreme ranges of certain conditions, but also demonstrate considerable overlap, and for most no good relationship with outcome.

Nevertheless, it is clear that quantitative evaluation of the pulmonary vasculature has an important contribution to make in the understanding of normal development and in the recognition of the vascular changes present in various conditions.

TABLE I. Morphologic parameters in normal lungs.

Age	Number	% media thickness to external diameter >200 µED	<200 µED	Range pulmonary arteries (µED) Terminal Bronchioles	Respiratory Bronchioles	Alveolar Ducts
21-25 w G		16.5-17.9				
28-27 w G	11	14.3-19.0				
0-3 d		15.7-19.2				
7-16 d	3	10.0-15.4				
4w-3m		6.8-11.0				
6m-4y	19	3.8-7.8				
Birth	1	3-6	5-19	40-101	31-72	
4m	1	2-4	4-7	87-296	53-169	
3y	1	2-3	2-4	172-380	87-296	
5y	1	2-4	2-4	325-600	73-404	
11y	1	2-3	2-4	300-705	176-450	
12 w G	1	3-5	8-11			
19 w G	1	3-5	6-15			
28 w G	2	3-5	4-11	35-62	25-50	
38 w G	1	3-5	6-15	50-82	40-85	
Birth	18 patients	-	-	-	-	-
3 d	in series,	3-6	3-7	87-175	45-145	60-70
4 m	number per	1-3	2-6	127-265	70-182	70-115
10 m	age not	1-3	2-6	175-360	98-250	75-145
18 m	specified	1-3	2-6	250-400	125-300	105-225
3y		1-3	2-6	320-530	112-320	130-165
4y		1-3	2-6	270-550	120-410	110-225
5y		1-3	2-6	430-600	80-530	100-280
10 y		1-3	2-6	220-430	105-415	75-177
11y		1-3	2-6	390-750	162-500	140-190
<25 h	8	6.7-10.4	14.7-29.8	28-90	13-55	10-32
6d	2	-	-	30-65	15-55	13-25
1-3m	11	5.7-8.5	9.1-15.2	35-113	18-100	15-45
3m-1y	5			43-105	25-105	13-60
1y-14y	23	5.8-7.6	7.2-9.6	75-445	23-300	20-175

G=gestational age
ED=external diameter
*=values taken from bar graph and corrected to cm^2

Smallest muscular artery (μED)	Range of partially muscular arteries (μ ED)	% Completely muscular arteries terminal bronchiole	bronchiole	Arteries <200 μ per unit area (cm2)	Alveolar to arterial ratio	Technique
						Noninjected Inflation not stated Ref 8
42	27-180	56	17	-		Arteries injected,
90	45-190	95	35	94*		100 cmH2O
160	100-300	98	26	255		pressure, 60° C
200	120-380	100	50	163		Inflation fixed
100	50-360	100	72	138		Ref 6
85	43-175					Arteries injected,
50	70-150					100 cmH2O
60&130	40-198					pressure, 60°C
75	30-150					Inflation fixed Ref 7
-	-			58	141	Arteries injected,
120	40-180			188	25	100 cmH2O
75	40-170			116	97.5	pressure, 60°C
112	55-220			287	43.3	Inflation fixed
185	100-300			364	28.7	Ref 2
77	52-295			250	51.6	
135	50-320			233	40.8	
155	50-370			195	46.8	
94	23-195			179	47.9	
148	50-320			-	-	
	All but 3		35-100		13.1	Noninjected
	(14 h, 4w, 5m)		41-45		9.2-13.7	Noninflated
	completely		42-94		9.7-14.6	Ref 9
	muscular		0-100		9.8-12.9	
			77-100		8.2-11.2	

REFERENCES

1. Hislop A and Reid L. (1977) *In* **Development of the Lung** (WA Hodson, ed) Marcel Dekker, Inc:NewYork.
2. Hislop A and Reid L. (1973) *Thorax* **28**:129.
3. Bucher U and Reid L. (1961) *Thorax* **16**:207.
4. Heath D, Wood EH, DuShane JW, *et al.* (1959) *J Pathol Bact* **77**:443.
5. Kay JM. (1983) *Am Rev Resp Dis* **128**:S53.
6. Davies G and Reid L. (1970) *Thorax* **25**:669.
7. Hislop A and Reid L. (1970) *J Anat* **113**:35.
8. Wagenvoort CA, Neufeld HN and Edwards JE. (1961) *Lab Invest* **10**:751.
9. Haworth SG and Hislop AA. (1983) *Am J Cardiol* **52**:578.
10. Pryce DM, Sellors TH and Blair LG. (1947) *Br J Surg* **35**:18.
11. Stocker JT and Malczak HT. (1984) *Chest* **86**:611.
12. Stocker JT. (1986) *Sem in Diag Path* **3**:106.
13. Holder PD and Langston C. (1986) *Pediatr Pulmonol* **2**:147.
14. Chen S and DeMello D. (1984) *Ped Res* **18**:338A.
15. Kitagawa M, Hislop A, Boyden EA, *et al.* (1971) *Br J Surg* **58**:342.
16. Areechon W and Reid L. (1963) *Br Med J* **1**:230.
17. Naeye RL, Shochat SJ, Whitman V, *et al.* (1976) *Pediatrics* **58**:902.
18. Geggel RL, Murphy JD, Langleben D, *et al.* (1985) *J Peds* **107**:457.
19. Chi TPL and Krovetz LJ. (1975) *J Peds* **86**:533.
20. Noonen JA and Walters LR. (1974) *Pediatr Res* **8**:353.
21. Greenwood RD and Nadas AS. (1976) *Pediatrics* **58**:893.
22. Cooney TP and Thurlbeck WM. (1982) *N Engl J Med* **307**:1170.
23. Janney CG, Askin FB and Kuhn C. (1981) *Am J Clin Pathol* **76**:722.
24. Haworth SG and Reid L. (1977) *Thorax* **32**:129.
25. Thiene G, Frescura C, Bini RM, *et al.* (1979) *Circulation* **60**:1066.
26. Haworth SG and Reid L. (1977) *Thorax* **32**:121.
27. Heath D and Edwards JE. (1958) *Circulation* **18**:533.
28. Heath D and Smith P. (1977) *Med Clinic N Amer* **671**:1279.
29. Haworth SG. (1983) *Am J Cardiol* **51**:265.
30. Yamaki S and Wagenvoort CA. (1981) *Am J Pathol* **105**:70.
31. Juaneda E and Haworth SG. (1984) *Am J Cardiol* **54**:1314.
32. Adams P, Lucas RV, Ferguson DK, *et al.* (1957) *Am J Dis Child* **94**:476.
33. Haworth SG and Reid L. (1978) *Br Heart J* **40**:825.
34. Wagenvoort CA. (1985) *Histopathology* **9**:417.
35. Rabinovitch M, Haworth SG, Vance Z, *et al.* (1980) *Human Pathol* **11**:499.

36. Takahashi T and Wagenvoort CA. (1983) *Arch Pathol Lab Med* **107**:23.
37. Hoffmeister HM, Fischbach H and Hoffmeister HE. (1981) *J Thorac Cardiovasc Surg* **29**:355.
38. Juaneda E, deGroot AG, Oppenheimer-Dekker A, *et al.* (1985) *Inter J Cardiol* **7**:223.
39. Rabinovitch M, Castaneda AR and Reid L. (1981) *Am J Cardiol* **47**:77.
40. Rabinovitch M, Keane JF, Norwood WI, *et al.* (1984) *Circulation* **69**:655.
41. Shapira N, Rosenthal A, Heidelberger K, *et al.* (1982) *J Thorac Cardiovasc Surg* **83**:650.
42. Hislop A and Reid L. (1973) *Br Heart J* **35**:1178.
43. Haworth SG and Hislop AA. (1981) *J Pediatr* **98**:915.
44. Murphy JD, Rabinovitch M, Goldstein JD and Reid LM. (1981) *J Pediatr* **98**:962.
45. Murphy JD, Vawter GF and Reid LM. (1984) *J Pediatr* **104**:758.
46. Morrow WR, Haas JE and Benjamin DR. (1982) *J Pediatr* **100**:117.
47. Levin DL, Weinberg AG and Perkins RM. (1983) *J Pediatr* **102**:299.
48. Arnold J, O'Brodovich H, Whyte R, *et al.* (1985) *J Pediatr* **106**:806.
49. Northway WH, Rosan RC and Porter DY. (1967) *N Engl J Med* **276**:357.
50. Taghizadeh A and Reynolds EOR. (1976) *Am J Pathol* **84**:241.
51. Bonikos DS, Bensch KG, Northway WH, *et al.* (1976) *Hum Pathol* **7**:643.
52. Tomashefski JF, Oppermann HC, Vawter GF, *et al.* (1984) *Pediatr Pathol* **2**:469.
53. Sobonya RE, Logvinoff MM, Taussig LM, *et al.* (1982) *Pediatr Res* **16**:969.
54. Anderson WR and Strickland MB. (1971) *Arch Pathol Lab Med* **91**:506.
55. Berman W, Yabek SM, Dillon T, *et al.* (1982) *Pediatrics* **70**:708.
56. Melnick G, Pickoff AS, Ferrer PL, *et al.* (1980) *Pediatrics* **66**:589.
57. Haworth SG, Sauer U and Bullmeyer K. (1980) *Br Heart J* **43**:306.
58. Dahms BB and Halpin TC. (1980) *J Pediatr* **97**:800.
59. Levene MI, Batisti O, Wigglesworth JS, *et al.* (1984) *Acta Pædiatr Scand* **73**:454.
60. Shulman RJ, Langston C and Schanler RJ. (in press) *J Pediatr.*
61. Lloyd TR and Boucek MM. (1986) *J Pediatr* **108**:130.
62. Ferencz C and Damman JF. (1957) *Circulation* **16**:1046.
63. Johnson AL, Wigglesworth FW, Dunbar JS, *et al.* (1958) *Circulation* **17**:340.
64. Haworth SG and Reid L. (1977) *Br Heart J* **39**:80.

65. Newfeld EA, Wilson A, Paul MH, *et al.* (1980) *Circulation* **61**:103.

66. Petersen RC and Edwards WD. (1983) *Histopathology* **7**:487.

67. Shinebourne EA, Jones ODH, Denison DM, *et al.* (1981) *In* **Paediatric Cardiology**, Vol. 4. (M Goodman ed) Churchill Livingston:London.

68. Edwards JE. (1960) *Lab Invest* **9**:46.

69. Shone JD, Amplatz K, Anderson RC, *et al.* (1962) *Circulation* **26**:574.

70. Kawashima Y, Ueda T, Naito Y, *et al.* (1971) *Ann Thorac Surg* **12**:196.

71. Sade RM, Freed MD, Matthews ECl. (1974) *J Thorac Cardiovasc Surg* **67**:953.

72. Wagenvoort CA, Wagenvoort N and Takahashi T. (1985) *Hum Pathol* **16**:1033.

73. Tinglestad JB, Alterman K and Lambert EC. (1969) *Am J Dis Child* **117**:219.

74. Stoler MH, Anderson VM and Stuard ID. (1982) *Arch Pathol Lab Med* **186**:645.

75. Cagle P and Langston C. (   ) *Arch Pathol Lab Med* **108**:338.

76. Wagenvoort CA and Wagenvoort N. (1977) **Pathology of Pulmonary Hypertension**. John Wiley and Sons Inc:New York.

77. Cooney TP and Thurlbeck WM. (1982) *Thorax* **37**:572.

78. Fernie JM, McLean A and Lamb D. (1985) *Arch Pathol Lab Med* **109**:843.

79. Wagenvoort CA. (1960) *Circulation* **22**:535.

80. Cook TA, Salno NA and Yates PO. (1970) *J Pathol* **117**:253.

Summary: The Morphology of the Pulmonary Vasculature

The symposium on the morphology of the pulmonary vasculature must be regarded as an unqualified success. As always, studies in human disease must take precedence and the two contributors to this topic, Dr. Wagenvoort and Dr. Langston, emphasised the importance of diagnostic pathology. Both also underlined the problem of methodology and obtaining normative data. Dr. Meyrick reviewed the microscopic appearance of the pulmonary vasculature, with emphasis on the microvasculature. Of particular interest was her discussion of the pericyte and its role in capillary growth, modification of the small pulmonary arteries, and perhaps its role in maintenance of alveolar architecture. Dr. Kay provided a masterly review, not only of the experimental pulmonary hypertension, but also of the comparative histology of the pulmonary vascular system.

As an outsider, I had not realised the problems and controversies about the assessment of normal and abnormal morphology of the pulmonary circulation. These derive in part from differences in methodology of preparation of the pulmonary vasculature (well covered by the participants) and measurements used to assess the morphology of the pulmonary vessels. The question of the value of distension of the pulmonary arterial system remains unresolved. The inter-relationship betwen such measurements as the thickness of the components of the arterial wall to assessments of area also remain unsolved. These are serious issues and should be resolved because of the clinical importance of pulmonary hypertension.

WILLIAM M. THURLBECK

Pharmacology

Pharmacology of the Pulmonary Circulation: Introduction

Compared with other vascular beds and segments, the pulmonary circulation has been less extensively examined by pharmacologists. This made it difficult to identify, as speakers, pharmacologists with a primary research focus on the pulmonary vasculature, a problem compounded by our desire to cover topics primarily related to pharmacodynamics. Furthermore, the limited amount of available symposium time precluded extensive coverage of pharmacological topics semingly relevant to the pulmonary circulation. Our final selection of topics was, to a large extent, guided by the availability of speakers with experience in pharmacodynamic studies of pulmonary vessels. We hope that the research presented at this symposium will stimulate a more widespread interest in pharmacological studies of the pulmonary circulation.

CARL K. BUCKNER

The Pulmonary Circulation
in Health and Disease

77

Pharmacology of the Pulmonary Circulation: An Overview[1]

BURTON M. ALTURA
*SUNY Health Science Center at
Brooklyn
Brooklyn, New York 11203*

I.   INTRODUCTION

The pulmonary vascular bed is noted for its complexity of microvascular structure, hemodynamic properties, and its liability to interference by extrinsic factors (1,2). It's unique in being the major site for inactivation of many vasoactive substances, which often obscures the effects of these substances, per se, on the pulmonary blood vessels (3,4,5). Therefore, in order to properly evaluate and analyze the direct pulmonary vascular actions of vasoactive agents, one needs to minimize the extraneous factors. In addition to this major problem, pulmonary vascular smooth muscle (VSM) possesses inherent heterogeneous properties, not only from one species to another, but with respect to different segments within the pulmonary vasculature (6-16).

If one could provide distinct answers to the above, and even reveal for certain the direct (or indirect) actions of the different ions, amines, peptides, drugs, etc., on the mammalian pulmonary micro- and macro- vasculature, there still would be the critical need to understand the mode(s) of action of vasoactive

[1]*The original studies described herein, were supported, in part, by USPHS Research Grants HL-18002, HL-18015, HL-29600 and DA-02339, as well as grants in aid from the Upjohn Company, Miles Laboratories and CIBA-GEIGY Corporation.*

79

substances on, and contractility of, these unique blood vessels. In this mini-review an attempt has been made to point out some of the major influences, and actions, of important factors and vasoactive substances on pulmonary blood vessels. Due to limitations of space, I had to be somewhat selective and apologize for areas, research and authors not considered.

II.   FACTORS INFLUENCING VASOMOTOR TONE

Table I lists a number of physiological, pharmacological, and experimental factors that could play important roles in the known, diverse actions of vasoactive substances and drugs on pulmonary blood vessels. Inasmuch as a number of these factors have been reviewed recently (1,2,4-6,16-32), I have elected to review here only some of these modifying influences. However, in addition to such modifying factors, we must keep in mind that endogenously released or synthesized vasoactive substances may interact with one another on vascular smooth muscle cells to effect either stronger contractile or inhibiting actions on blood vessels. For example, non-pressor doses of neurohypophyseal peptide hormones can potentiate catecholamine-induced contractions and vice versa (27,28). Non-vasodilator doses of histamine, bradykinin, prostanoids, and serotonin can attenuate contractile responses induced by a variety of amines and peptides on vascular smooth muscle (5,18,21,22,33).

A.   Fine Structure

The fine structure (ultrastructure) of blood vessels and type appear to be very important in dictating a particular type and strength of response (17). For example, rat mesenteric and cremaster (skeletal muscle) venules not only exhibit higher thresholds for both epinephrine and norepinephrine, but in addition, these venules only exhibit a 20-40% maximal luminal closure compared to the 80-100% observed in arterioles, metarterioles and precapillary sphincters (17). Recent evidence in rat mesenteric and cremaster venules suggest that the smallest microscopic venules (invested with both smooth muscle cells and pericytes) (approximately 30-40 μm) are more responsive (*e.g.*, lower threshold and greater maximal response) to the constrictor catecholamines than are venules 40-75 μm in size (17). Such findings, I believe are suggestive of the probability that the pericytes (primitive smooth muscle cells) are contributing to the overall response of these smallest venules. With respect to neurohypophyseal peptides, it has been shown for several regional microvasculatures that the muscular venules (40-70 μm

TABLE I. Physiological, pharmacological and experimental facts that can modify the tone and actions of vasoactive substances in pulmonary vascular smooth muscle.

Physiological factors	Pharmacological and experimental factors
Aging, development	Anesthetic (presence and type)
Sex hormones	Analgesics
Innervation	Buffers
Ionic milieu	Solvents, preservatives
Heterogeneity of smooth	Chlorobutanol
muscle elements	Alcohol
Endothelial cell integrity	Acetic acid
Physical	Presence of certain drugs
Length-tension (e.g.	Route of drug administration
blood pressure, wall	Purity of peptide, etc.
thickness, geometry, etc.)	Surgical manipulation
Temperature	
Tissue metabolism and osmolarity	
Local chemicals and hormones	
Physiologic state of host	
presence or absence of	
microorganisms	
presence or absence of	
certain diseases	
Species, strain	

in size) are often more sensitive to these hormones than are the precapillary microvessels (26,27). Whether such distinctions exist for the pulmonary vascular tree will have to await investigation.

B. Innervation, Synaptic Clefts and Cell-Cell Junctions

Although it is well known that pulmonary blood vessels can contract and relax in response to alpha-adrenergic and beta-adrenergic stimuli, respectively (6-10) it is not thought such adrenergic nerves or endogenous stimulation of these nerves play much of a role in controlling vasomotor tone of the pulmonary vasculature, despite the fact that the density of such nerves is great. Inasmuch as the innervation is dense here, what is their physiologic function and do they play a role in the pharmacologic responsiveness of these blood vessels to endogenous vasoactive humoral stimuli?

Since the synaptic (neuromuscular) cleft distance in pulmonary blood vessels is much longer than most other vascular regions (e.g., 7,000 - 30,000 Å compared to 400 - 2,000 Å) (7,32,34), it has been suggested that this is a major factor in the slower on set-time and lower magnitude of contraction of pulmonary vascular smooth muscle to adrenergic stimulation (7,34), despite the fact that pulmonary blood vessels demonstrate a high sensitivity of their effector smooth muscle cells to norepinephrine.

In many regions of the body, neighboring vascular smooth muscle cells along a vessel segment and from one layer of the media to another are excited, by numerous endogenous vasoactive stimuli, via an electrotonic spread of current from one cell to another via nexuses (or tight junctions) (35); *i.e.*, via low-resistance pathways. Action potentials are usually found in these spike-generating (or single unit) smooth muscle cells (36). However, the available evidence in pulmonary vascular muscle suggests that this does not readily take place in these blood vessels, although these cells do undergo graded depolarization often associated with the magnitude of the vasoactive stimulus.

C.   Pharmacologic Property of Unequal Maximal Responsiveness to Contractile and Relaxant Agents

Approximately 20 years ago, it was demonstrated that VSM exhibits different degrees of maximal contractile and relaxant responses to all types of vasoactive agents (36-39). This concept has now been extended to all types of pulmonary VSM, so far investigated (4,6,8-10,13,40). Although such a phenomenon has been observed on all types of pulmonary VSM from millimeters in diameter to μm in diameter, the mechanism(s) for these unequal maximal respones remain to be elucidated.

D.   Sensitivity and Receptor Distribution and Density

Although the constrictor catecholamines, norepinephrine and epinephrine are potentially potent endogenous substances on pulmonary blood vessels (threshold conc. $= 10^{-10}$ to 10^{-8}M), there are numerous additional hormonal and humoral agents that can elicit contractile responses on the pulmonary vasculature (*e.g.*, angiotensin II, dopamine, prostanoids, serotonin, histamine, acetylcholine, bradykinin, leukotrienes, opioid peptides, substances P, etc. (2,4,6-11,13-15,40-45). The wide differences in concentration-effect curves and slopes together with the fact that specific antagonists for most of these agonists inhibit specific agonists-induced responses suggest that there are specific receptors for each of these contractile substances. The evidence, so far, suggests that the number and distribution of these receptors differs with the location in the lung and species (46). A similar situation appears to exist with respect to hormonal and humoral dilator agents such as acetylcholine, bradykinin, vasoactive intestinal peptide, prostanoids, neuropeptide Y, and other neuropeptides, despite the fact that the evidence is sparse in nature (8-11,13-15,40,41). In addition, one should mention the fact that specific receptors which subserve relaxation for beta-adrenergic agents appear to exist in mammalian pulmonary blood vessels (8,41,42). Receptors for certain hormones such as the neurophypophyseal peptides may, however, either be very sparse or completely absent in the pulmonary vascular tree (8,27,28).

E.   Mechanisms for Hormonal Inactivation

1.   Adrenergic Amines

The contractile actions of catecholamines on VSM are thought to be inactivated by at least four different mechanisms: overflow, neuronal reuptake, deamination by nonoamine oxidase (MAO), and o-methylation by catechol-o-methyltransferase (C-O-MT) (5,7). In addition, binding by the elastin and collagen components may play a role in inactivation of catecholamines (47). With respect to pulmonary VSM, the available evidence appears to indicate that all of the previous mechanisms play a role in inactivation of the contractile action of the neurotransmitter (5,7,47). The endothelial lining also appears to play a role in the lung (3,48).

2.   Other Vasoactive Hormones

Here, it is clear that enzymes exist for the inactivation of angiotensin and some peptides (3,15). However, it is not certain as to whether mechanisms exist for inactivation of the contractile or relaxant actions of most other substances within the pulmonary vasculature, per se.

F.   Heterogeneity of Cellular Sources of Calcium Mobilization for Contractility in Pulmonary VSM

One of the currently unresolved issues in VSM physiology is the mechanism of.excitation-contraction coupling (49). At least three paths have been proposed to account for contraction of VSM. One proposes that the initial step is depolarization of the outer cell membrane by the vasoactive stimulant followed by bursts of action potentials, which are in turn followed by an influx of extracellular Ca^{2+}, which interacts with the actin and myosin filaments. This would be similar to observations obtained for many types of smooth, skeletal and cardiac muscles (35). A second concept is that, in certain types of VSM, the vasoactive stimulant causes graded depolarization, without induction of action potentials, followed in turn by either an influx of extracellular Ca^{2+} or a release of Ca^{2+} from some intracellular store (36). A third concept is that contraction can be initiated in certain types of VSM without a change in membrane potential; in this nonelectrical type of activation, Ca^{2+} is thought to be released from some intracellular store(s) (36,50,51). It is also possible that in certain types of VSM, different agonists utilize different mechanisms for activation and recruit several sources of cellular Ca^{2+} (38,52,53).

During the past decade, a new class of drugs have been brought forth which are thought to antagonize or block the entry of Ca^{2+} into cells, including VSM. These have been termed Ca^{2+} antagonists, Ca^{2+} entry blockers, or Ca^{2+} channel blockers (54). Several subclasses of these, e.g. 1,4-dihydropyridine derivatives (e.g., nitrendipine) have been suggested to act on, primarily, voltage-dependent Ca^{2+} channels in smooth muscle cell membranes (55), whereas others, e.g. verapamil, are thought to act on membrane receptor and voltage-operated Ca^{2+} channels in VSM (54). Tools such as these special drugs might, therefore, be useful in elucidating the source of activator Ca^{2+} ions for different vasoactive agents in pulmonary VSM. Using such drugs, we have recently examined their actions on canine intrapulmonary arteries and veins (28,56).

Although both nitrendipine and verapamil were able to attenuate in a dose-dependent manner (10^{-10} to 10^{-5}M) potassium-induced contractions in pulmonary VSM, with verapamil being about 100-1,000 times more potent, neither of these Ca^{2+} channel blockers were effective at attenuating vasoactive agonist (i.e., norepinephrine, phenylephrine, serotonin, angiotensin, prostanoid) –induced contractions until fairly high concentrations were used. In addition, both Ca^{2+} channel blockers were found to shift the potassium and vasoactive agonists contractile concentration effect curves to higher concentrations concomitant with progressive reductions in maximum responses when fairly high concentrations (e.g. 10^{-7} to 10^{-5}M) were used (28,56). Such data are consistent with the concept that although potassium probably induces contraction of pulmonary VSM primarily via an influx of Ca^{2+} from the extracellular compartment and/or membrane, and depolarization of the cell membrane, some of the Ca^{2+} is recruited from an intracellular compartment. With respect to the vasoactive agonists mentioned above, most of the Ca^{2+} required for contraction, particularly contractions of large magnitude, appears to be released or recruited from an intracellular compartment(s).

Whether these concepts will hold for all types of pulmonary VSM or different mammalian species must await further investigation.

G. Hypoxia-induced Contractions of Pulmonary VSM: Importance of Membrane Potential and Ca^{2+}

Although it has long been established that pulmonary hypertension develops in normal humans and animals during exposure to chronic hypoxia (57), there is still no adequate explanation of the mechanism. Several studies in rats and cats during the past four years lead one to now believe that the constrictor response to chronic hypoxia of pulmonary VSM may be multifactorial in etiology and may differ in the pulmonary vascular tree.

Recently, Madden and co-workers (16) have shown with cats, using isolated large (500 µm diam) *vs.* small (300 µm diam) pulmonary arteries that with the latter there is a consistent depolarization of the cell membrane as the oxygen in the bath was reduced from 400 to 50 Torr, concomitant with a progressive contraction, but a similar phenomenon was not observed in the large pulmonary arteries. In addition, this same group of investigators noted that the small vessel hypoxia-induced contractions increased in magnitude as the $[Ca^{2+}]$ was raised and blocked on addition of verapamil; concomitant with the contractions they also observed action potentials in the small vessels which could be aborted on addition of verapamil (58). Such data led these workers to conclude that hypoxia-induced pulmonary vasoconstriction is associated with an increase in Ca^{2+} conductance and is membrane potential dependent.

Other investigators (59), using rats and isolated main pulmonary artery and small pulmonary arteries, found that as chronic pulmonary hypoxia developed, pronounced differences between these types of pulmonary vessels were observed. Surprisingly, the resting membrane potential of the main pulmonary artery VSM underwent gradual depolarization, whereas the VSM of the small pulmonary artery underwent gradual hyperpolarization. They concluded that the former was due to an increased membrane permeability to Cl^-, whereas the hyperpolarization may be associated with an increased activity of an electrogenic Na^+,K^+pump.

One is thus left with the idea that either different pulmonary VSM may utilize several different mechanisms for the production of constriction upon exposure to prolonged hypoxia, or that there are species differences, or that both possibilities are probable. In any event, this only supports the idea that pulmonary VSM is heterogeneous in nature and that contractility is dependent upon a multiplicity of factors (Table I).

H.   Influences of Age and Development on Vascular Reactivity

Upon aging, there appears to be a generalized increase in peripheral vascular resistance and a decrease in perfusion of a number of critical organ regions (23). Data acquired, so far, in general, support the idea that arterial, arteriolar, and precapillary sphincter smooth muscle cells become hyporeactive to contractile agents in old age (18,22,23,26,60). Similar phenomena appear to be present in the pulmonary vasculature as well (Table II). Using piglets, we have found that receptors which subserve contraction for several agonists, e.g., norepinephrine, vasopressin, serotonin, and angiotensin, are already present in most peripheral blood vessels within 1-12 days after birth (22,61). Spontaneous mechanical activity (or vasomotion) appears within 2-4 days after birth in many piglet arteries and veins (61).

However, maturation of receptors for many contractile substances in piglet intrapulmonary arteries and veins appears to require at least 5-12 days after birth (62). For example, we have noted that although receptors which subserve contraction for norepinephrine are present witin 1-2 days after birth in intrapulmonary arteries, receptors for serotonin, angiotensin II and vasopressin are not present. With respect to piglet intrapulmonary veins, receptors for norepinephrine, serotonin, and acetylcholine are present within 1-2 days after birth. Such results suggest that not only is there a slow maturation of certain receptors in pulmonary blood vessels, but that there is a difference in development of receptors between pulmonary arteries and veins. Although these piglet pulmonary blood vessels demonstrated the presence of beta-adrenergic receptors which subserve

TABLE II. Contractile sensitivity of rat main pulmonary artery to vasoactive agents in young, mature and old Wistar rats.

Vasoactive Substance	ED 50 (Molar Conc.)*		
	Young	Mature	Old
Epinephrine	1.62 ± 0.25	3.80 ± 0.73	$9.4 \pm 0.83 \times 10^{-8}$
Serotonin	1.3 ± 0.4	2.66 ± 1.0	$6.23 \pm 0.72 \times 10^{-6}$
PGE$_2$	1.15 ± 0.23	4.65 ± 1.4	$12.24 \pm 2.47 \times 10^{-6}$

* All values (means $\pm$ SE) within each group are significantly different from one another (P <0.01).

relaxation within one day after birth, histamine H_2 receptors were not present even after 10 days after birth despite the fact that mature intrapulmonary blood vessels demonstrate such relaxation for histamine (9,62).

Such observations are beginning to make it clear that reactivity of pulmonary VSM can be influenced rather dramatically by the aging and maturation process.

I.   Influence of Ionic Environment on Responsiveness to Vasoactive Agents: Magnesium Concentration

Several years ago, we demonstrated that an alteration in the extracellular concentration of free Mg^{2+} can exert profound effects on contractility and reactivity of *in situ* and *in vitro* VSM (63-65). Such findings are particularly noteworthy because 1) Mg^{2+} is often omitted from physiologic salt solutions in many experimental designs, and 2) because the dietary intake of Mg^{2+} in the Western world is known to be sub-optimal (66-68). Furthermore, there is now evidence for a strong causal association between a high incidence of sudden death ischemic heart disease, strokes, hypertension and pre-eclampsia and low dietary intake of Mg^{2+} (69).

Briefly, it is now known that the contractile activity of all types of endogenous and exogenous contractile substances, so far investigated, is enhanced when the $[Mg^{2+}]_0$ is lowered. Conversely, an elevation of the $[Mg^{2+}]$, *i.e.*, above the normal plasma level (≥ 1.0 mM), will result in a nonspecific inhibition (in a concentration-dependent manner) of all types of contractile responses. Such effects have now been noted for all types of *in vivo* and *in vitro* mammalian VSM so far investigated, including pulmonary blood vessels (arterial and venous) (63-65,70). These vascular actions of Mg^{2+} are now known to be attributed to influences on Ca^{2+} content, intracellular binding and flux across VSM membranes. The findings suggest that membrane Mg sites may act, physiologically, to control and regulate content, entry and exit of Ca^{2+} in smooth muscle, including pulmonary VSM.

J.   Role of Vascular Endothelium

Approximately six years ago, it was reported that rabbit aortic rings contracted with various stimulants would relax when acetylcholine was added, provided the aortic rings were prepared with their endothelial cells (EC) left intact (71). We wondered whether selective removal of the endothelium from intrapulmonary arteries would result in a loss of these vessels to relax in response to certain neuro-humoral vasodilators and whether the vessels would contract, rather than relax, in response to these agents (41).

There is at present no agreement on the etiology of pulmonary hypertension although numerous mechanisms have been proposed (72). During the past decade, evidence has accumulated suggesting that circulatory shock induced by such factors as septicemia, trauma, and hypovolemia often results in a condition known as shock lung (72-74); the mortality in this syndrome often being around 50 percent. Shock lung syndrome is characterized by several pathologic findings that include massive vascular congestion, interstitial and intra-alveolar edema and hemorrhage, hyaline membrane formation, and—if the patient survives—pulmonary fibrosis. The pulmonary hypertension and shock lung syndromes both involve elevations in pulmonary vascular resistance and pulmonary congestion of unknown etiology. On autopsy, both of these syndromes reveal destruction of intrapulmonary arterial EC (72-74).

We reasoned that if intrapulmonary arteries and arterioles *in situ*, which are normally very distensible, develop constrictor responses to circulating neurohumoral agents that normally induce vasodilation in the lung, such as acetylcholine, kinins, and prostanoids, this mechanism could aid in explaining the etiology of shock lung and pulmonary hypertension.

Five years ago, we were the first to report that acetylcholine and bradykinin produce potent concentration–dependent relaxation of isolated intrapulmonary arteries, provided the endothelium is left intact (14,41,75). Selective removal of the EC causes a transformation in these effects so that only contractile actions are exerted on the intrapulmonary arteries. This concept has now been extended by our group to intact arterioles and metarterioles in the living microcirculation of rats (74,76).

Other studies from our laboratory have provided evidence that, in certain pulmonary blood vessels, an endothelium derived relaxing factor (or EDRF) (71) may not be involved in mediation of acetylcholine and bradykinin–EC relaxation (41). Our *in-vitro* studies rather suggest that these latter endogenous vasodilators may act by hyperpolarizing the pulmonary EC membrane to elicit the relaxation responses; myo-endothelial junctions could transfer the hyperpolarizing current to the underlying VSM cells and, thereby produce relaxation. Alternatively, some EDRF's may act by hyperpolarizing the underlying VSM cells to cause relaxation.

Irrespective of the exact mechanism, selective removal or pathological destruction of endothelium from intrapulmonary arteries and probably arterioles (76) can transform important circulating dilator agents into pulmonary vasoconstrictors. Obviously, such factors must be closely monitored in discerning responsiveness to vasoactive drugs or agonists in the pulmonary vasculature.

K.   Anesthetics Attenuate Actions of Vasoactive Agents on Pulmonary Blood Vessels

Most of the studies done on intact animals and the pulmonary vasculature employ a variety of substances in order to first anesthetize the animals. All general anesthetic agents (intravenous and volatile types) currently approved for clinical use in the USA, including even newer agents like ketamine and narcotic analgesics (*e.g.*, morphine, fentanyl) are known to compromise cardiovascular responses in intact animals, humans, and on isolated VSM (30,52,53,77). Up until recently, it was thought that the peripheral vasodilatation induced by general anesthetics was due exclusively to the effects these molecules exert on the cental and autonomic nervous systems and on the myocardium (78). Recent *in-vitro*, as well as direct microcirculatory, experiments are beginning to suggest that concentrations of anesthetics and analgesics used to induce surgical anesthesia can exert direct depressant and vasodilator effects on VSM. Evidence has accumulated which indicates that a variety of general anesthetics (barbiturates, halothane, isoflurane, ethanol, urethane, steroids, ether, propanidid, etomidate, ketamine, and even acetaldehyde) markedly, and dose dependently, attenuate contractile responses of isolated blood vessels to prostanoids, serotonin, histamine, catecholamines, angiotensins, vasopressin, kinins, substance P, and potassium ions (18,53,60,63,79). This is also observed on all pulmonary vessels so far investigated (rat main pulmonary artery, canine intrapulmonary arteries and veins; Altura, Carella and Altura, unpublished findings). A typical example is shown in Table III. None of the inhibitory effects induced by these anesthetics on peripheral or pulmonary blood vessels are modified or attenuated by known pharmacologic antagonists or PG synthetase inhibitors. A number of experiments on isolated VSM reveal that these anesthetic agents can, dose-dependently, prevent the uptake of radiolabeled Ca^{2+} into the VSM (30,63,80). It is important to emphasize that all of these inhibitory actions (*i.e.*, on contractility and ^{45}Ca uptake and distribution) are observed with plasma concentrations of the anesthetic agents that are associated with induction of anesthesia.

L.   Adverse Effects of Artificial Buffers on Contractility of Pulmonary Vascular Muscle

Due to the poor solubility and stablity of some prostanoids and other vasoactive drugs in bicarbonate buffered solutions, a variety of artificial buffers (*e.g.* Tris, HEPES, MOPS, etc.) are commonly employed to study the vasoactivity of these agents. Moreover, most studies investigating excitation-contraction coupling in VSM, including pulmonary VSM, employ these buffers

TABLE III. Anesthetics inhibit contractility of canine intrapulmonary arteries.*

Anesthetic Concentration (M)	Tension (Mg ± SEM)		
Pentobarbital, 2.5×10^{-4}			
Control	1200	±	175
Anesthetic	185	±	65**
Urethane, 5×10^{-2}			
Control	1350	±	202
Anesthetic	725	±	86**
Ketamine, 2×10^{-4}			
Control	1286	±	185
Anesthetic	370	±	40**

*Contracted with KCl, N = 6 - 10 each
**Significantly different from control (P <0.01).

so that high concentrations of various divalent cation-anion complexes will remain soluble in solution. It is rather common to utilize 10-30 mM concentrations of these artificial buffers to investigate VSM.

Several years ago, we reported that these artificial buffers, introduced by Good et al. in 1966, and Tris, when substituted for bicarbonate and phosphate anions and maintained at pH 7.3 to 7.4, attenuate, markedly, vasoactive drug (i.e,serotonin, histamine, amine, kinins, catecholamine, angiotensin II, vasopressin) and Ca^{2+}–induced contractions in VSM (29,31,81). In addition, we reported that these commonly used artificial buffers, such as Tris, HEPES and MOPS, exert significant inhibitory effects on exchangeability and transmembrane movement of Ca^{2+} in VSM (81-83). Similar findings on contractility and calcium exchange have now been observed in isolated rat and canine pulmonary VSM (Table IV).

M.   Influence of Tissue Injury and Shock on Responsiveness of Pulmonary Blood Vessels to Vasoactive Mediators

Even if all of the physiologic, pharmacologic, and experimental factors which can influence reactivity of pulmonary blood vessels to vasoactive hormones and mediators (Table I) are taken into consideration, one must still consider if tissue injury, handling, storage, pathophysiologic conditions and/or circulatory shock can alter vascular responsiveness. (Obviously, these considerations are over

TABLE IV. Adverse effects of artificial buffers* on contractile responses of pulmonary blood vessels.

	Vessel (species)		
	Tension (mg $\pm$ SE)		
Agonist, Buffer	Main Pulmonary Artery (Rat)	Intrapulmonary Artery (Dog)	Intrapulmonary Vein (Dog)
Phenylephrine			
Control	350 $\pm$ 28	1100 $\pm$ 123	305 $\pm$ 32
Tris	78 $\pm$ 12**	258 $\pm$ 43**	182 $\pm$ 24**
HEPES	85 $\pm$ 8**	185 $\pm$ 32**	166 $\pm$ 22**
MOPS	166 $\pm$ 36**	565 $\pm$ 129**	195 $\pm$ 28**
Serotonin			
Control	275 $\pm$ 18	1350 $\pm$ 148	325 $\pm$ 27
Tris	92 $\pm$ 8**	485 $\pm$ 110**	160 $\pm$ 16**
HEPES	86 $\pm$ 12**	566 $\pm$ 123**	142 $\pm$ 15**
MOPS	138 $\pm$ 18**	725 $\pm$ 142**	196 $\pm$ 15**
Potassium			
Control	365 $\pm$ 20	1402 $\pm$ 214	275 $\pm$ 41
Tris	14 $\pm$ 8**	275 $\pm$ 58**	152 $\pm$ 22**
HEPES	60 $\pm$ 25**	242 $\pm$ 44**	198 $\pm$ 36
MOPS	182 $\pm$ 65**	465 $\pm$ 78**	180 $\pm$ 25**

* All buffers used at 5mM concentrations; N=6-10 each.
** Significantly different from controls (P<0.01).

and above the destruction of the intimal EC mentioned above). A fairly large body of evidence has now accumulated which does indeed indicate that tissue injury, improper handling, the pathophysiologic state of the host and shock-trauma can greatly influence vascular reactivity (4,5,17,19,21,22,26,29,65,69,74). Recent unpublished studies from our laboratory have now clearly demonstrated that both the directions and magnitudes of the pulmonary VSM responses are altered by such pathophysiologic states. Often after circulatory shock and trauma in rats, reactivity of the main pulmonary artery and small intrapulmonary arteries (e.g. 300-400 μm od) to potassium and constrictor catecholamines is markedly and irreversibly reduced (Altura, Altura, Carella, Gebrewold and Weinberg, unpublished findings). Simple improper handling has been found to alter ionic equilibrium and reactivity. For example, Ca^{2+} and K^+ are lost and Na^+ is elevated in the latter situation. Quantitative studies which characterize receptors, hormone binding sites

and VSM smooth muscle biochemistry in tissue injury and shock with respect to
the pulmonary vasculature are, however, not available.

III.   CONCLUSIONS

In summary, the overview presented herein indicates that a wide variety of
physiologic, pharmacologic, and experimental factors can influence and modify the
tone and responsiveness of pulmonary blood vessels to endogenous and exogenous
vasoactive substances. The data reinforce the idea that heterogeneity of VSM
extends into the pulmonary vasculature. In addition, the data strengthen the
concept that some of the reported, diverse heterogeneous pharmacologic nature of
site-specific pulmonary blood vessels, and segments thereof, may be due to one or
more ofthese important, and often overlooked, factors. A great many of these
modifiers appear to influence the vascular actions of vascoactive agents, mediators
and local humoral substances by influencing the concentration of ionized activator
Ca^{2+} within the VSM cells. Finally, it is becoming apparent that many of the
pharmacologic, physiologic, and experimental agents discussed herein may be
useful tools in elucidating the mechanisms by which locally, and systemically,
generated vasoactive mediators induce relaxation and contraction of pulmonary
VSM.

REFERENCES

1.   Kaley G and Altura BM. (1977) **Microcirculation**, Vol 1, Univ Park
      Press:Baltimore.
2.   Abramson DI and Dobrin PI. (1984) **Blood Vessels**. Academic Press:New
      York
3.   Gillis CN and Roth JN. (1976) *Biochem Pharmacol* **25**:2547.
4.   Kaley G and Altura BM. (1978) **Microcirculation**, Vol II, Univ Park
      Press:Baltimore.
5.   Vanhoutte PM, Verbeuren TJ and Webb PC. (1981) *Physiol Rev*
      61:151.
6.   Somlyo AP and Somlyo AV. (1970) *Pharmacol Rev* **22**:249.
7.   Su C and Bevan JA. (1976) *Pharmacol Therap* **B:2**:275.
8.   Chand N and Altura BM. (1980) *J Appl Physiol* **49**:1016.
9.   Chand N and Altura BM. (1980) *Experientia* **36**:1186.
10.   Chand N and Altura BM. (1980) *Prostagland Med* **5**:59.

11.   Kadowitz PJ, Joiner PD and Hyman AL. (1975) *Am Rev Pharmacol* **15**:285.

12.   Kadowitz PJ, Spannhake EW, Levin EJ and Hyman AL. (1980) *In* **Advances in Prostaglandin and Thromboxane Research.** (B Samuelsson, PW Ramwell and E Paoletti, eds). Raven Press:New York.

13.   Altura BM and Chand N. (1981) *Brit J Pharm* **73**:819.

14.   Altura BM and Chand N. (1981) *Brit J Pharm* **74**:10.

15.   Dey RD and Said SI. (1985) *In* **The Pulmonary Circulation and Acute Lung Injury.** (SI Said ed) Futura Publ Co:Mt Kisco.

16.   Madden JA, Dawson CA and Harder DR. (1985) *J Appl Physiol* **59**:113.

17.   Kaley G and Altura BM. (1980) **Microcirculation,** Vol. III, Univ Park Press:Baltimore.

18.   Altura BM. (1978) *Microvascular Res* **16**:91.

19.   Altura BM. (1980) *Adv Shock Res* **3**:3.

20.   Altura BM. (1980) **Vascular Endothelium and Basement Membranes.** Karger:Basel.

21.   Altura BM. (1981)*In* **Microcirculation: Current Physiologic, Medical And Surgical Concepts.** (EM Effros, M Schmid-Schonbein and J Ditzel, eds). Academic Press:New York.

22.   Altura BM. (1981) *J Cardivasc Pharmacol* **3**:1413.

23.   Altura BM and Altura BT. (1977) *In* **Factors Influencing Vascular Reactivity.** (O Carrier Jr and S Snibata, eds). Igaku-Shain Ltd:Tokyo.

24.   Altura BM and Altura BT. (1977) *In* **Factors Influencing Vascular Reactivity.** (O Carrier Jr and S Shibata, eds). Igaku-Shoin Ltd:Tokyo.

25.   Altura BM and Altura BT. (1982) *Fed Proc* **41**:2442.

26.   Altura BM and Altura BT. (1982) *In* **Role of Chemical Mediators in the Pathophysiology of Acute Illness and Injury.** (R McConn ed). Raven Press:New York.

27.   Altura BM and Altura BT. (1984) *Fed Proc* **43**:80.

28.   Altura BM and Altura BT. (1984) *In* **Nitrendipine.** (A Scriabine, R Vanov and R Deck, eds). Urban and Schwarzenburg:Baltimore.

29.   Altura BM and Altura BT. (1986)*Alcoholism Clin and Exp Res* In press.

30.   Altura BM, Altura BT, Carella A and Turlapaty PDMV. (1980) *Brit J Pharmacol* **69**:207.

31.   Altura BM, Altura BT, Carella A, et al. (1980) *Fed Proc* **39**:1584.

32.   Altura BM, Carella A and Altura BT. (1980) *Prostaglandins Med* **5**:123.

33.   Bohr DF, Somlyo AP and Sparks HA Jr. (1980) **Handbook of Physiology, The Circulation: Vascular Smooth Muscle.** Am Physiol Soc:Washington DC.

34.   Altura BM and Altura BT. (1978)*In* **Mechanisms of Vasodilatation.** (PM Vanhoutte and I Leusen, eds). Karger:Basel.

35. Bevan JA and Su C. (1974) *J Pharmacol Exp Ther* **190**:30.
36. Prosser CL. (1974) *Am Rev Physiol* **36**:503.
37. Somlyo AP and Somlyo AV. (1968) *Pharmacol Rev* **20**:197.
38. Altura BM and Altura BT. (1970) *Eur J Pharmacol* **12**:44.
39. Altura BM and Altura BT. (1970) *Am J Physiol* **219**:1698.
40. Altura BM, Malaviya D, Reich CF and Orkin L R. (1972) *Am J Physiol* **222**:345.
41. Chand N and Altura BM. (1980)*Prostagland Med* **5**:469.
42. Hyman AL. (1969) *J Pharmacol Exp Ther* **168**:96.
43. Altura BM and Halevy S. (1978) *In* **Handbook of Experimental Pharmacology, Vol. 18. Histamine and Antihistaminics, Part II: Anti-Histaminics.** (M Roche e Silva ed) Springer Verlag:New York.
44. Chand N and Altura BM. (1980) *Artery* **7**:232.
45. Chand N and Altura BM. (1981) *Science* **213**:1376.
46. Suzuki HJ and Kou K. (1983) *Pflugers Arch* **399**:46.
47. Chand N and Altura BM. (1980) *Fed Proc* **39**:581.
48. Shepherd JT and Vanhoutte PM. (1975) **Veins and Their Control.** Saunders:Philadelphia.
49. Rorie DK. (1982) *Am J Physiol* **243**:H732.
50. Stephens NL. (1985). **Biochemistry of Smooth Muscle.** CRC Press:Boca Raton.
51. Bohr DF. (1969) *In* **The Pulmonary Circulation and Interstitial Space.** (AP Fishman and HH Mecht, eds). Univ. of Chicago Press:Chicago.
52. Hausler G. (1972) *J Pharmacol Exp Ther* **180**:672.
53. Altura BT and Altura BM. (1978) *In* **Microcirculation,** Vol II. (G Kaley and BM Altura, eds). Univ Park Press:Baltimore.
54. Altura BT and Altura BM. (1978) *In* **Mechanisms of Vasodilatation.** (PM Vanhoutte and I Leusen, eds). Karger:Basel.
55. Fleckinstein A. (1983) **Calcium Antagonists.** John Wiley & Sons, Inc:New York.
56. Scriabine A, Vanov R and Deck R. (1982) **Nitrendipine.** Urban L Schwarzenburg:Baltimore.
57. Altura BM, Altura BT, Carella A, Gablewold A, Murakawa T and Nishio A. (1986)*Canad J Physiol Pharmacol* In press.
58. Von Euler US and Liljestrand H. (1946) *Acta Physiol Scand* **12**:301.
59. Harder DR, Madden JA and Dawson C. (1985) *J Appl Physiol* **59**:1389.
60. Suzuki HJ and Twarog BM. (1982) *Am J Physiol* **242**:H907.
61. Altura BM and Altura BT. (1980) *In* **Vascular Neuroeffector Systems.** (JA Bevan, T Godfraind, RA Maxwell and P Vanhoutte, eds). Raven Press:New York.

62. Turlapaty PDMV, Altura BT, Gootman PM and Altura BM. (1979) *Fed Proc* **38**:437.
63. Chand N and Altura BM. (1979) Unpublished Findings.
64. Altura BM and Altura BT. (1981) *In* **New Perspectives in Calcium Antagonists.** (GB Weiss ed). Am Physiol Soc:Washington DC.
65. Altura BM and Altura BT. (1981) *Fed Proc* **40**:2672.
66. Altura BM and Altura BT. (1985) *Magnesium* **4**:244.
67. Marier JR, Neri LC and Anderson TW. (1979) *Natl Res Council Canada* Publ No. **17581**:1.
68. Turlapaty PDMV and Altura BM. (1980) *Science* **208**:198.
69. Seelig MS. (1980) **Magnesium Deficiency in the Pathogenesis of Disease.** Plenum Press:New York.
70. Altura BM and Altura BT. (1985) *Magnesium* **4**:226.
71. Altura BM, Altura BT, Carella A and Turlapaty PDMV. (1981) *Artery* **9**:212.
72. Furchgott RF and Zawadski J. (1980) *Fed Proc* **39**:581.
73. Moser KM. (1979) **Pulmonary Vascular Disease.** Marcel Dekker Inc:New York.
74. Thal AP, Brown EB Jr, Hermreck AS and Bell HM. (1971) **Shock: A Physiologic Basis for Treatment.** Year Book Med Publ:Chicago.
75. Altura BM, Lefer A M and Schumer W. (1983) **Handbook of Shock and Trauma, Vol. I: Basic Science.** Raven Press:New York.
76. Chand N and Altura BM. (1981) *Microcirculation* **1**:297.
77. Altura BM. (1986) *In* **Surgical and Critical Care of the Critically Ill Patient.** (RA Litte and R Frayn, eds). Manchester Univ Press:Manchester.
78. Altura BM and Halevy S. (1986) **Cardiovascular Actions of Anesthetics and Drugs Used in Anesthesia.** Karger:Basel.
79. Hug CC Jr. (1979) *In* **Cardiac Anesthesia.** (JA Kaplan ed). Grune & Stratton:New York.
80. Altura BT and Altura BM. (1975) *Anesthesiol* **43**:432.
81. Altura BT, Turlapaty PDMV and Altura BM. (1980) *Biophys Acta* **595**:309.
82. Turlapaty PDMV, Altura BT and Altura BM. (1978) *Am J Physiol* **235**:H208.
83. Turlapaty PDMV, Altura BT and Altura BM. (1979) *Biochim Biophys Acta* **551**:459.
84. Turlapaty PDMV, Altura BT and Altura BM. (1979) *J Pharmacol Exp Ther* **211**:59.

Vascular Smooth Muscle Metabolism and Mechanisms of Oxygen Sensing

RICHARD J. PAUL [1]
YUKISATO ISHIDA
GABOR RUBANYI
Department of Physiology &
Biophysics
University of Cincinnati
College of Medicine
Cincinnati, OH 45267-0576

I.   INTRODUCTION

The control of vascular smooth muscle contractility, the final effector in the regulation of circulation, has many dimensions. Much attention has been focused on the control of intracellular Ca^{2+}, which plays a central, though as yet not completely understood, role in the control of vascular contractility. Less well understood, vascular metabolism has received little attention as a possible control point. However, as will be argued here, vascular metabolism must be closely coordinated with contractile energy requirements for normal function. The potential role of metabolism as a control point for contractility is most clearly recognized in terms of the vascular response to changes in tissue oxygen levels. In this chapter, we would like to briefly review vascular metabolism, to consider vascular metabolism and energy limitations as a possible mechanism for the regulation of

[1] *Supported in part by NIH 23240 and an Established Investigatorship of the American Heart Association* .

vascular tone, particularly in response to hypoxia, and lastly to consider the
evidence for mechanisms of oxygen sensing in vascular tissue not related to energy
limitation.

II. RELATIONS BETWEEN VASCULAR METABOLISM AND CONTRACTILITY

In considering skeletal muscle performance one is readily aware that its
metabolic capacity can affect function, particularly in terms of fatigue. This is
less obvious for vascular smooth muscle (VSM), though like any muscle, it must
match contractile energy requirements with the appropriate ATP synthesis. It is
somewhat paradoxical that smooth muscle (which is characterized by a remarkable
low tension cost: its rate of ATP utilization per unit isometric force maintained
may be up to 1000-fold less than skeletal muscle) is even more immediately
dependent on a continuous supply of metabolic energy than skeletal muscle for
normal function. This is primarily due to the fact that the preformed pool of high
energy phosphagen (ATP + PCr) is an order of magnitude lower in smooth than in
striated muscle. As illustrated by the extents of the phosphagen pools and rates of
energy utilization for typical smooth muscles given in Table I, if solely dependent
on pre-formed phosphagen, smooth muscle could not achieve the peak force of an
isometric contraction. A consequence of this dependence on a continuous supply
of metabolic supply is shown in Figure 1, which shows the isometric force
response of typical smooth muscles to the inhibition of oxidative metabolism

TABLE I. Energy stores *vs.* energy flux in muscle.

| | Store* $\Delta \sim P$ $\mu mol/g$ | Utilization rate | | References |
| | | Basal | Contraction | |
		$\mu mol/min \cdot g$		
Skeletal muscle				
Dog semitendinosus	15-30**	1.3	50	Stainsby and Barclay (31)
Smooth muscle				
Hog carotid artery	1.2	0.6	1.2	Glück and Paul (19)
				Krisanda and Paul (1)
Guinea pig taenia coli	4.0	1.7	3.0	Ishida and Paul
				(unpublished)

*   ATP + PCr
** Range reported for skeletal muscle

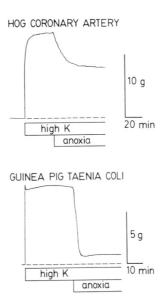

Figure 1. Contractile response to a high concentration of potassium (high K) under aerobic and anoxic conditions in the hog coronary artery and guinea pig tænia coli. Anoxia was achieved by vigourously bubbling bathing solutions with 95% N_2 - 5% CO_2 instead of 95% O_2 - 5% CO_2.

induced by anoxia. The question as to whether the observed loss of force can be quantitatively explained in terms of a limitation of energy metabolism will be assessed following the discussion of vascular metabolism.

In contrast to skeletal muscle, under normal oxygenated conditions little change in the phosphagen content of tonic VSM occurs during the transition from rest to fully stimulated conditions (1). This indicates that ATP synthesis is closely coupled to ATP utilization. Vascular tissue is primarily oxidative with more than 80% of the total ATP synthesis ascribable to oxidative phosphorylation (2,3). Due to the rapid achievement of a steady state of the phosphagen pools, non-tissue destructive techniques, such as continuous measurement of vascular oxygen consumption, can be used to assess contractile ATP requirements. An example of this is given in Figure 2 which shows the responses of isometric force and oxygen consumption of hog carotid artery following depolarization by added KCl. A striking feature of this response is that vascular smooth muscle can maintain isometric forces as large as those of skeletal muscle with only a two-fold increase in JO_2 over the basal rate. Skeletal muscle in contrast may increase JO_2 up to 40-

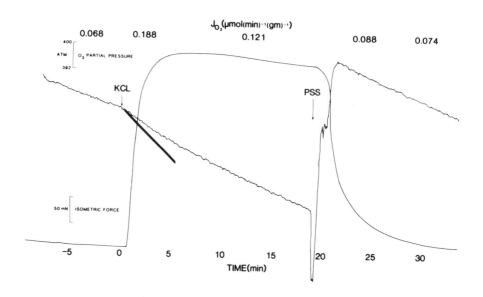

Figure 2. Record of O_2 tension and isometric force for a strip of porcine carotid artery media stimulated with 50 mM KCl. Passive tension was 50 mN and active isometric tension was 430 mN (147 mN/mm²). Slope of O_2 tension vs. time trace (determined by straight-edge fit) was used to calculate basal (0.068), and steady-state (0.121) levels of tissue O_2 consumption (JO_2) (μmol O_2/min/g). The peak suprabasal JO_2 was approximately twice steady-state suprabasal JO_2. Continuous dark line intersecting O_2 tension recording at 30 s poststimulation is calculated O_2 tension record assuming a peak suprabasal JO_2 that is 4 times steady-state rate. From Krisanda and Paul (4).

fold, which is still not adequate to maintain isometric force under similar conditions. In numerous experiments it has been shown that isometric force and the concomitant actomyosin ATPase underlie approximately 80% of the suprabasal oxygen consumption (2,3). A schematic outline of the experiments indicating that isometric force is the primary determinant of suprabasal vascular O_2 consumption is given in Figure 3. More recent experiments dealing with the time course of JO_2 and the effects of calcium relevant to those interested in the mechanisms of regulation and mechanochemical energy transduction have been reported (4,5,6).

Although most of the ATP synthesized in vascular smooth muscle (VSM) occurs via oxidative phosphorylation, an unusual feature of vascular metabolism is that under fully oxygenated conditions a substantial amount of lactate is produced. More than 90% of the glucose that enters the cell is

ENERGETICS OF ISOMETRIC CONTRACTION IN VASCULAR SMOOTH MUSCLE

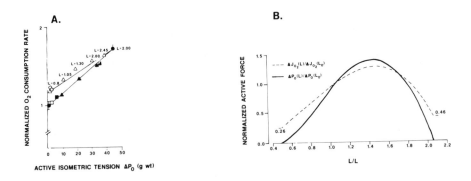

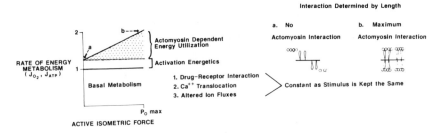

C. MAXIMAL ACTIVATION AT VARIOUS MUSCLE LENGTHS

D. FIXED MUSCLE LENGTH AT VARIOUS DEGREES OF ACTIVATION

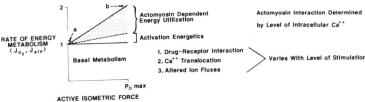

Figure 3. Schematic of experiments and interpretation of the major determinants of vascular smooth muscle oxidative metabolism. For details see text; adapted from 2,3.

catabolized to lactate. Such aerobic glycolysis is a characteristic of relatively few cell types, notably transformed cell lines such as the Ehrlich ascites tumor cells. While often viewed as some type of metabolic defect, we have shown that while oxidative metabolism is correlated with force, aerobic glycolysis in VSM is strongly correlated with the activity of the Na-pump (7,8). Although the degree of correlation of aerobic glycolysis and Na-pump activity varies among smooth muscles, it is quite clear that oxidative metabolism and the aerobic production of lactate can be varied independently. We have proposed that this functional compartmentation of metabolism reflects a cytosolic compartmentation of glycolytic and glycogenolytic enzymes, with a membrane bound glycolytic enzyme cascade positioned to support membrane pump function and a separate glycogenolytic cascade responsive to contractile energy requirements (9). Current work in this area focuses on the compartmentation of cyclic nucleotide effects potentially underlying the independent control of oxidative and glycolytic metabolism (10) and the possibility that high energy phosphagens are also compartmentalized in VSM (11).

With this overview of vascular metabolism, we are now in a position to test the hypothesis that the loss of force observed with anoxia (Fig. 1) can be attributed to a limitation of energy metabolism at the level of the contractile apparatus. The energy limitation hypothesis for the guinea pig taenia coli was based on the observation that an increase in media glucose can increase both force and the rate of ATP synthesis under anoxia (12). A major competing hypothesis is that the loss in tension is due to an inhibition of excitation-contraction coupling (13). For example, Ashoorie *et al.* (14) proposed that a decrease in membrane permeability to Ca is a major factor, when the tissue is exposed to metabolically suppressed conditions such as substrate (glucose) depletion. Altura and Altura (15) reported that the addition of Ca is not capable of restoring the contractile response of the rabbit aorta exposed to glucose-free conditions. This would support the energy limitation hypothesis; however, neither of these hypotheses is likely to be valid in a general sense, given the wide variety of responses to anoxia among various smooth muscles. We have studied the energy limitation hypothesis in detail for hog coronary artery and guinea pig taenia, by measuring their mechanical response, phosphagen levels, and rates of ATP synthesis under various conditions.

When the concentration of media K was increased (from 5.4 to 45.4 mM for the taenia or to 85.4 mM for the coronary), the muscles developed sustained tensions of 180 mN/mm² in the coronary and 200 mN/mm² in the taenia. Exposure of these muscles to anoxia (solutions vigorously bubbled with 95% N_2-5% CO_2) elicited relaxions of approximately 30% and 90% of the control isometric force in the coronary and taenia, respectively (Fig. 1). Increasing glucose concentration from 5.5 to 55mM under anoxia restored the tension to approximately 40% of control in the taenia, but did not affect tension in the coronary.

Phosphagen (ATP and PCr) content was measured using analytical isotachophoresis (1). Table II shows phosphagen levels under various conditions in the steady state. In the presence of oxygen, the phosphagen level was less in the coronary than in the taenia. Anoxia did not alter the phosphagen level of the

TABLE II. Phosphagen content and rate of ATP synthesis of hog coronary arteries and guinea pig taenia coli under aerobic and anaerobic conditions.

Conditions	Potassium*	Glucose	Phosphagen content (PCr + ATP)		Rate of ATP synthesis	
			Coronary	Taenia	Coronary	Taenia
			(μmol/g)		(μmol/min·g)	
Aerobic	5.4	5.5	0.41	3.96	1.18	1.71
Aerobic	85.4 or 45.4	5.5	0.47	3.65	1.71	3.01
Anoxic	85.4 or 45.4	5.5	0.44	0.99	0.62	0.90
Anoxic	85.4 or 45.4	55.0	0.58	1.37	0.63	1.50

* High concentrations of potassium were 85.4 mM for the coronary artery and 45.4 mM for the taenia coli.

coronary, but reduced the level in the taenia. Increasing the glucose concentration partially restored the ATP content without significantly affecting the PCr content of the taenia.

The rate of oxygen consumption and rate of lactate production of tissues were measured, as reported previously (16). When muscles were stimulated with high concentrations of potassium, the oxygen consumption was increased from 0.16 to 0.26 μmol/min/g in the coronary and from 0.22 to 0.45 in the taenia, and lactate production was also increased from 0.15 to 0.24 μmol/min/g in the coronary and 0.05 to 0.08 μmol/min/g in the taenia. From these results, the rate of ATP synthesis can be calculated, assuming that glycolysis and glycogenolysis contribute to the same extent to produce ATP (17; Table II). The rates of ATP synthesis of the unstimulated muscles were 1.2 μmol/min/g for the coronary and 1.7 for the taenia. When muscles were exposed to anoxia, the rate of ATP synthesis was solely attributable to lactate production. Under anoxia in the presence of high K, those rates were decreased to 0.6 μmol/min/g in the coronary and to 0.9 in the taenia. Increasing the glucose concentration in the presence of high K under anoxia did not alter the rate of ATP synthesis in the coronary, but augmented it to 1.5 μmol/min/g in the tænia.

From these results, the guinea pig tænia coli appears to be a limiting case in that even if all the ATP synthesis under anaerobic conditions were directly due solely to the actomyosin ATPase, isometric force could not be maintained at the levels observed under aerobic conditions. Furthermore, the maintained level of force is refractory to other agonists under anoxic conditions (Ishida & Paul, unpublished observations). The validity of the energy limitation hypothesis is not as clear for the coronary artery; however, maintenance of aerobic levels of isometric force would require that the entire anærobic metabolism be directed to the actomyosin system, which is unlikely. The lower degree of inhibition of tension by hypoxia in the coronary artery may be attributed to the lower tension cost of the coronary relative to the tænia: the apparent rate of ATP utilization per unit isometric force (tension cost) was estimated at 3 μmol/min/g per mN/mm^2 for the coronary and 12 for the tænia, based on the difference between the presence and absence of high K under aerobic conditions. Thus, it appears to be clear that in some cases metabolism can be limiting to smooth muscle function, and a mechanism by which the ambient oxygen level can be sensed by the tissue.

III.   OXYGEN SENSING MECHANISMS INDEPENDENT OF METABOLISM

The relaxation of isometric force in isolated vascular strips induced by decreasing bath PO_2's can be adequately explained by the progressive development on an anoxic core region (18,19). However, Duling (20) has argued that the low PO_2's required for inhibition are unlikely to be obtained *in vivo*. It is worth noting that under certain conditions, Wilson *et al.* (21) have reported that mitochondrial respiration can be altered at PO_2's in the physiological range, substantially higher than the 1-2 torr found for these *in vitro* studies on isolated vascular strips. There have been a number of hypotheses put forth to account for the oxygen sensitivity of mechanical force in VSM that are independent of the mitochondrial electron transport chain [for a short review of this literature, see (22)]. Strong evidence for an oxygen sensing mechanism was provided by Coburn *et al.* (23) who showed that mechanical tension in rabbit aorta was still affected by altering organ bath PO_2 after inhibition of detectible oxygen uptake by cyanide. A difficulty in the interpretation of these alternative O_2-sensing mechanisms is that they are based on experiments in which the response to decreasing PO_2 was a relaxation of isometric force. This is in the same direction as predicted by the energy limitation hypothesis and thus tends to make the separation of these proposed mechanisms less than straightforward.

We have investigated the responses of hog coronary to changes in bath PO_2's. This preparation is somewhat unusual amongst systemic vessels in that as shown in Figure 4, decreases in bath PO_2 from 95% to 40% or 12% O_2 results in a contraction, whereas a decrease to 0% O_2 results in an initial contraction followed by a relaxation (22). The vasoconstriction observed with the change in PO_2 from 95% to 40%is not only a range in which it is unlikely to be limiting to mitochondrial respiration but this increase in tension would, in fact, require an increase rather than be the consequence of a decrease in metabolic energy. The

PORCINE CORONARY ARTERY

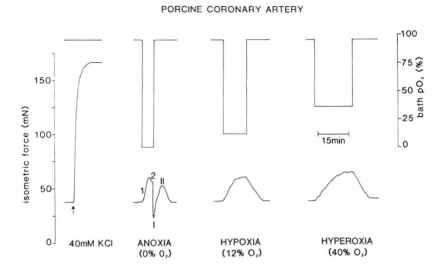

Figure 4. Responses of porcine coronary artery rings to changes in bath PO_2. Reduction in oxygen tension by gassing the bathing medium with 95% N_2, 5% CO_2 (anoxia) induced a transient contraction (phase 1) followed by relaxation (phase 2). Reoxygenation by 95% O_2, 5% CO_2 resulted in a relaxation (phase I) followed by contraction (phase II) above baseline. The decrease of bath PO_2 to 12% (hypoxia) or 40% elicited a sustained contraction (10-15% of 40 mM KCl-induced test contracture, lefthand side of the figure), which was reversible upon reoxygenation with 95% O_2. From Rubanyi and Paul (22).

response at high O_2 levels thus appeared to be distinct from that seen with anoxia, which as indicated above is likely to be due to energy limitation. Similar to the vasodilatation induced by changes in PO_2 at relatively high levels, observed by Kalsner (24) in bovine coronary artery, the vasoconstriction response observed in porcine coronaries was abolished by cyclooxygenase inhibitors. This sensitivity to cyclooxygenase inhibition was not observed for the relaxation induced by anoxia. We also found that the ß-agonist isoproterenol which decreased the overall coronary tone, paradoxically increased the response to O_2 in the high PO_2 range. In subsequent work (25) it was shown that the effects of oxygen were due to a shift in the sensitivity of the coronary artery to the relaxation induced by isoproterenol. As shown in Figure 5, the dose-response curve to isoproterenol measured at a PO_2 of 40% is shifted to the left when measured at 95% O_2. Furthermore, we showed that this shift in the dose-response curve to isoproterenol was likely mediated by eicosanoid metabolism. Interventions which inhibit eicosanoid synthesis,

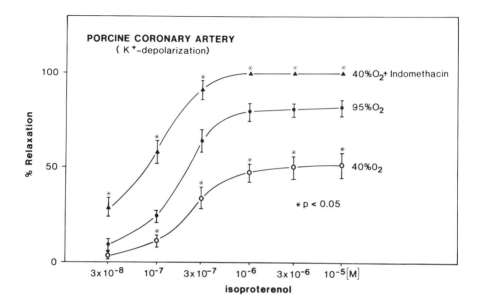

Figure 5. Effects of a decrease in bath PO₂ from 90 to 40% on ISO-induced relaxation in K⁺-depolarized (40 mM KCl) isolated porcine coronary artery rings. O₂ (40%) significantly inhibited beta adrenergic relaxation which was totally abolished by indomethacin (5.5 x 10⁻⁶M). Mean ± S.E. of six experiments. From Rubanyi and Paul (25).

indomethacin or high PO_2 (26), potentiated the response to isoproterenol, while those which stimulated eicosanoid metabolism, the addition of arachidonic acid or intermediate PO_2's, inhibited the response to isoproterenol (Fig. 5). Similar results were obtained when adenosine was the agonist used to elicit relaxation (27). Thus the vasoconstriction observed on decreasing PO_2's in a range where metabolism would not be affected appears to be due to an interaction between eicosanoid metabolism and ß-adrenergic mechanisms. Recent work suggests that the underlying mechanism is not simply a modulation of total cellular cAMP content in response to alterations in eicosanoid metabolism (10). This example of a vascular response to oxygen that is independent of metabolism may represent a more general class of mechanism whereby oxygen sensing is achieved by the modulation of response to vasoactive substances mediated by alterations in eicosanoid metabolism.

IV.   ROLE OF ENDOTHELIUM

Recently, much research activity has focused on the role of the endothelium in modulating vascular responses. Furchgott (28) has shown that the response to various pharmacological agents is dramatically dependent on the presence of an intact endothelium. We have recently shown in preliminary experiments on coronary arteries, that the metabolism of the vessel wall is not significantly dependent on the presence of endothelium *per se*, other than that mediated by the oxygen consumption related to isometric force, which in turn can be modulated by endothelium (29). An intact endothelium does inhibit the levels of basal tone (active isometric force produced in the absence of stimulation) and because of this can reduce the vasoconstriction due to alterations of PO_2 in the high PO_2 range (30). Though only speculative at this point, one might anticipate that endothelial energy metabolism might play a role in the oxygen sensing of intact vessels.

V.   SUMMARY AND CONCLUSIONS

The response of the pulmonary circulation to oxygen is complex and obviously multifactorial. In this brief review, we have attempted to show that the energy metabolism of vascular smooth muscle plays an important role in regulation of contractility and to more precisely define the conditions in which energy limitations can affect vascular responses. It is also clear that mechanisms in addition to metabolism can play a role in oxygen sensing. In particular, oxygen sensitivity in PO_2 ranges not limiting to metabolism can modulate contractile responses by a mechanism in which eichosanoid metabolism modulates the sensitivity to ß-agonists. Little is known about endothelial metabolism, and though it is not a major factor in the metabolism of the whole vessel, an intact endothelium can modulate responses to oxygen. The physiological significance of these potential oxygen sensing mechanisms to the response of whole vascular beds remains to be elucidated.

REFERENCES

1.   Krisanda JM and Paul RJ. (1983) *Am J Physiol* **244**:C385.
2.   Paul RJ. (1980) *In* **Handbook of Physiology, Section 2. The Cardiovascular System. Vol II: Vascular Smooth Muscle.** (DF Bohr, AP Somlyo and HV Sparks, eds) Amer Physiol Soc:Bethesda, Maryland.

3. Paul RJ. (1986) *In* **Physiology of the Gastrointestinal Tract.** 2nd edition. (LR Johnson ed) Raven Press:New York.
4. Krisanda JM and Paul RJ. (1984) *Am J Physiol* **246**:C510.
5. Hellstrand P and Paul RJ. (1983) *Am J Physiol* **244**:C250.
6. Paul RJ, Krisanda JM and Lynch RM. (1984) *J Cardiovascular Pharmacol* **6**:S320.
7. Paul RJ, Bauer JM and Pease W. (1979) *Science* **206**:1414.
8. Paul RJ. (1983) *Am J Physiol* **244**:C399.
9. Lynch RM and Paul RJ. (1983) *Science* **222**:342.
10. Rubanyi G, Galvas P, Di Salvo J and Paul RJ. (1986) *Am J Physiol* **250**:C406.
11. Ishida Y and Paul RJ. (1986) *Fed Proc* **45**:766.
12. Ishida Y, Takagi K and Urakawa N. (1984) *J Physiol* **347**:149.
13. Tomita T, Takai A and Tokuno H. (1985) *Experientia* **41**:963.
14. Ashoori R, Takai A, Tokuno H and Tomita T. (1984) *J Physiol* **356**:347.
15. Altura BM and Altura BT. (1970) *Am J Physiol* **219**:1698.
16. Paul RJ and Peterson JW. (1975) *Am J Physiol* **228**:915.
17. Peterson JW and Paul RJ. (1974) *Biochim Biophys Acta* **357**:167.
18. Pittman RN and Duling BR. (1973) *Microvasc Res* **6**:202.
19. Glück E and Paul RJ. (1977) *Pflügers Arch* **370**:9.
20. Duling BR. (1974) *Am J Physiol* **227**:42.
21. Wilson DF, Erecinska M, Drown C and Silver IA. (1979) *Arch Biochem Biophys* **195**:485.
22. Rubanyi G and Paul RJ. (1985) *Circ Res* **56**:1.
23. Coburn RF, Grubb B and Aronson RD. (1979) *Circ Res* **44**:368.
24. Kalsner S. (1975) *Can J Physiol Pharmacol* **53**:560.
25. Rubanyi G and Paul RJ. (1984) *J Pharmacol Exp Ther* **230**:692.
26. Kalsner S. (1976) *Blood Vessels* **13**:155.
27. Rubanyi G and Paul RJ. (1985) *Blood Vessels* **22**:209.
28. Furchgott R. (1983) *Circ Res* **53**:557.
29. Close L, Roth PS and Paul RJ. (1986) *Fed Proc* **45**:767.
30. Ngai JH and Paul RJ. (1985) *Fed Proc* **44**:1235.
31. Stainsby WN and Barclay JK. (1971) *Am J Physiol* **221**:1238.

Pharmacological Studies of Contractile and Relaxant Responses to Serotonin in Extralobar Pulmonary Arteries Isolated from the Guinea Pig

CARL K. BUCKNER
RICARDO SABAN
JAMES M. HAND[1]
RAYMOND B. LARAVUSO
JAMES A. WILL
*School of Pharmacy and Departments
of Anesthesiology and Veterinary
Science
University of Wisconsin
Madison, WI 53706*

I.   INTRODUCTION

Serotonin is known to cause contraction of isolated pulmonary vascular smooth muscle segments (arteries and veins) from several species (reviewed in 1). In contrast, the predominant response to serotonin in isolated sheep (2) and goat (3) pulmonary veins is relaxation. However, there is a relative paucity of information about the several potential responses and receptor subtypes for serotonin in the pulmonary vasculature.

---

[1] *Present address: Wyeth Laboratories, Inc., P.O. Box 8299,
Philadelphia, PA 19101*

The Pulmonary Circulation
in Health and Disease

109

Contractile responses of isolated guinea-pig pulmonary arteries to serotonin consist of two dose-dependent phases (1). Contractions seen at small concentrations, but not those seen at large concentrations, of serotonin are antagonized by methysergide (1). This communication describes further studies on the multiple effects of serotonin on these pulmonary arteries.

II.   METHODS

Albino guinea pigs (Department of Veterinary Science, University of Wisconsin, Madison, WI), weighing 300-700 g, were sacrificed by cervical dislocation. The proximal half of the main pulmonary artery (MPA) and the left main branch (LPA) were examined as isolated ring segments as previously described in detail (4). In most cases, animals were pretreated with reserpine, 5 mg/kg, i.p., 16-20 hr before sacrifice in order to minimize contribution to the responses by release of endogenous norepinephrine. In some cases, animals were pretreated with 6-hydroxydopamine, 200 mg/kg, i.p., for 2 days and used on day 3. Both treatments resulted in loss of contraction evoked by transmural electrical stimulation.

Dose-response curves were obtained by addition of agonist to the tissue bath in cumulative increments of about 3-fold. Transmural electrical stimulation (ES) was applied through platinum plate electrodes placed one each side of the tissue and monophasic square wave pulses generated from a Grass model S44 stimulator. Cumulative frequency-response effects were obtained using 10V stimuli of 1 msec duration. Each increment in concentration or pulse frequency (2-fold) was applied after the effect of the previous treatment reached a stable plateau.

Contractile response to each concentration of agonist was expressed as a percentage of the maximum contractile response to barium chloride, 3×10^{-2} M, added at the end of each experiment.

Relaxant responses were examined after incubation of the tissues for 35 min with phenoxybenzamine, 10^{-5} M. This was used to block all contractile responses to serotonin. Tone was induced in each tissue by prostaglandin $F_{2\alpha}$ ($PGF_{2\alpha}$) added 20 min before evoking relaxation. The concentrations of $PGF_{2\alpha}$ were 6×10^{-7} M and 3×10^{-6} M for the MPA and LPA, respectively. These produced 30-50% of the maximum contraction to barium in each segment. None of the pretreatments reported here altered the magnitude of the $PGF_{2\alpha}$-induced contractions. The contraction produced by $PGF_{2\alpha}$ was at its peak within 20 min (when relaxation was evoked) and was maintained for a period of time longer than that required to complete the experiments described here. Relaxant responses were expressed as a percentage of the maximum relaxant response produced by papaverine, 10^{-3} M, added at the end of each experiment.

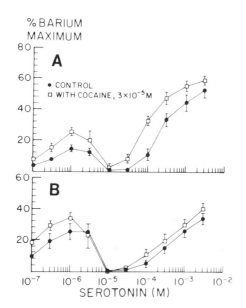

Figure 1. Log dose-response curves to serotonin in paired MPA (A) and LPA (B) segments. Cocaine was added 30 min before serotonin. Each curve is the average of 6 observations and vertical lines represent SEM.

Usually, only one dose-response curve was obtained on a single piece of tissue. Statistical comparisons were made using analysis of variance or Student's t test for unpaired samples.

III.   RESULTS

A.   Contractile Responses to Serotonin

Dose-response curves to serotonin exhibited two contractile phases (Figure 1). Contractions at small concentrations (10^{-7} to 3×10^{-6} M; phase I) were separated from those at large concentrations (3×10^{-5} to 3×10^{-3} M; phase II) by a slow return to baseline tension. The contraction existing at the peak of phase I gradually faded and basal tension was reached within 3 to 6 min. Subsequent increases in serotonin concentration resulted in the development of phase II contractions. Cocaine did not alter the shape of the dose-response curves (Figure 1).

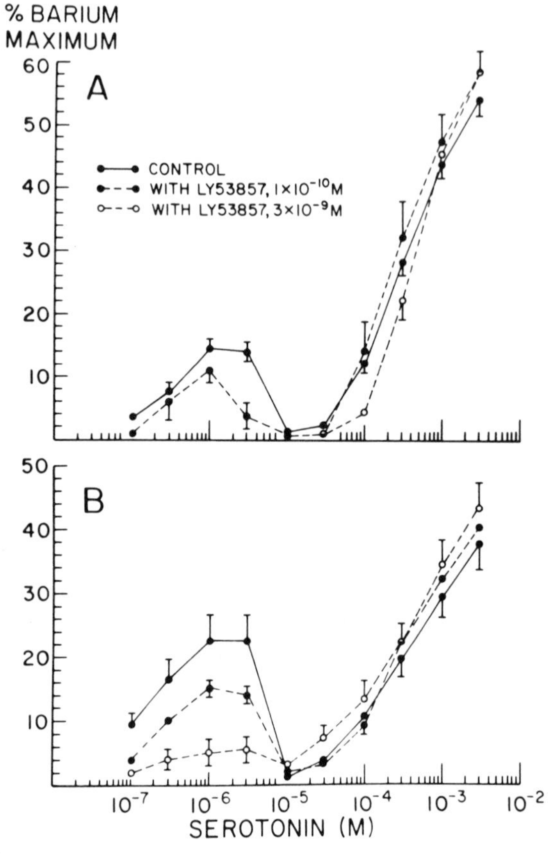

Figure 2. LY53857 was added 1 hr before serotonin. n = 13 (•—•), 3 (•---•) and 5 (°). See also Fig. 1 legend.

The selective 5-HT_2 receptor antagonist LY53857 (5) produced dose-dependent antagonism of phase I without alteration of phase II in the two segments (Figure 2). Spiperone, 10^{-6} M, abolished phase I contractions and shifted phase II in the MPA, but not the LPA, to the right by about 0.5 log units (Figure 3). The -log molar K_B (apparent dissociation constant) calculated for spiperone in antagonizing phase II in the MPA was 6.34. In the presence of mepyramine, 10^{-6} M (Figure 4), phase I was shifted to the right in both segments. Phase II of the MPA was not altered, but was markedly depressed by mepyramine in the LPA. Indomethacin, 5 X 10^{-6} M, added to the physiological salt solution and present throughout the experiments, did not alter either phase (n = 2, data not shown).

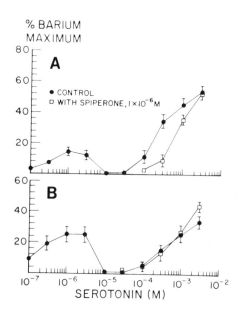

Figure 3. Spiperone was added 1 hr before serotonin. N = 6 (•) and 4 (º). See also Fig. 1 legend.

The effect of phentolamine was dose-dependent (Figure 5). With 10^{-6} M, there was antagonism of phase I in both segments, but the magnitude of this phase in the LPA was increased. Antagonism of phase II contractions was evident only in the MPA (-log molar K_B = 6.28). With 10^{-5} M, the shape of the serotonin dose-response curves was altered so that the curves assumed more of a monophasic appearance in both segments. A similar change in the shape of the serotonin dose-response curves was obtained in the presence of dansylcadaverine, 3 X 10^{-5} M (Figure 6). In the presence of cocaine and phentolamine, LY53857, 3 X 10^{-9} M (which abolished phase I in the absence of other treatments, see Fig. 2), antagonized serotonin only in the MPA (Figure 7).

Tachyphylaxis to the contractile effects of serotonin was observed in both arterial segments (Figure 8). When two consecutive dose-response curves to serotonin were obtained in the same tissue, there was selective diminution of phase I responses. When the tissues were first exposed to a large dose of serotonin, there was complete loss of phase I and reduction of phase II contractions in both segments. Neither treatment resulted in inhibition of dose-response curves for contraction produced by methoxamine or histamine.

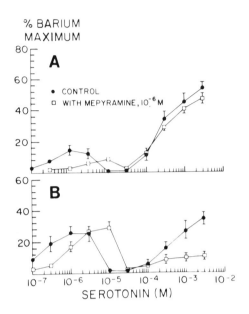

Figure 4. Mepyramine was added 1 hr before serotonin. N = 6 (•) and 7(°) See also Fig. 1 legend.

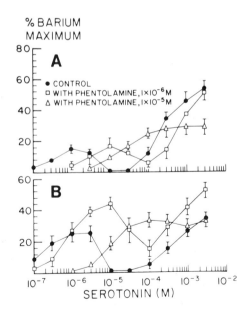

Figure 5. Phentolamine was added 1 hr before serotonin. n = 6 (•), 5 (°) and 4 (Δ). See also Fig. 1 legend.

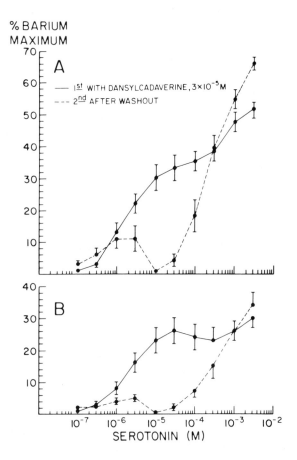

Figure 6. Dansylcadaverine (DC) was added to the physiological salt solution and in contact with the tissues from the time of extirpation. At the peak of response to serotonin, tissues were washed for 15 min in the presence of DC and then for 45 min in DC-free solution before obtaining the second dose-response curve to serotonin. n = 8. *See also Fig. 1 legend.*

B.   Relaxant Responses to Serotonin

Serotonin produced dose-dependent relaxation in the MPA without causing substantial relaxation in the LPA (Figure 9). The maximum relaxant response to serotonin, 10^{-5} M, in the LPA was $6 \pm 1\%$ (n = 9) of that produced by papaverine. The dose-response curve to serotonin in the MPA had a biphasic

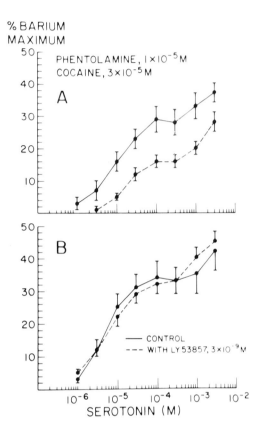

Figure 7. Phentolamine and LY53857 were added 1 hr and cocaine 30 min before serotonin. n = 9 (•—•) and 10 (•---•). See also Fig. 1 legend.

appearance with a plateau of phase I occurring between 10^{-7} and 3×10^{-7} M and stabilizing at about 20% of the maximum to papaverine.

When the tissues were exposed to serotonin, 10^{-3} M, 30 min, and washed for 1 hr, there was significant reduction of the relaxant effect of subsequently administered serotonin (Figure 9). This appeared more prominent for phase I.

Capsaicin also produced dose-dependent relaxation of the MPA and not of the LPA (Fig. 9). Relaxant responses to capsaicin were markedly reduced after prior exposure to capsaicin.

ES produced frequency-dependent relaxation of both arterial segments, but the MPA was about 10-fold more sensitive than the LPA (Figure 10). Prior application of ES resulted in reduction of the relaxant responses to subsequent ES. Tetrodotoxin, 10^{-6} M, antagonized relaxant responses to ES in both segments, but did not alter relaxant responses to serotonin or capsaicin.

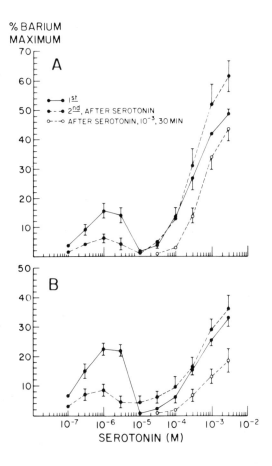

Figure 8. Two consecutive dose-response curves to serotonin obtained on
the same tissue (•, n = 6). Dose-response curves to serotonin after addition of a
single concentration of serotonin followed by 30 min wash (°). See also Fig. 1
legend.

When the MPA was first exposed to capsaicin or ES in protocols which
produced homologous tachyphylaxis, only capsaicin pretreatment produced cross-
tachyphylaxis to serotonin (Figure 11). This was observed only for phase II of the
relaxant response to serotonin. Capsaicin also produced cross-tachyphylaxis to the
relaxant effect of ES in the MPA, but not in the LPA (Figure 12). Serotonin
produced a smaller degree of cross-tachyphylaxis to ES, also observed only in the
MPA (Fig. 12).

Drugs that were found to antagonize serotonin-induced relaxation of the
MPA are listed in Table I. Of these, cocaine, imipramine, d-tubocurarine and

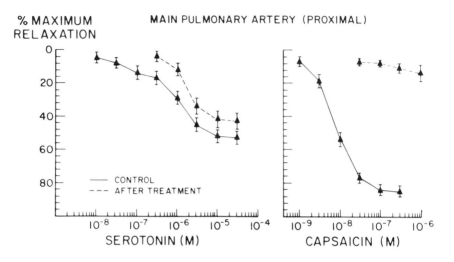

Figure 9. Log dose-response curves for relaxation by serotonin or capsaicin in the MPA (control n = 16 and 12, respectively). Treatment (---) consisted of serotonin, 10^{-3} M, 30 min (left, n = 8), or capsaicin, 3 x 10^{-6} M, 30 min (right, n = 6), both followed by 1 hr wash.

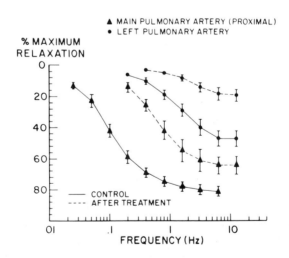

Figure 10. Log frequency-response curves for relaxation by ES in MPA and LPA (control n = 10). Treatment (---, n = 8) consisted of ES at 16 Hz for 30 min followed by 1 hr wash before obtaining frequency-response curves.

TABLE I. Relaxant responses of the proximal half of the guinea-pig main pulmonary artery in the absence or presence of drugs that significantly antagonized serotonin.

% Relaxation with SEM

Treatment[1]	Serotonin (10^{-5} M)	n	Capsaicin (10^{-7} M)	n	ES (1 HZ)	n
Control	60 ±2	40	81 ±2	11	73± 3	6
Cocaine						
3 x 10^{-5} M	36 ±5*	7	80 ±4	6	68 ±2	6
10^{-4} M	17 ±3*	8	81 ±2	6		
Imipramine						
10^{-6} M	33 ±7*	4	82 ±2	6	65 ±3	6
d-Tubocurarine						
10^{-5} M	39 ±7*	7	87 ±2	6	73 ±5	5
10^{-4} M	17 ±3*	9	87 ±2	6	73 ±5	5
Metoclopramide						
10^{-5} M	34 ±6*	9	87 ±2	6	66 ±5	6
10^{-4} M	3 ±2*	7				
MDL72222						
10^{-6} M	63 ±4	7				
10^{-5} M	20 ±4*	9	72 ±6*	7	54 ±7*	6
10^{-4} M	2 ±1*	8	50 ±7	7	0*	3

[1] Drugs were added 30 min before relaxant treatments.
* Denotes values statistically different (p< 0.05) from control.

metoclopramide produced blockade of serotonin, but did not alter responses to capsaicin or ES. MDL72222, an antagonist of serotonin-induced excitation of certain peripheral neurons (6), blocked relaxant responses to serotonin non-selectively and only at relatively large concentrations of the antagonist. Antagonism of serotonin-induced relaxation appeared non-competitive (Figure 13).

Antagonism of serotonin by these drugs appeared unrelated to local anesthetic actions since neither lidocaine, 10^{-6} M (n = 3) and 10^{-5} M (n = 3), nor procaine, 10^{-4} M (n = 3) produced blockade. Also, catecholamine uptake mechanisms are probably not involved since the serotonin-induced relaxation was not altered by hydrocortisone, 10^{-4} M (n = 6), norepinephrine, 10^{-5} M (n = 3) and 10^{-4} M (n = 3), or epinephrine, 10^{-5} M (n = 3), the latter examined in the presence

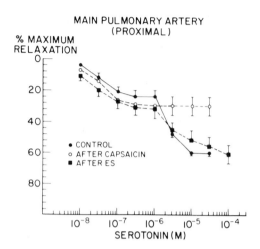

MAIN PULMONARY ARTERY
(PROXIMAL)

Figure 11. *Log dose-response curves for relaxation of MPA by serotonin without pretreatment (n = 8) and after exposure to capsaicin (n = 8) or ES (n = 9). Treatments were as described for Fig. 9 and 10. Control curves were matched for treatment and washing schedules.*

of propranolol 10^{-6} M. Furthermore, pretreatment of the animals with 6-hydroxydopamine to destroy adrenergic neurons did not alter the serotonin-induced relaxation (n = 7). Several other drugs or treatments that were ineffective in modifying the relaxant response to serotonin are listed in Table II.

Neither 5-methoxytryptamine nor 8-hydroxydipropylaminotetralin (8-OH-DPAT) in concentrations from 10^{-8} M to 10^{-4} M produced relaxation of the MPA. Relaxation of the MPA by ATP, 10^{-5} M (84 ±2%, n = 8), was markedly reduced after removal of endothelial cells (23 ±5%, n = 3). In the absence of endothelial cells, the maximum relaxation of the MPA to substance P, 10^{-5} M, was 15 ±2% (n = 9).

IV.   DISCUSSION

The guinea-pig extralobar pulmonary arteries contain several receptors and sites for the pharmacological actions of serotonin.

1) Contractile responses to small concentrations of serotonin (phase I) in both the MPA and LPA appear to be mediated by the 5-HT_2 subtype of serotonin receptor. This suggestion is based primarily on blockade by LY53857. Support for this classification is also provided by previous observations that phase I

TABLE II. Treatments that did not significantly ($p < 0.05$) alter the ability of serotonin, 10^{-5} M, to cause relaxation of the proximal half of the guinea-pig main pulmonary artery.

Treatment[1]	% Relaxation with SEM	n
Control	60 ± 2	40
Methysergide		
10^{-8} M	62 ± 5	6
10^{-6} M	60 ± 4	6
LY53857		
3×10^{-9} M	59 ± 4	6
10^{-6} M	59 ± 4	6
Ketanserin, 10^{-7} M	66 ± 7	3
Propranolol, 10^{-6} M	57 ± 9	5
Phentolamine, 10^{-5} M	55 ± 4	5
Atropine, 10^{-6} M	61 ± 6	5
Hexamethonium		
10^{-5} M	61 ± 5	7
10^{-4} M	52 ± 5	8
Morphine, 10^{-6} M	61 ± 2	3
Naloxone		
10^{-5} M	62 ± 5	7
10^{-4} M	63 ± 3	8
Metiamide, 10^{-4} M	59 ± 7	4
Picrotoxin, 3×10^{-5} M	58 ± 7	7
D-Pro[4], D-Trp[7,9]-SP(4-11)*	53 ± 4	10
Indomethacin, 5×10^{-6} M	52 ± 5	6
Endothelium removed	57 ± 2	13

[1] Drugs were added 30 (or 5*) min before serotonin.

contractile responses to serotonin were sensitive to antagonism by methysergide (1). Blockade by spiperone is also suggestive, but the concentrations used in these experiments (10^{-6} M) is too non-selective to provide definitive information about serotonin receptor subtypes (7,8). Phenoxybenzamine and phentolamine, while having the capability of binding to 5-HT$_2$ receptors (7,9), also exert multiple non-selective actions, especially as demonstrated in these arterial segments. Similar considerations of non-selective behavior may apply for mepyramine (10).

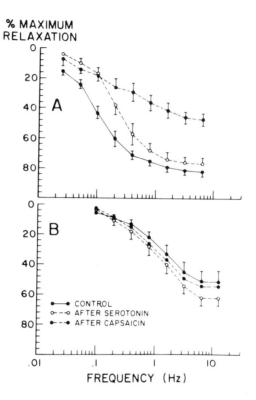

Figure 12. *Frequency-response effects of ES obtained without pretreatment (n = 10). Treatments (---) consisted of serotonin (n = 9) or capsaicin (n = 9) as described for Fig. 9. See also Fig. 1 legend.*

The apparent non-competitive antagonism by LY53857 of phase I contractions to serotonin precludes definitive receptor classification at the present time. It is possible that combined receptor antagonism and ongoing receptor desensitization by the agonist results in the reduction of peak contractions of phase I. In the MPA, the active relaxant response to serotonin, which was unaffected by LY53857, probably contributes as well to the reduction of contractile maximum of phase I.

2) Contractile responses to large concentrations of serotonin (phase II) in the MPA and LPA do not appear to be mediated by $5-HT_2$ receptors, since they were resistant to blockade by LY53857 at a concentration (3×10^{-9} M) that is almost 100 times its apparent dissociation constant at $5-HT_2$ receptors (5). While the mechanisms and receptor types for phase II contractions to serotonin remain obscure, data with antagonists used in this study provide support for involvement of different receptors mediating these responses in the two segments. Antagonism

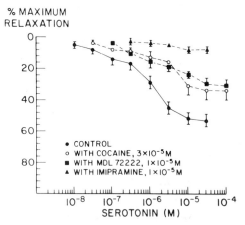

MAIN PULMONARY ARTERY (PROXIMAL)

Figure 13. Log dose-response curves for relaxation of MPA by serotonin in the absence (n = 16) and presence of cocaine (n = 7), MDL72222 (n = 7), or imipramine (n = 6), each added 30 min before serotonin.

of phase II contractions by phentolamine and spiperone only in the MPA might implicate an involvement of activation of alpha adrenergic receptors by serotonin in this segment. Since the tissues were taken from reserpine pretreated animals, any action of serotonin on alpha receptors would be direct rather than indirect (11,12). However, the calculated -log molar K_B values for phentolamine and spiperone were 10 to 100 times smaller than these values for antagonism of alpha agonists in other vascular segments (8,13). Therefore, it appears that serotonin produces phase II contractions in the MPA by acting on a receptor with similarities to that in the dog saphenous vein (where the -log molar K_B for phentolamine is similar to that found here; 13), or that these contractile responses are mediated by more than one type of pharmacological receptor. Antagonism of phase II contractions by mepyramine only in the LPA suggests an involvement of histamine H_1 receptors in the action of serotonin in this segment. A potential histamine releasing action of serotonin (14,15) in the guinea-pig pulmonary arteries has not been examined. However, if histamine were released by serotonin in this segment, a relatively large relaxant response should have been noted in relaxation experiments (4). Alternatively, the action of mepyramine could be unrelated to histamine H_1 receptor antagonism (10).

   3) Relaxant responses to serotonin appear to be mediated, at least in part, by receptors that have some relationship to certain serotonin receptors on peripheral neurons described in other mammalian systems (16,17). Receptors or mechanisms of action for the two phases of the relaxant response may be different,

especially in light of the observation that capsaicin pretreatment resulted in selective reduction of phase II. The small magnitude of response in phase I makes quantitation difficult and we have yet to examine this phase independent of the larger phase II relaxation.

The relationship between serotonin and capsaicin is of particular interest. Both substances are known to stimulate sensory neurons (16-19), release peptides (most commonly substance P, 20-23) and elicit the Bezold-Jarisch reflex (24-28). Furthermore, capsaicin pretreatment of rats has been shown to attenuate the serotonin-induced Bezold-Jarisch reflex (26). Since the relaxant responses to serotonin (phase II) and capsaicin were confined to the MPA and capsaicin pretreatment markedly reduced the magnitude of serotonin-induced relaxation, it is tempting to suggest a similar cellular site of action for the two, perhaps involving release of a vasodilating substance from afferent neurons located in the MPA (25).

Support for the release of vasodilating substances was obtained from the demonstration of tetrodotoxin-sensitive relaxant responses to ES in these segments. The greater sensitivity and magnitude of relaxation in the MPA to ES suggests release of different or additional vasodilator substances in this segment. Furthermore, capsaicin pretreatment resulted in a marked reduction of the relaxation produced by ES only in the MPA. The smaller amount of inhibition of relaxation to ES caused by serotonin pretreatment was also confined to the MPA. Since prior ES did not alter subsequent relaxant responses to serotonin, this pretreatment does not appear to exert a "capsaicin-like" effect.

If there exists a single vasodilating substance released in common by serotonin, capsaicin and ES, the identity of this substance is unknown. Our studies to date have been largely confined to the examination of drug effects on serotonin-induced relaxation. The data indicate that the putative vasodilator substance is not substance P, since the substance P antagonist D-Pro[4], D-Trp[7,9]-SP (4-11) did not alter the relaxant response to serotonin (nor to capsaicin and ES). Also, exogenously-added substance P produced only a small relaxation. Since the relaxant responst to ATP, but not that to serotonin, was endothelial-dependent, the effect does not appear to involve the "purinergic" system (29). Absence of effect of morphine and naloxone tends to discount a role for endogenous opioid mechanisms (23,30). Release by serotonin of vasodilating prostanoid (31) also appears unlikely in light of the lack of effect of indomethacin. Metiamide, to block histamine H_2 receptors, was also ineffective in modulating serotonin-induced relaxation.

The conclusion that serotonin causes relaxation of the MPA by interacting with receptors similar to certain neuronal receptors is supported primarily by observations of antagonism by cocaine and metoclopramide. Both drugs are known to antagonize several peripheral actions of serotonin, including excitation of postganglionic sympathetic neurons of the rabbit heart (32,33), rabbit superior cervical gangion (34) and vagal afferent neurons involved in the Bezold-Jarisch reflex (17). Furthermore, 5-methoxytryptamine, which did not relax the MPA, does not mimic these neuronal effects of serotonin (27). The actions of imipramine on peripheral neuronal responses to serotonin have not been adequately defined and antagonism by d-tubocurarine is usually reported to be non-selective (16,17,34,35).

The low potency and non-selective nature of the antagonism of serotonin-induced relaxation by MDL72222 is inconsistent with this suggested classification of the serotonin receptors. Selective blockade by this antagonist of neuronal responses to serotonin that are also susceptible to cocaine and metoclopramide usually occurs in the range of 10^{-9} to 10^{-7} M (6,36). Also, effective concentrations of cocaine and metoclopramide in the MPA were larger than those found to be effective in peripheral neuronal systems. The low potency of the antagonists in the MPA could be due to release by serotonin of a substance with a high intrinsic efficacy for producing relaxation, or to a species difference in the receptor subtype. Alternatively, only part of the serotonin-mediated relaxation might involve specific receptors, the remainder related to direct displacement of a vasodilator substance (e.g., 6,12). Apparent noncompetitive blockade by these antagonists could be related to combined receptor antagonism and ongoing tachyphylaxis during cumulative addition of serotonin.

The concentration of phenoxybenzamine employed in relaxation experiments (10^{-5} M) is adequate to produce nonequilibrium blockade of several pharmacological receptors, including alpha adrenergic, histamine H_1, cholinergic (muscarinic and ganglionic nicotinic), 5-HT_1, 5-HT_2, and serotonin D receptors. Therefore, the use of some of the competitive, reversible antagonists listed in Table II (e.g., methysergide, LY53857, ketanserin, atropine and hexamethonium) represents redundant treatment and the absence of an effect is not particularly surprising. Propranolol, in addition to antagonizing beta adrenergic receptors, is known to bind to 5-HT_1 receptors and to antagonize neuronal responses to serotonin (37-39). Absence of relaxation by 8-OH-DPAT, a 5-$HT_{1\alpha}$ receptor agonist (40), also tends to exclude an involvement of this receptor subtype. It should be noted, however, that absence of an effect of an agonist could be related to a low intrinsic efficacy and independent of receptor subtype. The same consideration applies for the inability of 5-methoxytryptamine to evoke a relaxant response in the MPA. For these several reasons, subclassification of the serotonin receptors involved in producing relaxation of the MPA must await additional information about antagonist and agonist selectivity and mechanisms involved in this response.

The case of phentolamine deserves special mention in light of the effects of this drug on the contractile dose-response curves to serotonin in both vascular segments. Since phentolamine did not inhibit the relaxant response and a substantial relaxant response was seen only in the MPA, the change in shape of the serotonin dose-response curves for contraction could not be related to a change in relaxation. Furthermore, cocaine, which antagonized the relaxant response, did not produce a change in the shape of the serotonin dose-response curves for contraction. Since dansylcadaverine, which is known to inhibit receptor-mediated endocytosis and specific desensitization in other systems (41,42), produced a similar change in the shape of the serotonin dose-response curve, it is reasonable to suggest a similar mechanism for phentolamine. However, if these two substances act to inhibit desensitization of receptors for phase I contractions, LY53857 should have been a potent antagonist of the contractile responses in both segments in the presence of phentolamine. Since antagonism was not observed in the LPA, that observed in the MPA could be related to the functionally antagonistic relaxant response in this segment, still evident in the presence of cocaine, 3×10^{-5} M.

In light of these considerations, the effect of phentolamine could result from potentiation of serotonin responses mediated by resistant phase II receptors or from an action to "unmask" LY53857-resistant receptors for serotonin. Alternatively, LY53857 could produce antagonism of phase I contractions by facilitating serotonin-induced desensitization and therefore, be ineffective if the desensitization process is inhibited by phentolamine. The latter postulate is supported by observations of an apparent non-competitive antagonism by LY53857 of phase I contractile responses to serotonin.

Regardless of the lack of precise information about the effect of phentolamine, it appears that the return to basal tension at the end of phase I of the contractile dose-response curve to serotonin in both segments is a result primarily of desensitization of receptors culminating in failure to produce a sustained contraction. In the MPA, part of this return to basal tension could be related to active relaxation, but this is not predominantly seen in the LPA. The presence of active relaxation in the MPA probably accounts for some of the quantitative differences in contractions between the two segments.

V.   ACKNOWLEDGEMENTS

The authors thank Mr. Kevin Duerson for technical assistance. We also thank Drs. M.L. Cohen (Eli Lilly & Co., Indianapolis, IN), J.R. Fozard (Merrell Dow Research Institute, Strasbourg, France) and J.M. Van Neuten (Janssen Pharmaceutica, Beerse, Belgium) for generous supplies of LY53857, MDL72222 and ketanserin, respectively.

REFERENCES

1. Will JA, Keith IM, Buckner CK, Chacko J, Olson EB and Weir EK. (1984)*In* **The Endocrine Lung in Health and Disease** (KL Becker and F Gazder, eds) W.B. Saunders Co:Philadelphia.
2. Eyre P. (1975) *Br J Pharmacol* **55**:329.
3. Chand N. (1981) *Br J Pharmacol* **72**:233.
4. Hand JM, Will JA and Buckner CK. (1982) *J Pharmacol Exp Ther* **220**:526.
5. Cohen ML, Fuller RW and Kurz KD. (1983) *J Pharmacol Exp Ther* **227**:327.
6. Fozard JR. (1984) *Naunyn-Schmiedeberg's Arch Pharmacol* **326**:36.
7. Leysen JE, Awouters F, Kennis L, Laduron PM, Vandenberk J and Janssen PAJ. (1981) *Life Sci* **28**:1015.
8. Feniuk W, Humphrey PPA, Perren MJ and Watts AD. (1985) *Br J Pharmacol* **86**:697.
9. Hoyer D, Engel G and Kalkman HO. (1985) *Eur J Pharmacol* **118**:13.
10. Lombroso M and Nicosia S. (1981) *Life Sci* **28**:705.
11. Innes IR. (1962) *Br J Pharmacol* **19**:427.
12. Pluchino S. (1972) *Naunyn-Schmiedeberg's Arch Pharmacol* **272**:189.
13. Humphrey PPA. (1978) *Br J Pharmacol* **63**:671.
14. Feldberg W and Smith AN. (1953) *Br J Pharmacol* **8**:406.
15. Bunag RD and Walaszek EJ. (1962) *J Pharmacol Exp Ther* **135**:151.
16. Wallis D. (1981) *Life Sci* **29**:2345.
17. Fozard JR. (1984) *Neuropharmacol* **23**:1473.
18. Virus RM and Gebhart GF. (1979) *Life Sci* **25**:1273.
19. Fitzgerald M. (1983) *Pain* **15**:109.
20. Furness JB, Papka RE, Della NG, Costa M and Eskay RL. (1982) *Neurosci* **7**:447.
21. Chahl LA. (1983) *Eur J Pharmacol* **87**:485.
22. Theodorsson-Norheim E, Hua X, Brodin E and Lundberg JM. (1985) *Acta Physiol Scand* **124**:129.
23. Buchheit K-H, Engel G, Mutschler E and Richardson B. (1985) *Naunyn-Schmiedeberg's Arch Pharmacol* **329**:36.
24. Bevan JA and Verity MA. (1961) *J Pharmacol Exp Ther* **132**:42.
25. Bevan JA. (1962) *Circ Res* **10**:792.
26. Makara GB, Hyorgy L and Molnar J. (1967) *Arch Int Pharmacodyn Ther* **170**:39.
27. Fozard JR. (1983) *Eur J Pharmacol* **95**:331.
28. Jancso G and Such G. (1983) *J Physiol (London)* **341**:359.
29. Al-Humayyd M and White TD. (1985) *Br J Pharmacol* **84**:27.

30.   Lemaire I, Tseng R and Lemaire S. (1978)*Proc Natl Acad Sci USA*
       75:6240.
31.   Coughlin SR, Moskowitz MA, Antoniades HN and Levine L. (1981)
       Proc Natl Acad Sci USA **78**:7134.
32.   Fozard JR and Mobarok Ali ATM. (1978) *Eur J Pharmacol* **49**:109.
33.   Fozard JR, Mobarok Ali ATM and Newgrosh G. (1979) *Eur J Pharmacol*
       569:195.
34.   Nash HL, Wallis DI and Ash G. (1984) *Gen Pharmacol* **15**:339.
35.   Bisgard GE, Mitchell RA and Herbert DA. (1979) *Resp Physiol* **37**:61.
36.   Azami J, Fozard JR, Round AA and Wallis DI. (1985) *Naunyn-
       Schmiedeberg's Arch Pharmacol* **328**:423.
37.   Adler-Graschinsky E. (1983) *J Auton Pharmacol* **3**:303.
38.   Middlemiss DN. (1984) *Eur J Pharmacol* **101**:289.
39.   Hoyer D, Engel G and Kalkman HO. (1985) *Eur J Pharmacol* **118**:1.
40.   Doods HN, Kalkman HO, De Jonge A, Thoolen MJMC, Wilffert B,
       Timmermans PBMWM and Van Zwieten PA. (1985) *Eur J Pharmacol*
       112:363.
41.   Davies PJA, Davies DR, Levitzki A, Maxfield FR, Milhaud P,
       Willingham MC and Pastan IH. (1980) *Nature* **283**:162.
42.   Siegel H and Triggle DJ. (1983) *J Pharmacol Exp Ther* **225**:534.

Pulmonary Vascular Responses to Eicosanoids

PHILIP J. KADOWITZ
DENNIS B. MCNAMARA
ALBERT L. HYMAN
*Departments of Pharmacology and
Surgery
Tulane University School of Medicine
New Orleans, Louisiana 70112*

I. INTRODUCTION

The leukotrienes are a family of biological active eicosanoids formed from arachidonic acid by way of the 5-lipoxygenase pathway (1-5). In the lipoxygenase pathway, the substrate is converted to 5-hydroperoxyeicosatetraenoic acid which is oxygenated to the labile epoxide intermediate leukotriene (LT) A_4 (3). This labile epoxide intermediate which is analogous to the pivotal prostaglandin (PG) endoperoxide intermediate, PGH_2, in the cyclooxygenase pathway, is transformed enzymatically to LTB_4 which has potent chemotactic activity (3). LTA_4 can also be converted to LTC_4 by the addition of glutathione. Leukotriene C_4 can be further metabolized to LTD_4 by a γ-glutamyl transpeptidase and subsequently to LTE_4.

It has been recently reported that LTC_4, LTD_4, and LTE_4 are the main components of the slow reacting substance of anaphylaxis (SRSA; 4-6). Since SRSA is a contractile substance which is released by immunologic challenge from the lung, it has been postulated that SRSA is an important mediator in bronchial asthma and other immediate-type hypersensitivity reactions (1,7-9). The effects of the leukotrienes on the lung are of considerable interest because of their postulated role as mediators (1,2,8,10-13). Leukotrienes C_4 and D_4 have potent contractile

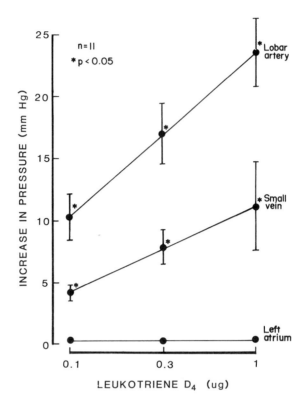

Figure 1. Dose-response curves showing the increases in lobar arterial and small intrapulmonary vein pressures in response to intralobar injections of LTD_4, 0.1-1 µg. Left atrial pressure was not changed by intralobar injections of LTD_4 in the group of 11 intact-chest sheep.

activity on preparations of airway and vascular smooth muscle from the lung (1,2,8,10,14-16). These agents have significant bronchoconstrictor activity in a variety of species (10,12,13,15-19). However, little has been written about the effects of the leukotrienes on the pulmonary vascular bed. In the monkey, the predominant response to injection of LTC_4 is a fall in pulmonary arterial pressure; whereas, aerosol administration of LTC_4 caused a marked rise in pulmonary arterial pressure (19). In the rat, injections of LTC_4 decreased pulmonary arterial pressure and may mediate hypoxic pulmonary vasoconstriction (20,21). In contrast to studies with LTC_4 in the rat and monkey, LTD_4 caused a marked increase in pulmonary vascular resistance in the newborn lamb when injected into the pulmonary artery (22). However, less is known about responses to LTD_4 on the pulmonary vascular bed of the mature animal (23-31). The purpose of this report is to describe responses to LTD_4 in the pulmonary vascular bed of cat and sheep under conditions of controlled blood flow using recently described methods. The effects of LTD_4 are also compared in the pulmonary vascular bed and in the airways.

II.   RESULTS

Pulmonary lobar vascular responses to LTD_4 in the intact-chest sheep were studied in 11 animals; these data are presented in Figure 1. Under constant flow conditions, intralobar injections of LTD_4 in doses of 0.1-1 μg caused significant dose-related increases in lobar arterial and small vein pressures without changing left atrial pressure. In the range of dose employed in the study in the sheep, LTD_4 had no significant effect on systemic arterial pressure. The increases in lobar arterial and small vein pressures were rapid in onset, and mean vascular pressures returned to baseline value over a 0.5-4 min period, depending on the dose of the leukotriene. The lobar arterial to small vein pressure gradient and the gradient from small vein to left atrium pressure increased significantly at all doses of LTD_4 studied (Table I).

TABLE I. Influence of intralobar injections of leukotriene D_4 (LTD_4) on mean vascular pressure gradients in the sheep lung.

	Pressure Gradient (mmHg)		
	Lobar artery – Left atrium	Lobar artery – Small vein	Small vein – Left atrium
Control	10 ±1	4 ±1	6 ±3
LTD_4, 0.1 μg	21 ±4*	11 ± 2*	10 ±2*
Control	12 ±1	5 ±1	7 ±2
LTD_4, 0.3 μg	29 ±4*	14 ±3*	15 ±4*
Control	10 ±2	4 ±1	6 ±3
LTD_4, 1 μg	34 ±5*	17 ±4*	17 ±5*

n = 10-11

* $P < 0.05$, when compared to corresponding control; paired for comparison

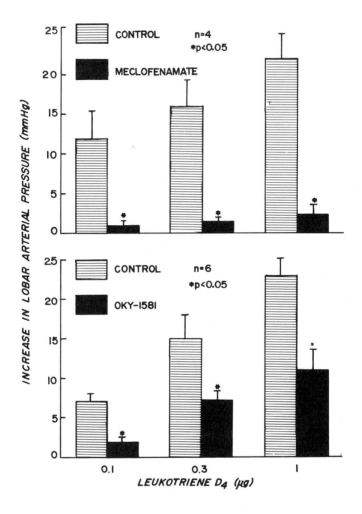

Figure 2. Top panel, effect of sodium meclofenamate, a cyclooxygenase inhibitor, on increases in lobar arterial pressure in response to intralobar injections of LTD$_4$ in the intact-chest sheep. Responses to LTD$_4$ were compared before and 10-15 min after administration of meclofenamate, 2.5 mg/kg iv. Lower panel, influence of OKY1581, a thromboxane synthesis inhibitor, on increases in lobar arterial pressure in response to LTD$_4$ in the sheep. Responses were obtained before and 15-30 min after administration of OKY1581, 5-10 mg/kg iv. n indicates number of animals.

In order to ascertain if pulmonary vascular responses to LTD_4 in the sheep are dependent on formation of products in the cyclooxygenase pathway, the effects of sodium meclofenamate, a cyclooxygenase inhibitor, and of OKY1581, a thromboxane synthesis inhibitor, were investigated. After administration of sodium meclofenamate, 2.5 mg/kg iv, the increases in lobar arterial pressure in response to LTD_4 were reduced markedly at each dose of the leukotriene studied (Figure 2). The thromboxane synthesis inhibitor, OKY1581, in doses of 5-10 mg/kg iv, also significantly reduced the increases in lobar arterial pressure in response to LTD_4 (Figure 2). However, the inhibitory effects of the cyclo-oxygenase inhibitor on responses to LTD_4 were greater than were the inhibitory effects of the thromboxane synthesis inhibitor. Neither OKY1581 nor meclofenamate had significant effect on pulmonary vascular or systemic arterial pressure in the sheep. The effects of meclofenamate and OKY1581 on pulmonary vascular responses to an agent whose actions mimic those of thromboxane A_2 were also investigated. U46619, an agent whose actions are similar to those of thromboxane A_2 on smooth muscle, caused dose-dependent increases in lobar arterial and small vein pressures without affecting left atrial or systemic arterial pressure. The increases in lobar arterial pressure in response to U46619 were not altered after administration of sodium meclofenamate, 2.5 mg/kg iv, or OKY1581, 5-10 mg/kg iv. In biochemical studies (32-34), the effects of OKY1581 on the metabolism of arachidonic acid and of the prostaglandin endoperoxide, PGH_2, by microsomal fractions from sheep lung were investigated. The addition of $1\text{-}^{14}C$-arachidonic acid (10 μM) to the microsomal fraction (200 μg protein) resulted in the formation of 6-keto-$PGF_{1\alpha}$, the stable breakdown product of PGI_2, 255 ±21 picomoles and TXB_2, the stable breakdown product of TXA_2, 230 ±19 picomoles per hr in the absence of the inhibitor. Prostaglandins $F_{2\alpha}$, E_2, and D_2 were also formed. However, when OKY1581 was added to the incubation medium in concentrations of 10^{-9} M or greater, the formation of TXB_2 was reduced to 37% of control at 10^{-7} M and 31% of control at 10^{-6} M. Moreover, the synthesis of 6-keto-$PGF_{1\alpha}$ was not decreased at concentrations of OKY1581 up to 10^{-6} M. The formation of $PGF_{2\alpha}$, PGE_2, and PGD_2 was not decreased by OKY1581 in concentrations up to 10^{-6} M. The effects of OKY1581 on thromboxane synthesis were also studied in two sheep. In these animals the lungs were removed after the animals were treated with OKY1581, 10 mg/kg iv. When thromboxane synthesis activity was compared in homogenates from the treated animals, it was found to be markedly depressed when compared to control animals.

The influence of OKY1581 on endoperoxide metabolism by sheep lung microsomal fraction was also investigated. In the absence of inhibitor, 166 ±15 picomoles of 6-keto-$PGF_{1\alpha}$ and 161 ±17 picomoles of TXB_2 were formed per two

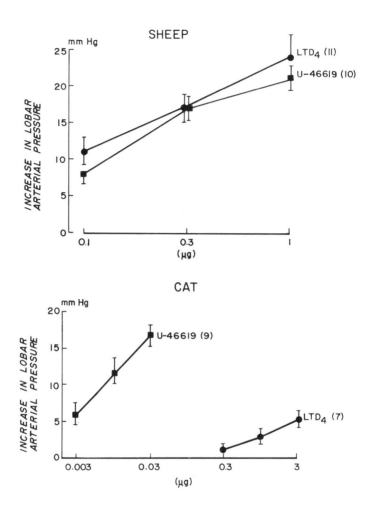

Figure 3. Dose response relationships comparing increases in lobar arterial pressure in response to LTD$_4$ and U46619 in the sheep (top panel) and in the cat (lower panel). Responses to the thromboxane mimic and LTD$_4$ were not significantly different at the 0.1, 0.3 and 1 µg doses in the sheep. Number in parenthesis indicates number of animal.

min period when 10 µM PGH$_2$ was added to 200 µg microsomal protein. PGF$_{2\alpha}$, PGE$_2$, and PGD$_2$ were not reduced by OKY1581.

The effects of the cyclooxygenase and thromboxane synthesis inhibitors on lobar vascular responses to arachidonic acid were also investigated in the sheep. Intralobar injections of arachidonic acid in doses of 30 and 100 µg caused a significant dose-dependent increase in lobar arterial pressure without affecting left atrial pressure. The increases in lobar arterial pressure in response to arachidonic acid were also decreased significantly after administration of OKY1581, 5-10 mg/kg iv.

The relationship between the effects of LTD_4 on ventilation and on the pulmonary vascular bed was also studied in the sheep. In these experiments, responses to LTD_4 were obtained when the left lower lobe was ventilated and when lobar ventilation was arrested at end-expiration by inflating a balloon catheter in the left lower lobe bronchus. In these experiments, the left lower lobe was perfused with arterial blood to lessen the effects of hypoxia on the lung and 1-3 ml of a 2% lidocaine viscous solution was instilled into the lobar bronchus to prevent coughing. The correlation between the increases in lobar arterial pressure in responses to intralobar injections of LTD_4 (0.1-1 µg) when the lobe was ventilated and when lobar ventilation was arrested was very good. The correlation of coefficient of the regression line was 0.90 ($p \leq 0.05$) with a slope (0.83) that was not significantly different from the line of identity. These data indicate that responses to LTD_4 are similar when the lobe is ventilated and when ventilation is arrested. These results suggest that the effects of LTD_4 on vascular airway smooth muscle in the lung occur independently.

In order to ascertain if responses of LTD_4 varied with species, the effects of LTD_4 on the pulmonary vascular bed were investigated in the intact-chest cat; these data are summarized in Figure 3. Intralobar injections of LTD_4 in doses of 0.3, 1 and 3 µg caused small but significant dose-related increases in lobar arterial pressure without affecting left atrial pressure. Systemic arterial pressure was increased significantly in response to intralobar injections of the 1 and 3 µg doses of LTD_4. Although lobar vascular responses to LTD_4 were small in the cat, U46619 had marked vasoconstrictor activity (Fig. 3). As described earlier, both LTD_4 and U46619 had marked vasoconstrictor activity in the sheep pulmonary vascular bed and the dose-response curves for both substances in this species were similar. However, in the cat, U46619 had far greater vasoconstrictor activity than did LTD_4 (Fig. 3).

In other experiments in the sheep and in the cat, responses to LTD_4 were similar when the lung was perfused with blood or with low molecular weight dextran. The role of the cyclooxygenase pathway in the mediation of pulmonary vascular responses to LTD_4 was also investigated in the cat. Administration of indomethacin or sodium meclofenamate, 2.5 mg/kg iv, had no significant effect on pulmonary vasoconstrictor responses to U46619 or LTD_4 in the cat. The increases in systemic arterial pressure in response to the 1 and 3 µg doses of LTD_4 were not altered by the cyclooxygenase inhibitors. However, the cyclooxygenase inhibitors, in the doses employed, significantly reduced the increases in lobar arterial pressure in response to intralobar injections of arachidonic acid. The cyclooxygenase inhi-

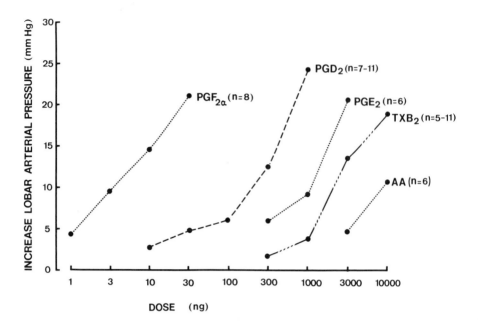

Figure 4. Dose-response curves comparing the effects of PGF$_{2\alpha}$, PGD$_2$, PGE$_2$, TXB$_2$ and arachidonic acid (AA) in the feline pulmonary vascular bed.

bitors had no significant effect on pulmonary vascular or systemic arterial pressure in the cat. The effects of the cyclooxygenase products of arachidonic acid are shown in Figure 4. It can be seen that all products in this pathway had far greater vasoconstrictor activity than did LTD$_4$ in the feline pulmonary vascular bed.

Airway and aortic blood pressure responses to LTD$_4$, as well as AA and U46619, were also investigated in the cat before and after cyclooxygenase blockade with sodium meclofenamate. Intravenous injections of LTD$_4$ in doses of 3, 10 and 30 μg caused significant increases in P$_{TP}$, R$_L$, and P$_{Ao}$ as well as decreases in C$_{dyn}$ (Figure 5). C$_{st}$ was decreased in response to LTD$_4$ (10 μg) in the 4 animals in which it was studied. These responses were slow in onset (usually greater than 10 seconds). Administration of meclofenamate, 2.5 mg/kg iv, had no significant effect on baseline P$_{TP}$, R$_L$, C$_{dyn}$, or P$_{Ao}$. Meclofenamate blocked the broncho-pulmonary responses to LTD$_4$, but did not significantly alter the increase in aortic pressure (Figure 5).

Intravenous injections of AA in doses of 300 and 1000 μg caused dose-dependent increases in P$_{TP}$, while C$_{dyn}$ and P$_{Ao}$ decreased. These responses were blocked by meclofenamate. U46619, a TXA$_2$ mimic, injected intravenously in

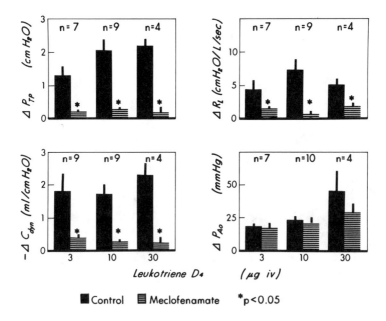

*Figure 5. Effects of LTD$_4$ on P$_{TP}$, R$_L$, C$_{dyn}$, and P$_{Ao}$ in the intact cat before and after cyclooxygenase blockade with meclofenamate. n indicates the number of animals. * indicates response significantly different from control response.*

doses of 0.1 and 0.3 μg, also caused increases in P$_{TP}$ and decreases in C$_{dyn}$. These airway responses were not blocked by meclofenamate (Figure 6).

The onset of airway effects was delayed an average of 2-4 seconds after injection of U46619 and AA.

In three of the animals, a small rise in P$_{TP}$ and R$_L$ and fall in C$_{dyn}$ were observed 7-8 minutes after iv injection of LTD$_4$, whether or not meclofenamate had been given. This late change in bronchopulmonary parameters was not observed after iv injections of AA or U46619. Four of fourteen cats showed little or no bronchopulmonary response to LTD$_4$ and reacted minimally to AA. These cats were not included in the study.

III.   DISCUSSION

Experiments in the intact-chest sheep demonstrate that intralobar injections of LTD$_4$ increase pulmonary lobar arterial pressure in a dose-related manner (31). Since pulmonary blood flow was maintained constant and left atrial

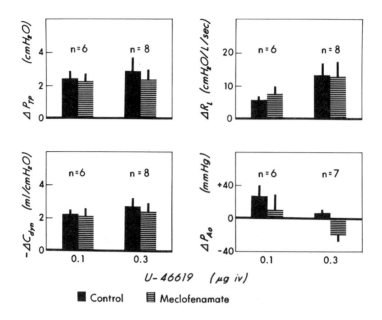

Figure 6. Influence of sodium meclofenamate, 2.5 mg/kg iv, on airway and aortic responses to U46619 in the cat.

pressure was unchanged, the increase in pressure gradient across the lung lobe suggests that pulmonary lobar vascular resistance was increased by LTD_4. The increases in lobar arterial pressure in response to LTD_4 were associated with dose-related increases in small intrapulmonary vein pressure. In addition to increasing lobar arterial and small vein pressures, LTD_4 increased the pressure gradient from lobar artery to small vein. These experiments in the sheep suggest that LTD_4 increases pulmonary vascular resistance by constricting intrapulmonary veins and segments upstream to the small vein (believed to be small arteries). Results obtained in mature animals are consistent with results in the newborn lamb in which LTD_4 increased pulmonary and systemic vascular resistance and decreased cardiac output (22,35). It has been reported that LTD_4 has potent coronary vasoconstrictor activity in the sheep that can be associated with left ventricular impairment (35). However, in the sheep, LTD_4 had no significant effect on systemic arterial or left atrial pressures in the range of doses studied. The effects of LTD_4 on left atrial pressure in the newborn lamb were not measured so that the mechanism of the fall in cardiac output is uncertain (22). The effects of LTD_4 on systemic vascular resistance of the newborn lamb appear to be greater than those observed in the mature animal.

In terms of relative pressor activity in the pulmonary vascular bed of the sheep, LTD_4 was very potent with activity paralleling that of U46619, a stable prostaglandin analog whose actions are thought to mimic those of thromboxane A_2. Moreover, when compared to other vasoactive hormones whose effects have been studied in the sheep, LTD_4 is far more active than other arachidonic acid metabolites, alveolar hypoxia, or histamine, which acts over a similar portion of the pulmonary vascular bed and is released along with the leukotrienes in immediate hypersensitivity reactions (23,29-31).

It has been reported that LTD_4 has potent contractile activity on isolated airway smooth muscle and lung parenchyma and that it increases bronchomotor tone (1,2,8,10,13,15,16,36-38). However, in the intact-chest sheep, the effects of LTD_4 on the pulmonary vascular bed appear to be independent of alterations in ventilation or those that occur as a consequence of changes in bronchomotor tone or lung volume, since similar responses were obtained when the lobe was ventilated or when lobar ventilation was arrested by obstruction of bronchial airflow. In previous studies, responses to a number of vasoactive substances including cyclooxygenase metabolites of arachidonic acid and histamine, were similar when the lobe was ventilated or lobar ventilation was arrested, suggesting that the actions of these vasoactive hormones on pulmonary vascular resistance appear to be independent of alterations in bronchomotor tone (25,27-29,31). In both the cat and in the sheep, pulmonary hypertensive responses to LTD_4 appear similar when the lung was perfused with blood or low molecular weight dextrans. Thus, responses to LTD_4 in both species are dependent on the interaction with formed elements in blood.

In the sheep, pulmonary vasoconstrictor responses to LTD_4 were markedly attenuated after treatment with sodium meclofenamate suggesting that responses to this lipoxygenase product are dependent on the formation of products in the cyclooxygenase pathway. In addition, vasoconstrictor responses to LTD_4 were decreased by OKY1581, a thromboxane synthesis inhibitor. These data suggest that a substantial portion of the pulmonary vasoconstrictor response to LTD_4 is due to the release of thromboxane A_2. The observation that meclofenamate had greater inhibitory effect on responses to LTD_4 than did OKY1581 suggests that pulmonary vasoconstrictor responses to this lipoxygenase metabolite are dependent on the formation of thromboxane A_2 and other cyclooxygenase products such as prostaglandins (PG) D_2 and $F_{2\alpha}$ which have substantial pressor activity in the pulmonary vascular bed (25,27-29,31). It has been shown that injections of SRSA or synthetic LTC_4 and LTD_4 cause the release of prostaglandins and TXA_2 from isolated guinea pig lung (11,36,38-41). The results of the present experiments in the sheep are consistent with data obtained with isolated guinea pig parenchyma and on bronchoconstrictor responses in the guinea pig indicating that responses to LTD_4 are dependent on the release of TXA_2 and prostaglandins.

A similar relationship between these inhibitors and responses to arachidonic acid was also observed, in that there was a greater reduction in response to LTD_4 after treatment with meclofenamate than after OKY1581. These data confirm previous studies showing that pulmonary vasoconstrictor responses to arachidonic acid are due to formation of products in the cyclooxygenase pathway, and extend these findings by showing that a portion of the response is due to TXA_2 formation (25-28,43).

Although responses to LTD_4 and arachidonic acid were markedly reduced by meclofenamate, this cyclooxygenase inhibitor had no significant effect on pulmonary vasoconstrictor responses to U46619, an analog whose actions are thought to mimic those of thromboxane A_2 (44). These data indicate that meclofenamate inhibited cyclooxygenase activity in the pulmonary vascular bed, and that the cyclooxygenase inhibitor did not influence vascular responses to the thromboxane mimic. In addition, vasoconstrictor responses to U46619 were not altered by OKY1581 in doses that inhibited responses to LTD_4 and arachidonic acid. These results also suggest that the thromboxane synthesis inhibitor did not alter thromboxane receptor-mediated responses and that the effects of the inhibitor were due to inhibition of the formation of thromboxane A_2. These data also suggest that thromboxane A_2 would have marked vasoconstrictor activity in the sheep pulmonary vascular bed, and that U46619 actually does mimic responses to this labile hormone (44). The inhibition of thromboxane A_2 synthesis was also investigated in microsomal fractions from sheep lung. The results of these studies show that OKY1581 inhibited the formation of TXA_2 as measured by formation of its stable breakdown product, TXB_2. TXB_2 formation was inhibited over a wide range of concentration of OKY1581 when either arachidonic acid or the endoperoxide PGH_2 was employed as substrate. Although TXB_2 formation was decreased by OKY1581, PGI_2 formation as measured by the production of 6-keto-$PGF_{1\alpha}$ was not inhibited even at very high concentrations of the thromboxane synthesis inhibitor. Prostaglandins E_2, $F_{2\alpha}$, and D_2 were formed when PGH_2 or arachidonic acid was added to the microsomal fractions. It is not known if this prostaglandin synthesis was enzymatic; however, the amount of these substances formed was not decreased by OKY1581, and in the case of PGE_2, was enhanced by the inhibitor. Since the total amount of product formed from arachidonic acid (6-keto-$PGF_{1\alpha}$, TXB_2, $PGF_{2\alpha}$, PGE_2, and PGD_2) was not decreased, although TXB_2 formation was reduced, it is unlikely that OKY1581 had a significant inhibitory effect on sheep lung cyclooxygenase activity. These experiments suggest that effects of OKY1581 on responses to LTD_4 and arachidonic acid are due to inhibition of thromboxane synthetase activity, and not to an effect on cyclooxygenase activity or on thromboxane receptor-mediated activity in the pulmonary vascular bed of the sheep. In other experiments in lung homogenates taken from sheep receiving OKY1581, 5-10 mg/kg iv, TXB_2 formation was greatly reduced.

The results of studies in the sheep demonstrate that LTD_4 has very potent vasoconstrictor activity in the pulmonary vascular bed of this species, and that this activity is due, for the most part, to release of products in the cyclooxygenase pathway. However, the effects of LTD_4 in the pulmonary vascular bed of the sheep and the cat are different. In the cat, LTD_4 had only modest pressor activity equal to that of arachidonic acid and far less than that of $PGF_{2\alpha}$, PGD_2, or PGE_2 in that species (28). Furthermore, in this species, cyclooxygenase blockers did not modify responses to this lipoxygenase product. Although the relative magnitude of responses to LTD4 as well as the mechanism of action differs in the sheep and the cat, both species were extremely sensitive to the effects of U46619. Thus, there appears to be true species variation in the pulmonary vascular response to this lipoxygenase metabolite. This variation was not observed with U46619, which may operate via TXA_2 receptors in the pulmonary vascular bed. In addition to demonstrating marked species variation in the response to LTD_4, the present data may be interpreted to suggest that LTD_4 itself does not have potent vaso-constrictor activity in the lung when the cyclooxygenase system is blocked. Moreover, the remaining pressor activity of LTD_4 in the sheep after cyclo-oxygenase blockade and the pressor activity in the cat, which were very similar, suggest that the activity of this lipoxygenase metabolite is far less than that of products of the cyclooxygenase pathway such as TXA_2, $PGF_{2\alpha}$, or PGD_2 (25-28, 31). The data from the present study suggest that it would be difficult to formulate a unified hypothesis on the role of LTD_4, a major component of SRSA, on the pulmonary circulation since species variation is so marked. The present data, however, suggest that LTD_4 could have pronounced effects on lobar arterial and small vein pressures, could contribute to an increase in capillary pressure and may alter fluid balance in the sheep lung. These hydrostatic effects, along with altera-tions in capillary permeability that could occur as a consequence of lung injury, could result in pulmonary edema and marked abnormalities in gas exchange.

The effects of LTD_4 on lung mechanics were also investigated in the cat. The observation that LTD_4 increased R_L and decreased C_{dyn} suggests that this agent constricts smooth muscle in central airways and in peripheral portions of the cat lung. U46619 and AA caused similar changes, and presumably act on similar segments of the lung. These observations, along with the finding that responses to LTD_4 are blocked by meclofenamate, support the hypothesis that LTD_4 causes bronchoconstriction by releasing products in the cyclooxygenase cascade (11,17, 36-42). Since changes in C_{dyn} and C_{st} were similar in response to LTD_4,

AA and U46619, these data suggest that the effects of these agents on peripheral portions of the lung were independent of changes in the distribution of ventilation.

Leukotrienes cause bronchoconstriction via direct smooth muscle stimulation and indirectly by the release of cyclooxygenase products (11,17,36-42). Scianterelli et al. (38) found that intravenous injections of LTC_4 inguinea pigs resulted in bronchospasm and hypertension followed by marked and long-lasting hypotension. These effects were inhibited by atropine. Ueno's group (38) reported similar inhibition of the bronchopulmonary responses to intravenous LTD_4 in guinea pigs as well as to bradykinin following blockade with both indomethacin or OKY1581, a thromboxane synthesis inhibitor. In vitro studies of guinea pigs parenchymal strips superfused with LTC_4, LTD_4, and LTB_4 by Piper and Samhoun (36,40) revealed that TXA_2 was generated via phospholipase activation.

Vargaftig et al. (41) reported that aspirin inhibited the bronchoconstriction induced by intravenous injections of LTC_4 and LTD_4 in propranolol-treated guinea pigs. Guinea pig lungs sensitized by ovalbumin will release more TXA_2 following leukotriene administration than non-sensitized lungs. The release of TXA_2 is inhibited by FPL-55712, suggesting the presence of specific receptors for leukotrienes in the lung (39).

These reports would appear to be inconsistent with leukotrienes playing an important role as mediators in acute hypersensitivity reactions and the nonsteroidal antiinflammatory drugs do not block allergen-induced bronchoconstriction. In fact, aspirin may precipitate an asthmatic attack in certain individuals. Dahlen (8), Weichman et al. (42), as well as Hamel et al. (18) explained these apparent discrepancies on the basis that the the route of administration plays a pivotal role in determining whether the actions of leukotrienes will be direct or indirect. The indirect bronchoconstriction associated with TXA_2 release occurs when the exposure to leukotrienes has been brief, such as with intravenous administration in vivo or superfusion or perfusion in vitro techniques. The indirect effects of the leukotrienes will be inhibited by cyclooxygenase blockers as well as by thromboxane synthesis inhibitors. The directly induced bronchoconstriction occurs with longer exposure to leukotrienes such as with aerosol administration or in organ baths. Cyclooxygenase blockade potentiates the direct effects of leukotrienes (39).

Smedegard et al. (19) compared intravenous and aerosolized LTC_4 in artificially ventilated monkeys. LTC_4 was equipotent with histamine when injected intravenously, whereas it was 1000 times more potent than histamine given as an aerosol. The bronchoconstriction following aerosolized LTC_4 lasted nearly an hour and was associated with a fall in PaO_2. C_{dyn} was more affected than R_L, indicating greater effects in the peripheral airways. Hamel et al. (18) found similar direct and indirect bronchopulmonary responses to LTC_4 and LTD_4 in the guinea pig.

The vascular effects of the leukotrienes appear also to be directly as well as indirectly induced (31,45). The differentiation between whether these effects occur directly or indirectly is not as clear cut as with the leukotriene-induced bronchopulmonary effect. Species differences may play an important role. For instance, LTD_4 is a very potent pulmonary vasoconstrictor similar to U46619 (2,44). Furthermore, LTD_4-induced pulmonary vasoconstriction was blocked by cyclooxygenase inhibitors in the sheep but not in the cat (31). Lippton *et al.* (45) reported that intra-arterial injections of LTC_4 and LTD_4 in the feline mesenteric vascular bed under conditions of controlled flow caused a dose-related increase in perfusion pressure that was not inhibited by meclofenamate. Weichman *et al.* (42) commented on the marked intraspecies variability they saw in response to the leukotrienes. Mongrel dogs do not respond to aerosolized LTD_4, whereas Basenji Greyhounds develop a pronounced bronchospasm (12). Four of fourteen cats in the present study did not respond to LTD_4. Although tachyphylaxis occurs readily with the leukotrienes (19), it is an unlikely explanation of the above differences, which occurred with the first administration. Inter- and intra-species differences in AA and its metabolism might explain the variability in responses seen with the leukotrienes. Or possibly, there may be differences in the leukotriene-induced release of histamine between species. Antihistamines will block antigen-induced changes in R_L, but not in C_{dyn}, whereas FPL-55712 will block both (46). LTB_4 is a considerably less potent bronchoconstrictor than LTC_4 or LTD_4, and induces essentially all of its effects via TXA_2. A species-specific distribution of enzyme could result in the preferential formation of LTB_4 rather than LTC_4, LTD_4, and LTB_4.

IV.   SUMMARY

Pulmonary vasoconstrictor responses to leukotriene (LT) D_4 were compared to intact-chest sheep and cats under conditions of controlled lobar blood flow. Intralobar injections of LTD_4 in the sheep caused dose-dependent increases in lobar arterial and small vein pressures without altering left atrial systemic arterial pressure. LTD_4 was very potent in increasing pulmonary vascular resistance in the sheep with activity similar to U46619, a thromboxane A_2 receptor mimic. Pulmonary vascular responses to LTD_4 in the sheep were similar when the lung was ventilated and when lobar ventilation was arrested, and when the lobe was perfused with blood or with artificial perfusate. Pulmonary vasoconstrictor responses to LTD_4, but not the thromboxane mimic, in the sheep were reduced by inhibitors of thromboxane and cyclooxygenase synthesis. In contrast, LTD_4 had modest vasoconstrictor activity in the pulmonary vascular bed of the cat, whereas

U46619 had marked activity in this species. Responses to LTD_4 were independent of changes in ventilation, but were dependent on the formation of cyclooxygenase products, including TXA_2, or the interaction with formed elements. However, in the cat, LTD_4 had very weak pressor activity and this activity was not dependent on the integrity of the cyclooxygenase system. In this species, LTD_4 had far less vasoconstrictor activity than did prostaglandins E_2, $F_{2\alpha}$, or D_2. These studies indicate that there is considerable species difference in responses to LTD_4, a major component of the slow reacting substance of anaphylaxis in the pulmonary vascular bed. These studies additionally show that there is a marked difference in the actions of LTD_4 on vascular and airway function in the cat lung.

REFERENCES

1.   Dahlen SE, Hedqvist P, Hammarström S and Samuelsson B. (1980) *Nature* **288**:484.
2.   Dahlen SE, Hedqvist P and Hammarström S. (1983) *Eur J Pharmacol* **86**:207.
3.   Hammarström S. (1983) Ann Rev Biochem 52:355.
4.   Morris HR, Taylor GW, Piper PJ and Tippins JR. (1980) *Nature* **285**:104.
5.   Murphy RC, Hammarström S and Samuelsson B. (1979) *Proc Natl Acad Sci USA* **76**:4275.
6.   Lewis RA, Austen KF, Drazen JM, Clark DA, Marfat A and Corey EJ. (1980) *Proc Natl Acad Sci USA* **77**:3710.
7.   Brocklehurst WE. (1960) *J Physiol* **151**:416.
8.   Dahlen SE, Hansson G, Hedqvist P, Bjorck T, Granstrom E and Dahlen B. (1983) *Proc Natl Acad Sci USA* **80**:1712.
9.   Kellaway CH and Trethewie EF. (1940) *Quart J Exp Physiol* **30**:121.
10. Drazen JM, Austen KF, Lewis RA, Clark DA, Goto G, Marfat A and Corey EJ. (1980) *Proc Natl Acad Sci USA* **77**:4354.
11. Engineer DM, Morris HR, Piper PJ and Sirois P. (1978) *Br J Pharmacol* **64**:211.
12. Hirshman CM, Darnell M, Brigman T and Peters J. (1983) *Prostaglandins* **25**:481.
13. Holroyde MD, Altounyan REC, Cole M, Dixon M and Elliot EV. (1981) *Lancet* **II**:17.
14. Hand JM, Will JA and Buckner CK. (1981) *Eur J Pharmacol* **76**:439.
15. Jones TR, Davis C and Daniel EE. (1982) *Can J Physiol Pharmacol* **60**:638.

16. Krell RD, Osborn R, Vickery L, Falcone K, O'Donnell M, Gleason J, Kinzig C and Bryan D. (1981) *Prostaglandins* 22:387.
17. Graybar GB, Harrington JK, Cowen KH, Spannhake EW, Hyman AL and Kadowitz PJ. (1984) *Prostaglandins* (submitted).
18. Hamel R, Masson P, Ford-Hurchinson AW, Jones TR, Brunet G and Piechuta H. (1982) *Prostaglandins* 24:419.
19. Smedegard G, Hedqvist P, Dahlen SE, Revenas B, Hammarström S and Samuelsson B. (1982) *Nature* 295:327.
20. Iacopino VJ, Fitzpatrick TM, Ramwell PW, Rose JC and Kot PA. (1983) *J Pharmacol Exp Ther* 227:244.
21. Morganroth ML, Reeves JT, Murphy RC and Voelkel NF. (1984) *J Appl Physiol* 56:1340.
22. Yokochi K, Olley PM, Sideris E, Hamilton F, Huhtanen D and Coceani F. (1982) *In* **Leukotrienes and Other Lipoxygenase Products.** (B Samuelsson and R Paoletti, eds) Raven Press:New York.
23. Hyman AL and Kadowitz PJ. (1975) *Am J Physiol* 228:397.
24. Hyman AL and Kadowitz PJ. (1979) *Circ Res* 45:404.
25. Hyman AL, Mathe AA, Leslie CA, Matthews CC, Bennett JT, Spannhake EW and Kadowitz PJ. (1978) *J Pharmacol Exp The*r 207:388.
26. Hyman AL, Spannhake EW and Kadowitz PJ. (1980) *Am J Physiol* 239:H40.
27. Kadowitz PJ and Hyman AL. (1977) *Circ Res* 40:282.
28. Kadowitz PJ and Hyman AL. (1980) *J Pharmacol Exp Ther* 213:300.
29. Kadowitz PJ and Hyman AL. (1983) *Am J Physiol* 244:H423.
30. Kadowitz PJ, Joiner PD and Hyman AL. (1974) *Proc Soc Exp Biol Med* 145:1258.
31. Kadowitz PJ and Hykan AL. (1984) *Circ Res* 55:707.
32. Lowry OH, Rosenbrough NJ, Farr AL and Randall RS. (1951) *J Biol Chem* 193:265.
33. She HS, McNamara DB, Spannhake EW, Hyman AL and Kadowitz PJ. (1981) *Prostaglandins* 21:531.
34. Spannhake EW, Colombo JL, Craigo PA, McNamara DB, Hyman AL and Kadowitz PJ. (1983) *J Appl Physiol* 54:191.
35. Michelassi F, Landa L, Hill RD, Lowenstein E, Watkins WD, Petkau AJ and Zapol WM. (1982) *Science* 217:841.
36. Piper PJ and Samhoum MN. (1981) *Prostaglandins* 21:793.
37. Schianterelli P, Bongrani S and Folco G. (1981) *Eur J Pharmacol* 73:363.
38. Ueno A, Tanaka K and Katori M. (1982) *Prostaglandins* 23:865.
39. Folco G, Hansson G and Granstrom E. (1981) *Biochem Pharmacol* 30:2491.

40. Piper PJ and Samhoum MN. (1982) *Br J Pharmacol* **77**:267.

41. Vargaftig BB, Lefort J and Murphy RC. (1981) *Eur J Pharmacol* **72**:417.

42. Weichman BM, Muccitelli RM, Osborn RR, Holden DA, Bleason JG and Wasserman WA. (1982) *J Pharmacol Exp Ther* **222**:202.

43. Spannhake EW, Hyman AL and Kadowitz PJ. (1980) *J Pharmacol Exp Ther* **212**:584.

44. Coleman RA, Humphrey PPA, Kennedy I, Levy GP and Lumley P. (1981) *Br J Pharmacol* **73**:773.

45. Lippton HL, Armstead WM, Hyman AL and Kadowitz PJ. (1984) *Prostaglandins* **27**:233.

46. Lamm WJE, Lai YL and Hildebrandt J. (1984) *J Appl Physiol* **56**:1032.

Relationship of Pharmacologic Agents, Pulmonary Endothelial Cells and Pulmonary Circulation

NARESH CHAND
WILLIAM DIAMANTIS
R. DUANE SOFIA
Department of Pharmacology
Wallace Laboratories
Cranbury, New Jersey   08512

I.   INTRODUCTION

A vast amount of literature has been published on various aspects of the biochemistry, structure-function, pharmacology and pathology of vascular endothelial cells (EC) in health and disease states. Endothelial destruction has been implicated in the pathophysiology of hypoxic pulmonary hypertension, adult respiratory distress syndrome ('shock lung syndrome'), primary pulmonary hypertension, thrombosis, diabetes mellitus, atherosclerosis and vascular spastic diseases (1-7). The endothelial layer not only provides a barrier in the lumen of blood vessels, but represents a vital, active and functional biochemical factory for the synthesis, metabolism, uptake, storage and destruction of many biologically active substances. For example, uptake and biodegradation of catecholamines, serotonin, ATP and kinins; enzymatic conversion of inactive angiotensin I to angiotensin II (a potent vasopressor agent), and biosynthesis/secretion of metabolites of arachidonic acid metabolism, *e.g.*, prostacyclin (PGI_2), 15-HPETE, 5-HETE, diHETE (8), neutrophil chemotactic factor (NCF; 4), platelet activating factor (PAF; 9), superoxide free radicals ($\cdot O_2^-$, H_2O_2, OH^-, etc.; 10), endothelial-

Copyright © 1987 by Academic Press, Inc.
All rights of reproduction in any form reserved.

TABLE I. Endothelium-dependent relaxants in isolated pulmonary arterial smooth muscles.

Species	Endothelial cell dependent relaxant	Inhibitor/antagonist
Dog	Ach (1)	Atropine
	BK (21,22,37,38)	—
	AA (37,38)	Indomethacin
Rabbit	Ach (16,28)	Atropine, p-BPB
	A23187 (28)	p-BPB, Hemoglobin, Methemoglobin, Methylene blue (28)
	Substance P (39), ATP (13)	Atropine (39)
	AA (15)	SKF-525A (15)
Guinea Pig	Ach (17), Carbachol (41)	Atropine
	A23187 [17,41]	—
	BK [17]	—
	Histamine (40)	Diphenhydramine
	Substance P (41)	
Cattle	Ach (23,27)	Methylene Blue (27)
	BK (23)	
Man	Ach (30)	Quinacrine, NDGA (30)
	ATP (30)	

derived relaxant factors (EDRFs) and endothelial-derived contractile factors (EDCFs; 1,3,11,12). PGI_2 is a potent inhibitor of platelet aggregation and an endogenous vascular relaxant and PAF is a powerful platelet and PMN aggregating agent. The biologically active substances such as HPETEs, HETEs, PAF, LTB_4, NCF (NCF-A), ECF (ECF-A), and EDRFs/EDCFs could play important roles in the control, regulation and maintenance of pulmonary vascular reactivity and pulmonary circulation in health and disease states. The products derived from pulmonary endothelium cells (EC) may also play a significant role in capillary permeability changes, chemotaxis, chemokinesis and edema in the lungs. Endothelial cells possess receptors for numerous neurohumoral and vasoactive/bronchoactive substances. By virtue of the strategic location of the lungs and enormous surface area of pulmonary endothelial layer, they constantly interact with blood constituents (leukocytes, erythrocytes, platelets), coagulation factor, complement system and pulmonary vascular smooth muscles and may help to maintain homeostasis in the lung circulation.

During the past five years it has been shown that pulmonary arteries of several species react with potent and concentration-dependent relaxation to several pharmacologic agents provided they were precontracted and endothelium was left intact (Table I). Depending upon the species, diet (13), site of blood vessel (intrapulmonary vs. extrapulmonary rings), tone (15), oxygen supply (3) and nature of constrictor agents (1) as well as several other factors (Table II), some of the endothelial-dependent vasodilators could produce vasoconstriction (14,15).

The objective of this chapter is to briefly review (i) the pharmacology of the pulmonary endothelial cells and their interactions with lung blood vessels especially in the light of our own work; (ii) to discuss the putative mechanism of

TABLE II. Possible factors responsible for the heterogeneity of endothelial-dependent relaxations in pulmonary arteries.

- species, age, sex
- state of health (lung parasites, toxemia, bacterial and viral infections, immune complexes), stress
- diet (hypercholesteremia)
- method of euthanasia (air emboli)
- preparation (segments vs. strips; intrapulmonary vs. extrapulmonary blood vessels); storage; intravascular clots
- expertise (isolation, dissection, mounting of blood vessels), amount of attached lung or adipose tissues
- composition of physiological solution (Ca^{++}, Mg^{++}, K^+), pH, temperature, and oxygen tension
- constrictor agent ($PGF_{2\alpha}$, catecholamines, KCl)
  - concentration
  - mechanism of constriction (intracellular vs. extracellular Ca^{++} utilization)
  - duration of exposure
  - magnitude of induced tone
- nature, dosage and frequency of administration of relaxants (single vs. cumulative)
- method of endothelial destruction
  - mechanical
  - enzymatic
  - chemical
- concentration, duration of contact with antagonists/inhibitors (pH, temperature, dilution, solvents, storage)

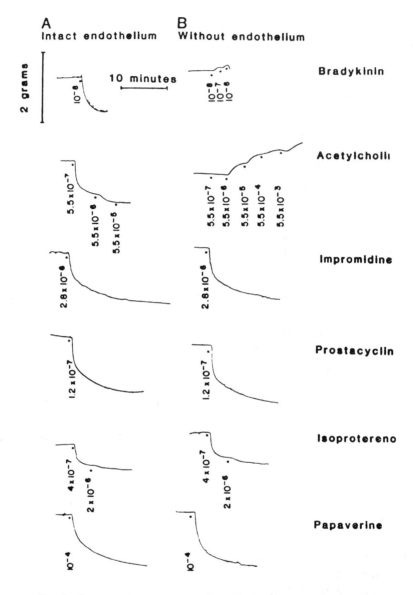

Fig. 1. Comparative responses of canine intrapulmonary arteries contracted with serotonin (2.6x10⁻⁸ to 1.3x10⁻⁷ M) to bradykinin, acetylcholine, impromidine, PGI₂, isoproterenol, and papaverine in the presence (left column) and in absence (right column) of endothelium. Dots indicate points at which agonists (M) were added. Removal of endothelium results in a complete loss of relaxant responses to acetylcholine and bradykinin, whereas relaxant responses to other agonists are not altered by endothelial destruction. (Taken from Science (ref. 1) with permission of the American Asociation for the Advancement of Science).

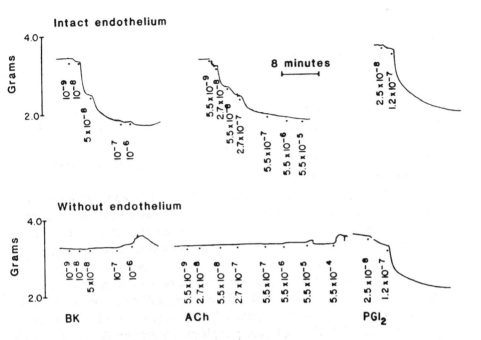

Fig. 2. *Responses of canine intrapulmonary arteries contracted with phenylephrine to cumulative concentrations (moles per liter) of bradykinin (BK), acetylcholine (Ach), and prostacyclin (PGI$_2$). All three agents induce concentration-dependent relaxation in the presence of intact endothelial cells. Mechanical destruction of the endothelium results in the obliteration of relaxant responses to bradykinin and acetylcholine but not to prostacyclin. The vertical bars on the left represent tension; time marker, 8 minutes. Dots indicate points at which cumulative concentrations of agonists were added. [Taken from Science (ref. 1) with permission of the American Association for the Advancement of Science].*

EDRF synthesis/secretion from pulmonary EC and the mode of EDRF-induced pulmonary vascular relaxation; and (iii) to correlate these *in vitro* observations to the pathophysiology of lung vascular diseases.

II.   PHARMACOLOGY OF PULMONARY ENDOTHELIUM

Acetylcholine (Ach), methacholine, substance P, bradykinin (BK), calcium ionophore (A23187), ATP and arachidonic acid (AA) have been reported to produce endothelial-dependent relaxation of the pulmonary arteries of dogs, rats, cattle, guinea pigs, rabbits and man (Table I, Figures 1,2). The mechanical destruction of the EC obliterates the relaxation induced by the aforementioned agents without influencing relaxation exerted by sodium nitroprusside, isoproterenol, PGI_2, dimaprit or impromidine (H_2-agonists) and papaverine (1,2,16,17; Figures 1,2,).

Atropine selectively antagonizes Ach-induced, EC-dependent, relaxation of the pulmonary arteries of dogs (1), rabbits (14,16), rats, guinea pigs (17), and cattle (18) as well as Ach-induced EC-dependent contractile responses in rabbit intrapulmonary arteries (14). The existence of specific muscarinic cholinergic receptors on the pulmonary EC is well established. Atropine could act by blocking muscarinic receptors on EC, thus preventing the synthesis/secretion of EDRF/EDCF. Alternatively, the EDRF-induced relaxation (in response to Ach) is selectively reversed by atropine (Figure 3). This suggests that EDRF receptors (guanylate cyclase/EDRF receptor complex) in pulmonary vascular smooth muscle exhibit selectivity to atropine blockade.

The perfusion of rat lung with collagenase impairs Ach-induced (EC-mediated) pulmonary vasodilator responses (19). *In vivo* exposure to hyperoxia for a period of one week increases the sensitivity of rat isolated proximal intrapulmonary arteries to vasoconstrictor $PGF_{2\alpha}$ and attenuates EC-dependent relaxation to Ach (20).

Bradykinin (BK) produces concentration-dependent, EC-dependent relaxation in isolated pulmonary arteries of dogs (1,21,22) and cattle (23; Figures 1,2). This effect is not influenced by indomethacin, suggesting noninvolvement of prostaglandins (PGI_2; 1,21,22). EC destruction attenuates BK (10^{-7} M)-induced relaxation in pulmonary arteries of old rabbits (16). Indomethacin (1.4×10^{-5} M, 30 min) as well as p-bromophenacylbromide (5×10^{-6} M, 30 min) inhibited BK (10^{-8}-10^{-7} M)-induced relaxation in rabbit pulmonary arteries (24). Interestingly, in extrapulmonary arterial segments of young rabbits in which the endothelial layer was damaged (unintentionally or intentionally) and which failed to relax to Ach (10^{-7} M), addition of the single doses of BK (10^{-10}-10^{-8} M) were found to produce a strong relaxant response (24). These observations suggest that Ach-induced relaxation is extremely sensitive and entirely dependent on the integrity of the EC, whereas BK still relaxes rabbit pulmonary arteries either by acting on some undamaged EC cells, or by stimulating the production of PGI_2 by acting on other cell types, *e.g.*, vascular smooth muscle cells.

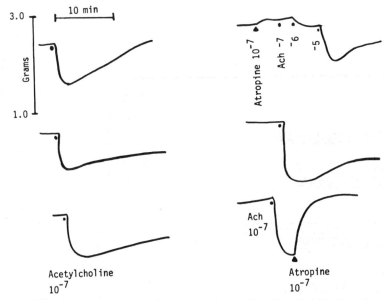

Fig. 3. Antagonism and reversal of acetylcholine (Ach)-induced, endothelial-dependent relaxation by atropine in the phenylephrine (PE: 1.5x10⁻⁷ M) contracted rabbit pulmonary arterial segment.

Indomethacin potentiated the relaxant responses to Ach (Fig. 4) and A23187 in rabbit pulmonary arteries, perhaps by inhibiting the synthesis of endogenous PGI_2 in pulmonary EC (25). Endogenously released PGI_2 might be exerting a negative feed-back (inhibitory) influence on the secretion (synthesis/release) of EDRFs. The indomethacin-induced potentiation of Ach- and A23187-induced EC-dependent relaxation may also be explained by the inhibition of EC-derived contractile substances (EDCFs: e.g., PGH_2/G_2, thromboxane A_2/B_2) in response to Ach (14) and A23187.

p-Bromophenacylbromide [5x10⁻⁶ M, p-BPB, a potent phospholipase A_2 (PLA_2) inhibitor] exerted a slowly developing tension (500-1000 mg) over a period of 30-60 min in some rabbit pulmonary arterial segments. This p-BPB-induced contraction was not reversible even after several washings. Such a response may be associated with its endothelial damaging effect (26) or to its unknown Ca^{++} mobilizing properties in vascular smooth muscles.

p-Bromophenacylbromide (5x10⁻⁶ M, 30-60 min) selectively inhibited relaxant responses to Ach, BK and A23187 (10⁻⁷ M of each) in rabbit pulmonary arterial segments without influencing papaverine-, isoproterenol-, or sodium nitroprusside-(EC-independent relaxants)-induced relaxation (Figure 5). These

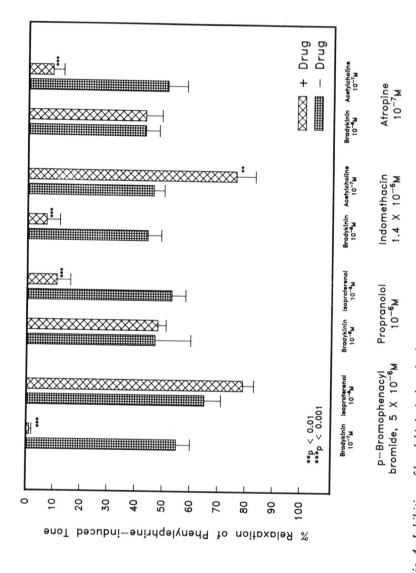

Fig. 4. Inhibition of bradykinin-induced relaxation by indomethacin (1.4x10⁻⁵ M, 30 minutes preincubation) in a phenylephrine-contracted rabbit pulmonary arterial segment. The acetylcholine (endothelial-dependent)- induced relaxation was enhanced by indomethacin.

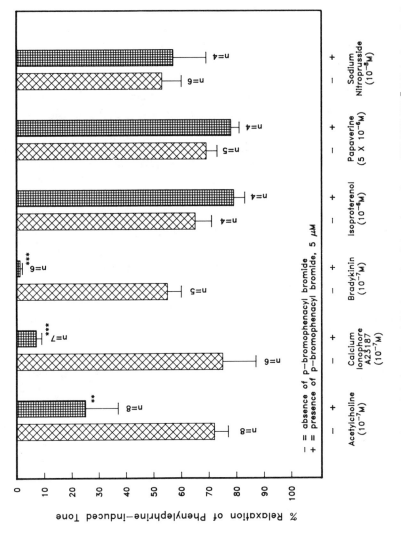

Fig. 5. Abolition of acetylcholine, bradykinin, and calcium ionophore A23187 (10^{-7} M)-induced relaxations by p-bromophenacylbromide (5×10^{-6} M, 30-60 min).

observations suggest that EC-dependent relaxants stimulate PLA_2 in EC, initiating a cascade of a series of biochemical reactions leading to synthesis/release of EDRF (which may be PAF, superoxide free radicals: $\cdot O_2^-$, H_2O_2, OH^-, etc., or lipid peroxide, a metabolite of arachidonic acid other than PGI_2; 16,25).

Removal of EC produced a shift to the left of the concentration-effect curves to epinephrine, norepinephrine and UK 14,304 (a selective α_2-adrenoceptor agonist) in canine pulmonary arteries and veins. EC destruction did not influence phenylephrine (a selective α_1-agonist) concentration-effect curves. Norepinephrine-induced relaxation in canine pulmonary veins was also abolished by de-endo-thelization (29).

In rabbit pulmonary arterial segments contracted with KCl (a depolarizing agent), the relaxant responses to Ach, papaverine, BK, A23187, and sodium nitroprusside were significantly attenuated as compared to arterial segments contracted with phenylephrine (16,17). It is possible that EDRFs (released by Ach and A23187) directly produce relaxation by hyperpolarization of pulmonary vascular smooth muscles (1).

In rabbit pulmonary arterial rings with a low basal tension (1.5 g), arachidonic acid (AA) produces weak contractile responses which were obliterated by EC removal or by indomethacin (10^{-6} M). Thus, EC-dependent, AA-induced contractile responses were mediated via a product of the cyclooxygenase pathway (*e.g.*, endoperoxide PGH_2, G_2 or TXA_2/TXB_2). The rings precontracted to 3.5 - 4 g tension with phenylephrine (7×10^{-7} M) respond with concentration-dependent relaxation to AA. EC-independent, AA-induced relaxation was attenuated by indomethacin, whereas EC-dependent relaxation to AA was selectively inhibited by SKF-525A, an inhibitor of cytochrome P-450-dependent monooxygenase. Induction of vascular cytochrome P-450-dependent monooxygenases with 3-methylchloanthrene and -napthoflavone (40 mg/kg/day, i.p., for 3 days) enhanced EC dependent relaxation to AA 10 fold, a response reversed by SKF-525A. On the other hand, depletion of cytochrome P-450-dependent enzymes with cobalt chloride (24 mg/kg/day, s.c., for 2 days) suppresses AA (EC-dependent) relaxation. Based on these data, Pinto and his associates concluded that a cytochrome P-450-dependent monooxygenase localized in the EC may play an important role in the mediation of relaxation to AA in rabbit pulmonary arteries (15) and perhaps other blood vessels.

Hypercholesterolemia has been reported to attenuate Ach and ATP-induced relaxation (EC-dependent) in rabbit pulmonary arteries. The reduction of EC-dependent relaxation in hypercholesterolemic arteries may be due to thickening of the internal layers which could then inhibit the diffusion of EDRF to the vascular smooth muscle cells (13).

ATP and Ach exerted concentration-dependent relaxation of 5-HT or phenylephrine contracted human pulmonary arterial segments, provided the EC were intact. Ach-induced relaxation was inhibited by quinacrine (3×10^{-5} M) as well as by nordihydroguiaretic acid (NDGA, a lipoxygenase inhibitor, 10^{-4} M) but not by propranolol or indomethacin (30). Based on the susceptibility of Ach-induced relaxation to NDGA, these investigators suggested the involvement of a product of the lipoxygenase pathway. However, it must be emphasized that high concentrations of lipoxygenase inhibitors (NDGA, ETYA, BW 755c, etc.) could exert nonspecific pharmacological activities (*e.g.*,antioxidative properties, inhibition of phospholipases, cytochrome P-450-dependent monooxygenases, cyclooxygenases and Ca^{++}-influx, free radical scavengers, etc).

III.   MECHANISM OF ENDOTHELIAL DEPENDENT RELAXATIONS

The exact chemical nature of EDRF is not yet known. EDRF could produce vasodilation by one or more of the following mechanism(s) (Fig 6; 16):

1. EDRF could produce hyperpolarization of contracted pulmonary arteries by some unknown mechanism (1). This view is supported by the observations that elevated concentrations of K^+ (10-40 mM) attenuate or inhibit EC dependent relaxation in canine and rabbit pulmonary arteries (1,16,17).

2. Platelet activating factor (PAF: 10^{-6}-10^{-5} M) produces weak and inconsistent relaxation of rabbit pulmonary arteries (17). EC can generate PAF in response to several stimuli including A23187, histamine, bradykinin and ATP (9). Recently, PAF has been reported to blunt vasopressor stimuli in rat lung possibly by mechanisms that may relate to PAF-induced edema and/or vasodilation (32). PAF (10^{-9} M) relaxes norepinephrine-contracted, sodium-meclofenamate treated rat pulmonary arteries with intact endothelium (33). I.V. injection of PAF (0.01 pM) depresses hypoxic pulmonary vasoconstrictor responses (33). It remains to be established if endogenously released PAF could act as a mediator/modulator of pulmonary vascular reactivity and pathophysiology of lung diseases.

3. The role of the products of the lipoxygenase pathway of arachidonic acid in the mediation of EDRF-induced vascular relaxation is controversial (1,26). EC synthesize 5-, 12-, 15-HPETE, 5-HETE, di-HETE (8) and perhaps leukotrienes. The lipoxygenase inhibitors (LI) such as NDGA and BW755C exert little or no effect on Ach-induced relaxation in canine pulmonary arteries. NDGA reverses Ach and BK-induced relaxation in canine renal arteries (2) and inhibits Ach-induced relaxation in human pulmonary arteries (30). LI may act as antioxidants and scavengers for superoxide free radicals. It remains to be established whether EDRF is a product of the lipoxygenase pathway of AA metabolism (*e.g.*, HPETE, HETE) in pulmonary blood vessels.

4. Endothelial cells are capable of releasing superoxide free radicals (10). BK, Ach, histamine, A23187, substance P and other vasoactive agents may

Receptors on Pulmonary Endothelial Cells

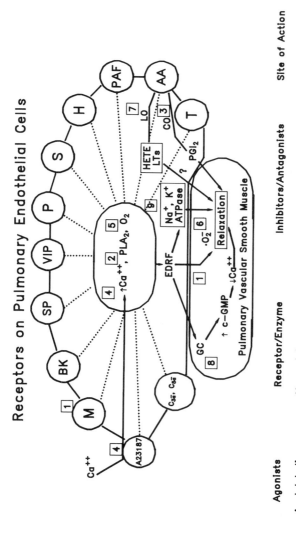

Agonists	Receptor/Enzyme	Inhibitors/Antagonists	Site of Action
Acetylcholine	Muscarinic Receptor	Atropine	[1]
	Phospholipase A_2	p-Bromophenacyl bromide, Sterolds	[2]
Bradykinin	BK Receptor	Indomethacin (Rabbit)	[3]
A23187	Ca^{++} Channels	Ca^{++} -antagonists	[4]
	Oxidative Enzymes	Hypoxia; Antioxidative Drugs	[5]
	Overshoot Phenomenon	Methylene Blue, Hemoglobin	[6]
	Catalase Competition	Methemoglobin	
	Lipoxygenases	NDGA, BW755c, Antioxidative	[7]
	(Lipid Peroxidation)	Agents	
	Guanylate Cyclase	Methylene Blue, Hemoglobin	[8]
	Na^+-K^+-ATPase	Ouabain, K^+-free Solution	[9]

generate superoxide free radicals ($\cdot O_2$, OH^-, H_2O_2, etc.). H_2O_2 (10^{-5} to 10^{-3} M) produces concentration-dependent relaxation in endothelial-denuded intrapulmonary arteries of cattle (34), and extrapulmonary arteries of the rabbit (17). In rabbit extrapulmonary arteries with intact endothelium, H_2O_2 (10^{-6}-10^{-4} M) induces moderate to strong, but transient (superimposed) constriction (200 to 700 mg) (17). H_2O_2 activates guanylate cyclase in bovine intrapulmonary arteries (34). Lipid or oxygen radicals may be the candidate for EDRF, and subsequent vascular relaxation. Such a view is supported by the following observations (i) methylene blue (MB), hemoglobin (Hb) and methemoglobin (MHb) (10^{-7}-10^{-6} M) do not appear to interfere with the production of EDRF (released by Ach and BK) and (ii) MB, Hb and MHb not only produce rapid 100-300% reversals 'overshoot phenomenon' (Fig. 7) of relaxation induced by Ach, BK, A23187 but also exert similar reversals of H_2O_2 (0.5-1×10^{-4} M) and sodium nitroprusside (10^{-8}-10^{-7} M)-induced relaxations in rabbit pulmonary arteries (28; Fig. 6). The rapid reversals of EDRF-induced relaxations by MB and Hb may be related to their electron accepting properties and thus chemically inactivating EDRF [lipid peroxides, lipid hydroperoxides (34), ROOH, ROO^-, superoxide free radicals: $\cdot O_2^-$, H_2O_2, OH^-, etc.]

Fig. 6. Possible mechanism of endothelial-dependent relaxation in pulmonary vasculature. Endothelial cells possess receptors for acetylcholine (M=muscarinic receptor), bradykinin (BK), substance P (SP), vasoactive intestinal peptide (VIP), purine nucleotides (P: ATP, ADP, adenosine), serotonin (S: 5-HT receptors), histamine (H_1-receptors), platelet activating factor (PAF), arachidonic acid (AA), thrombin (T), anaphylatoxins (C_{3a}-, C_{5a}-), and calcium ionophore (A23187). The activation of these receptors by circulating neurohumoral substances and their respective agonists cause the influx of Ca^{++} into the pulmonary endothelial cells, which stimulate phospholipase A_2 (a Ca^{++} and O_2-dependent biochemical step) leading to the generation of endothelial derived relaxant factors (EDRFs: for example, $\cdot O_2^-$, H_2O_2, OH^-, lipid peroxides, PAF, etc.). These factors stimulate soluble guanylate cyclase in pulmonary vascular smooth muscles and increase the level of C-GMP which lowers intracellular Ca^{++} and ultimately produces vasodilation under normal physiological conditions. Under abnormal conditions, e.g., adult respiratory distress syndrome, 'shock lung syndrome', hypoxia (which may cause functional or morohological abnormality in endothelial cells), the vasoactive substances may act directly on pulmonary vascular smooth muscle and induce vasoconstriction.

at the vascular smooth muscle level, or to the easy inactivation of EDRF-, H_2O_2-, and sodium nitroprusside-activated guanylate cyclases (guanylate cyclase/EDRF receptor complex) by lower concentrations of MB, Hb and MHb, causing 100-300% reversal of relaxation into contractions. It should be mentioned that MB, Hb and MHb (10^{-7}-10^{-6} M) exert weak or no contractile responses under resting conditions. However, the addition of MB, Hb and MHb (10^{-6} M) produces strong (500-2000 mg) superimposed contractile responses in contracted rabbit pulmonary arteries. This may relate to the chemical inactivation of endogenous EDRF and/or to pharmacological antagonism of the activated guanylate cyclase (intracellular receptor for EDRF) (28). Higher concentrations of MB (27), Hb and MHb (>10^{-6} - 5×10^{-5} M) inhibit soluble guanylate cyclase (an enzyme or receptor activated by EDRF) thereby inhibiting the formation of C-GMP which lowers intracellular Ca^{++} and relaxes vascular smooth muscles. In addition, Hb has been reported to promote the autooxidative breakdown of HPETEs to hydroxy, epoxy and peroxy derivatives (35). Hæm proteins are also known to be capable of destroying lipid peroxide (ROOH, ROO⁻) and breaking the autooxidation chain. Hb, hæmin and cytochrome C (10^{-5}-10^{-4} M) also strongly inhibit lipid peroxide formation and oxygen uptake by microsomes (36). Therefore, inactivation of EDRF (HPETE, lipid peroxides, ROOH, ROO⁻) by Hb, MH and MB may explain the overshoot phenomenon observed during reversal of EDRF relaxation in rabbit pulmonary arteries.

The rapid reversal of EC dependent relaxation by HB and MHb may represent an endogenous regulatory (homeostatic) mechanism in blood vessels. The interactions between erythrocytes (containing catalase for the destruction of H_2O_2, and Hb and MHb for inactivation of EDRF), EC, and smooth muscle cells could play a vital role in the control of pulmonary circulation. Under hypoxic conditions, the synthesis of EDRF may be abolished or altered, and now EC may even generate EDCFs responsible for hypoxic pulmonary vasoconstriction.

The role of enzymes (*e.g.*, peroxidases, lipoxygenases, monoxygenases; NADPH/NADH, reductase/oxidases, xanthine oxidase, hydroxylases; cytochrome P-450 as electron acceptors/donors; Na^+-K^+ ATPase, Na^+-Ca^{++} exchanges) in the metabolism (synthesis/secretion/inactivation) of EDRF/EDCF in endothelial cells and pulmonary vascular smooth muscles remains to be studied.

IV.   PULMONARY ENDOTHELIUM AND PATHOPHYSIOLOGY OF LUNG VASCULAR DISEASES

Pulmonary vascular endothelium is exposed to the varying oxygen tension of mixed venous blood. This variation may be an important stimulus for hypoxic pulmonary vasoconstriction. Holden and McCall showed that an EC-derived mediator is responsible for hypoxia-induced pulmonary vasoconstriction in the main pulmonary arteries of swine. This EC-derived mediator was not PG, TXA_2 or B_2, catecholamine or Ach (3). It is possible that pulmonary EC sense a reduced O_2 tension and alter their biochemical process to generate some unknown excitatory mediator(s).

In pulmonary vascular diseases where the endothelium is damaged, for example, hypoxic pulmonary vasoconstriction, pulmonary hypertension, adult respiratory distress syndrome 'shock lung syndrome', endotoxemia and several other related conditions (1-6,31), the endogenous substances, such as Ach, BK, AA, histamine, thrombin, ATP, etc. (which normally release EDRFs and counteract pulmonary vasoconstriction) could themselves directly act on pulmonary vascular smooth muscle and could increase pulmonary vascular resistance (pulmonary hypertension). In intact animals, the effect of EC dependent relaxants on pulmonary arterioles, venules, capillaries and veins of different species may be quite different from those observed in isolated pulmonary arterial segments bubbled with 95% O_2 and 5% CO_2 mixture. Therefore, caution must be exercised in extending and interpreting *in vitro* experimental observations to explain the pathophysiology of pulmonary vascular diseases in animals and man.

Complement derived factors (anaphylotoxins, C_{5a}-, C_{3a}-), coagulation factors (plasminogen, thrombin, etc.), endotoxins, mediators released from PMN (lysosomal enzymes, superoxide free radicals: $\cdot O_2^-$, H_2O_2, OH^-), eosinophils (leukotrienes, major basic proteins), platelets (PAF, endoperoxides, TXA_2, TXB_2, 5-HT), mast cells, basophils (PGD_2, LTs, PGs, histamine, chemotactic factors, PAF) and endothelial cells themselves (lipid peroxides, ROOH, ROO^-, PGI_2, EDRF/EDCF, PAF, chemotactic factors, NCF-A, ECF-A?, etc.) and their interactions could play important and critical roles in the initiation of the inflammatory process, *i.e.*, margination of PMN and adherence of platelet etc. Acute systemic anaphylaxis and adult respiratory distress syndrome are associated with sequestration of PMN (leukocytes: neutropenia) and platelets (thrombo-cytopenia) in the lung. The synthesis/release of mediators/ modulators such as chemoattractant stimuli (such as LTB_4, 5-HETE, NCF, PAF, lipid peroxides, ROOH, ROO^-, EDRF, etc.) in pulmonary EC may have a profound effect on the pathogenesis of pulmonary vascular diseases.

In conclusion, pulmonary arterial endothelial cells generate EDRFs under normal resting conditions, as well as in response to vasoactive/ bronchoactive agents and thus oppose pulmonary vasoconstriction due to pathophysiological stimuli, such as sympathetic discharge, epinephrine, norepinephrine, $PGF_{2\alpha}$, endoperoxides, thromboxanes, hypoxia, etc. Endothelial cells and their products (EDRF, PGI_2, free radicals, lipid peroxides, ROOH, ROO^-, NCF, ECF, PAF, etc?) in conjunction with blood constituents (leukocytes, platelets and their

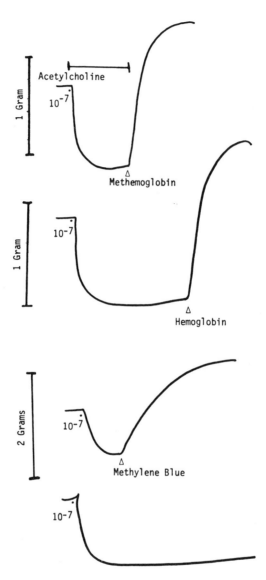

Fig. 7A+B. Typical tracings depicting the reversal 'overshoot phenomenon' of acetylcholine- and A23187-induced relaxation by methylene blue, hemoglobin, and methemoglobin in rabbit isolated pulmonary arterial segments.

products, erythrocytes, coagulation factors and complement system) and circulating vasoactive substances could play a vital role in the control and regulation of homeostasis in the pulmonary circulation in health and disease states. EDCFs can

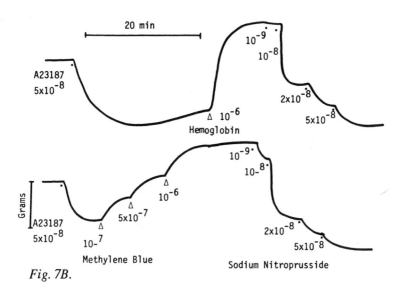

Fig. 7B.

also be generated by pulmonary endothelial cells especially under hypoxic (anoxic) conditions. Thus, the EDRFs/EDCFs production/secretion could modulate the pulmonary circulation.

ACKNOWLEDGMENTS

The authors gratefully acknowledge Mr. T.P. Mahoney for technical assistance, Mrs. J. Rittman for secretarial assistance and Mr. J. Pillar for graphics.

REFERENCES

1. Chand N and Altura BM. (1981) *Science* **213**:1376.
2. Chand N and Altura BM. (1981) *Microcirculation* **1**:297.
3. Holden WE and McCall E. (1984) *Experimental Lung Res* **7**:101.
4. Rounds S, Farber HW, Hill NS and O'Brien RF. (1985) *Chest* **88**:213S.
5. O'Brien RF and McMurtry IF. (1984) *Am Rev Resp Dis* **129**:A337.
6. Barst RJ and Stalcup SA. (1985) *Chest* **88**:216S.
7. Altiere RJ, Olson JW and Gillespie MN. (1986) *J Pharm Exptl Therap* **236**:390.
8. Kuhn H, Ponicke K, Halle W, Weisner R, Schewe T and Forster W. (1985) *Prostaglandins, Leukotrienes and Medicine* **17**:291.

9. Camussi G, Pawlowski I, Bussolino F, Caldwell PR, Brentjens, J and Andres G. (1983) *J Immunol* **131**:1802.

10. Rosen GM and Freeman BA (1984) *Proc Natl Acad Sci* **81**:7269.

11. Furchgott RF and Zawadzki JV. (1980) *Nature* **288**:373.

12. Furchgott RF, Cherry PD, Zawadzki JV and Jothianandan, D. (1984) *J Cardiovasc Pharmacol* **6**:S336.

13. Coene MC, Herman AG, Jordaens F, Van Hove C, Verbeuren TJ and Zonnekeyn L. (1985) *Br J Pharmacol* **85**:267P.

14. Altiere RJ, Kiritsy-Roy JA and Catravas JD. (1986) *J Pharm Exp Ther* **236**:535.

15. Pinto A, Abraham NG and Mullane KM. (1986) *J Pharm Exp Ther* **236**:445.

16. Chand N, Mahoney TP, Diamantis W and Sofia RD. (1986) *J Critical Care* **1**:122.

17. Chand N, Diamantis W, Mahoney TP and Sofia RD. (recent unpublished observations)

18. Ignarro LJ, Burke TM, Wood KS, Wolin MS and Kadowitz PJ. (1984) *J Pharm Exp Therap* **228**:682.

19. Fedderson CO, McMurtry IF, Henson P and Voekel NF. (1986) *Am Rev Resp Dis* **133**:197.

20. Coflesky JT and Evans NJ. (1986) *Am Rev Resp Dis* **133**:A159.

21. Altura BM and Chand N. (1981) *Br J Pharmacol* **74**:10.

22. Cherry PD, Furchgott RF, Zawadzki JV and Jothianandan D. (1982) *Proc Natl Acad Sci* **79**:2106.

23. Gruetter CA and Lemke SM. (1986) *Eur J Pharmacol* **122**:363.

24. Diamantis W, Chand N, Mahoney TP and Sofia RD. (1986) *Pharmacologist* **28**:187.

25. Sofia RD, Chand N, Mahoney TP and Diamantis W. (1986) *Pharmacologist* **28**:152.

26. Furchgott RF. (1984) *Ann Rev Pharmacol Toxicol* **24**:1.

27. Ignarro LJ, Harbison RG, Wood KS and Kadowitz PJ. (1986) *J Pharm Exp Ther* **236**:30.

28. Chand N, Mahoney TP, Diamantis W and Sofia RD. (1986) *Pharmacologist* **28**:187.

29. Miller VM and Vanhoutte PM. (1985) *Eur J Pharmacol* **118**:123.

30. Barnes PJ, Greenberg B and Rhoden KJ. (1986) *Br J Pharmacol* **87**:198P.

31. Welsh CH, McMurtry IF and Weil JV. (1986) *Am Rev Resp Dis* **133**:A276.

32. Gillespie MN and Bowdy BD. (1986) *J Pharm Exp Ther* **236**:396.

33. McMurtry IF and Morris KG. (1986) *Am Rev Resp Dis* **133**:A227.

34. Burke TM and Wolin MS. (1985) *Circulation* **72**:177.

35.   Hamberg M. (1975) *Lipids* **10**:87.
36.   Willis ED. (1969) *Biochem J* **113**:315.
37.   Chand N and Altura BM. (1981) *Fed Proc* **40**:452.
38.   Chand N and Altura BM. (1981) *Clin Res* **29**:493.
39.   Tanaka DT and Grunstein MM. (1985) *J Appl Physiol* **58**:1291.
40.   Satoh H and Inui J. (1984) *Eur J Pharmacol* **97**:321.
41.   Bolton TB and Clapp LH. (1986) *Br J Pharmacol* **87**:713.

Pharmacology of the Pulmonary Circulation: Summary

Posters presented in the pharmacology session helped to reemphasize that marked differences in pharmacological responsiveness can be seen between the pulmonary and systemic circulations. The discussion also highlighted the need for more extensive mechanistic information concerning the actions of several drugs and their differential effects.

Burchfield and Drummond described the hemodynamic actions of halothane administration to lambs. In the absence of other anesthetic drugs, halothane caused a decrease in systemic artery pressure (SAP), an effect primarily related to a decrease in stroke volume. Pulmonary artery pressure (PAP) did not change and this was attributed to an increase in pulmonary vascular resistance (PVR) concomitant with the decrease in cardiac output. Systemic vascular resistance (SVR) did not change during halothane administration. All effects of halothane were the same in neonatal *vs.* juvenile lambs.

Ethanol caused an increase in PAP and PVR with a 55% increase in the ratio of PVR/SVR in newborn lambs (Drummond, Polak and Dailey). Cardiac output and SVR were not altered. All vascular effects of ethanol were abolished by indomethacin (7-8 mg/kg) and attenuated by meclofenamate (4 and 8 mg/kg). It was suggested that the smaller magnitude of effect of the latter drug is related to a smaller degree of absorption from the oral route of administration. The implication is that the vascular effects of ethanol are caused by the release of cyclooxygenase metabolites of arachidonic acid.

Small doses of ATP (1-2 μmoles/kg) were shown to produce selective pulmonary vasodilation in patients with chronic obstructive pulmonary disease (Gaba, Trigui, Michel, *et al.*). As the dose of ATP was increase up to 5 μmoles/kg, SAP also decreased. At this dose of ATP, ΔPVR/ΔSVR (%) was 0.86. The reversal of this ratio was suggested to be due to saturation of pulmonary endothelial cell uptake of ATP at the larger dose.

A selective dopamine DA_1 receptor agonist, fenoldopam, was shown to produce markedly different effects in pulmonary and systemic circulations of lambs (Polak and Drummond). While this compound produced a ΔSVR of -16%, the ΔPVR rose to a maximum of 68%. The rise in PVR, but not the fall in SVR, was attenuated by SCH-23390, a selective DA_1 receptor antagonist. It was also reported that dopamine can attenuate hypoxic pulmonary vasoconstriction in the dog (Lejeune, Maeije, Leeman *et al.*). Dobutamine, at an equivalent dose of 20 μg/kg/min, was more effective than dopamine in blocking the hypoxic response. These reports suggest a potential importance of dopamine receptors in the pulmonary circulation, an area that has yet to be extensively examined.

The clinical effectiveness of vasodilator therapy in pulmonary hypertension was noted in two studies. One (Jezek, Michaljanic, Fucík, *et al.*) showed that isosorbide dinitrate, given to patients with pulmonary hypertension due to interstitial lung fibrosis, significantly decreased mortality rate within a 2 year period. The drug decreased PAP, PVR and right ventricular work in patients with stabilized blood gases, but was ineffective in patients with progressive hypoxemia. Another (Long, Barst, Fishman, *et al.*) examined the acute effects of prostacyclin in 65 patients with primary pulmonary hypertension. A decrease in PVR was noted in the majority, but seven patients demonstrated an increase in PVR with prostacyclin. Both clinical studies emphasized that some patients with pulmonary hypertension do not benefit from vasodilator therapy.

The role of endothelial cells in responses of isolated pulmonary vascular smooth muscle to several substances was examined by Chand, Mahoney, Diamantis, *et al.* Most of these data were presented earlier in the session. There is clearly a need for additional studies in this area.

CARL K. BUCKNER

Hemodynamics

Pulmonary Hemodynamics: Introduction

Measurements of blood flows, pressures, and volumes are often used to detect and quantify the vasomotor and structural changes which occur in the pulmonary vascular bed in response to various physiologic, pathophysiologic and pharmacologic stimuli. The hemodynamic consequences of these pulmonary vascular responses can be important in regard to control of pulmonary gas exchange, lung fluid balance, nonrespiratory functions of the pulmonary endothelium, and right heart function. Therefore interpretation of the information content of the data in terms of what they reveal about the organ function is of practical experimental and clinical importance (1,2). These data, which can be obtained from the lungs *in vivo* and/or from isolated lungs, without damaging the lungs, typically include pressures such as pulmonary arterial and venous pressures, pulmonary artery wedge pressure (3), and airway and pleural pressures. Pressures in small arteries and veins have also been obtained using small catheters inserted through the pulmonary artery or vein (4) or by micropuncture of subpleural vessels (5,6). Mean flows are commonly measured using the indicator dilution method, and pulsatile flows are measured using flow meters and plethysmographic methods (7,8). Vascular volumes are also measured using indicator dilution (11) and diffusing capacity methods (9). Measurements of lung weight have been used to determine changes in lung blood volume and to estimate capillary pressure from the rate of fluid filtration (10,11).

Physiological interpretation of the above-mentioned data is generally based on analyses which imply structural and functional relations that are not accessible to direct observation at the time the measurements are made. Thus, the methods of data analysis might be referred to as black box approaches[1]. For the sake of comparison, one might classify these approaches into several categories.

---

[1]*For this discussion the term "black box" model will mean that the data analysis (the assignment of parameter values) does not require the use of any quantity measured inside the organ. This is as apposed to a "deterministic" model in which parameter values are assigned on the basis of direct measurement of some aspect(s) of the internal organ structure.*

In the first, the steady or mean values of pressures, flow and/or volumes are measured and the values compared with normal or preintervention values. Pulmonary vascular resistance is a calculated parameter commonly used to make such comparisons. Because of the complex interaction between active and passive events in the pulmonary circulation such data can be difficult to interpret (1,2). Thus, in the second category, the same kind of steady or mean data are collected. However, in addition, one or more of the measured variables is changed to a new steady level and the measurements repeated. The differences between two or more steady states provide additional information and allow the calculation of additional parameters [e.g., vascular compliance, segmental resistance (10,11), etc.]. The pressure versus flow curve falls into this second category (1,13-15). The use of the pressure-flow curve to interpret changes in pulmonary hemodynamics has been motivated by the fact that active changes in the pulmonary vascular bed can be difficult to detect in the face of concurrent passive mechanical effects. For example, pulmonary vasoconstriction can be accompanied by an increase, decrease or no change in pulmonary vascular resistance (calculated as pulmonary artery pressure minus left atrial pressure divided by pulmonary blood flow) depending on the accompanying changes in flow and vascular transmural pressures. A shift in the pressure-flow curve can provide information for separating active and passive responses which is less ambiguous than a measurement of vascular resistance alone. In an attempt to learn more about the responses of the pulmonary vascular bed from pressure versus flow data, different models of the pulmonary vascular bed have been used to explain the shape of the pulmonary-pressure flow curves. In one, the pulmonary vascular bed is viewed as a large number of parallel nondistensible flow pathways. Flow through each pathway is then controlled by a critical closing pressure and the open pathway conductance. The closing pressures vary from pathway to pathway such that the shape of the pressure flow curve is determined by the distribution of closing pressures and the sum of the open pathway conductances (14). In another model the conductance of the whole vascular bed is controlled by the distensibility of the individual vessels (14,22,23). Each of these models can explain the data, but it is not entirely clear whether pressure and flow data alone can establish superiority of one model over the other (14). In a third category, the pulsatile pressures and flows are measured and the data analyzed in the frequency domain. The phasic data contain more information about the geometric and physical properties of the vascular bed than do the steady or mean data. Models of varying degrees of complexity have been used to interpret the pulmonary artery input impedance spectrum calculated from such data (8,16,17). These have provided important hemodynamic insights, primarily about the pulmonary arterial tree. A fourth category utilizes the transient pressure data obtained when a bolus of saline or plasma having a viscosity less than that of blood is introduced into the pulmonary artery (18,19). As the bolus passes through the pulmonary vascular bed there is a transient fall in the arterial-venous pressure difference due to the decrease in vascular resistance as the bolus moves through the vascular bed. The time course for this decrease follows a pattern that can be analyzed to obtain the longitudinal or series distribution of vascular resistance with respect to vascular volume from pulmonary artery to vein. In a fifth category a rapid occlusion of short duration (*e.g.*, 1-2 seconds) is performed on the arterial inflow, venous outflow, or both (24). The transient pressure data obtained contain information about the viscoelastic properties of the pulmonary vascular bed and about the arterial to venous distribution of vascular resistance relative to the distribution of vascular resistance relative to the distribution of vascular compliance.

The black box models upon which the interpretations of these categories of data are based vary in the complexity of structure and function they attribute to the vascular bed. Each includes some implicit view of the anatomy of the pulmonary vascular bed, but requires no specific anatomic data. An alternative to these black box approaches is more deterministic modeling based on detailed data on the morphometry of the vascular bed and the properties of the individual vessels. To data this approach has required destructive methods of measurement (*e.g.*, elastomer casts, etc.), and therefore cannot replace the black box approaches for following responses in many experimental or in clinical situations. On the other hand, models based on detailed morphometric and viscoelastic data combined with fluid dynamic principles offer the opportunity to help put various assumptions involved in the black box analyses into perspective (8,14,16,22, 23,25,26). There are obviously many problems involved in attempting to develop a completely deterministic model. In constructing such a model, one, in a sense, takes the vascular bed apart and measures the number, size, and properties of each order of vessel and then puts the vessels back together in a model by connecting them in a manner that is plausible and mathematically tractable. This approach has tended to make use of simple branching patterns which may not fully address the problem of having to package the functional capillary units in a reasonably compact organ having a single inlet and outlet. This issue may have been avoided to some extent because of its complexity and because interest in flow distribution in the normal lung has centered mainly on the effects of gravity (21) which may be largely independent of the vessel branching pattern. However, the demonstration that there is also gravity independent flow heterogeneity in the lungs, such that flow decreases centrifugally from the hilum (20), emphasizes the problem of the manifolding required to distribute the flow to capillaries situated at different distances from the hilum. Thus, the question may be asked: how are the vessels connected together to minimize the energy cost of perfusing the lungs over a wide range of flow rates while at the same time minimizing perfusion heterogeneity at the alveolar capillary level?

The major vasomotor control in the lungs is that directed at minimizing the influence of perfusion heterogeneity on gas exchange, namely, hypoxic vasoconstriction (2). The pulmonary hemodynamic consequences of alveolar hypoxia depends on the degree and duration of the hypoxia and on whether it is regional or pan-alveolar (22). Deterministic modeling of vasomotor responses such as hypoxic vasoconstriction is hindered by the difficulty of obtaining detailed morphometric and elasticity data under such conditions. However, plausible manipulations of the model parameters are likely to improve understanding of the hemodynamic data under conditions of altered vasomotor tone as well (14,22).

C. A. DAWSON

REFERENCES

1. Fishman AP. (1985) *In* **Handbook of Physiology. Section 3, The Respiratory System Vol 1.** (AP Fishman and AB Fishman, eds). Amer Physiol Soc:Bethesda, MD.

2. Grover RF, Wagner WW, McMurtry IF and Reeves JT. (1983) *In* **Handbook of Physiology. Section 2, The Cardiovascular System Vol III.** (JT Shepherd and FM Abboud, eds). Amer Physiol Soc:Bethesda, MD.

3. O'Quin R and Marini JJ. (1983) *Am Rev Resp Dis* **128**:319.

4. Hyman AL. (1969) *J Appl Physiol* **27**:179.

5. Bhattacharya J and Staub NC. (1980) *Science* **210**:327.

6. Nagasaka Y, Bhattacharya J, Nanjo S, Gropper MA and Staub NC. (1984) *Circ Res* **54**:90.

7. Lee G de J and DuBois AB. (1955) *J Clin Invest* **34**:1380.

8. Milnor WR. (1982) **Hemodynamics.** Williams and Wilkins:Baltimore.

9. Wanner A, Begin R, Conn M and Sackner MA. (1978) *J Appl Physiol* **44**:956.

10. Gaar KA, Taylor AE, Owens LJ and Guyton AC. (1967) *Am J Physiol* **213**:910.

11. Taylor AE and Parker JC. (1985) *In* **Handbook of Physiology. Section 3: The Respiratory System Vol I.** Amer Physiol Soc:Bethesda, MD.

12. McDonald IG and Butler J. (1967) *J Appl Physiol* **23**:467.

13. Janicki JS, Weber KT, Likoff MJ and Fishman AP. (1985) *Circulation* **72**:1270.

14. Mitzner W. (1987) In this chapter.

15. Murray PA, Lodata RF and Michael JR. (1986) *J Appl Physiol* **60**:1900.

16. Lucas CL. (1984) *CRC Crit Rev in Biomed Engineering* **10**:317.

17.   McDonald DA. (1974) **Blood Flow in Arteries.** Williams and
       Wilkins:Baltimore, MD.
18.   Brody JS, Stemmler EJ and DuBois AB. (1968) *J Clin Invest* **47**:783.
19.   Grimm DJ, Linehan JH and Dawson CA. (1977) *J Appl Physiol*
       43:1093.
20.   Hakim TS. (1987) In this chapter.
21.   Hughes JMB, Glazier JB, Maloney JE and West JB. (1968) *Resp Physiol*
       4:58.
22.   Marshall BE. (1987) In this chapter.
23.   Fung YC. (1987) In this chapter.
24.   Dawson CA, Linehan JH, Bronikowski TA and Rickaby DA. (1987) In
       this chapter.
25.   Wiener F, Morkin E, Skalak R and Fishman AP. (1966) *Circ Res*
       19:834.
26.   Attinger EO. (1963) *Circ Res* **12**:623.

Pulmonary Microvascular Hemodynamics: Occlusion Methods[1]

CHRISTOPHER A. DAWSON
Research Service
Zablocki VA Medical Center
Milwaukee WI 53295

JOHN H. LINEHAN
THOMAS A. BRONIKOWSKI
Depts. of Mechanical
Engineering,Mathematics,
Statistics and Computer
Science
Marquette University
Milwaukee, WI 53233

DAVID A. RICKABY
Research Service
Zablocki VA Medical Center
Milwaukee, WI 53295

I.   INTRODUCTION

The transient pressure and flow data obtained following rapid occlusion of the arterial inflow and/or venous outflow from a lung lobe contain information about both the viscoelastic properties of the pulmonary vascular bed and about the arterial to venous distribution of vascular resistance relative to the distribution of

[1]*Supported by NHLBI grant HL-19298 and by Veterans Administration Medical Research Funds.*

vascular compliance (1-6). Interest in this approach has, to a large extent, centered around the potential for following changes in microvascular pressure and determining the arterial or venous site of action of vasomotor stimuli. In the following we will present some of our ideas on the information content of occlusion data as interpreted using black box models in an attempt to provide useful parameters descriptive of the pulmonary microvascular bed.

II.   THE SIMPLE RC MODEL

Following rapid occlusion of the venous outflow from an isolated dog lung lobe perfused with constant flow, the venous pressure jumps to a pressure somewhere between the preocclusion arterial and venous pressures and then the arterial and venous pressures begin to rise more slowly as the vascular bed fills with blood at the constant inflow rate (Figure 1; 3). Originally, the step-like increase in venous pressure at the instant of occlusion suggested that the rapid jump represented a pressure drop across a relatively noncompliant but resistive portion of the lobar vascular bed downstream from a much more compliant region. The initial model of the response to venous occlusion was a simple resistance-

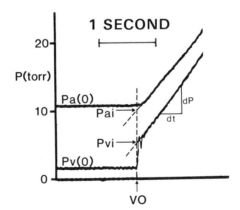

Figure 1. The arterial, P_a, and venous, P_v, pressures in response to sudden occlusion of the venous outflow, VO, from an isolated dog lung lobe perfused with a constant inflow rate. P_{ai} and P_{vi} are pressures obtained by linear extrapolation of the arterial and venous pressure curves, respectively, back to the instant of occlusion. The slope of the post occlusion pressure curves (dP/dT) is a measure of vascular compliance (see text).

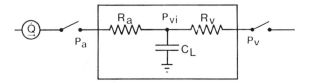

Figure 2. A simple resistance and compliance (RC) T section model which can explain the most obvious features of the post occlusion pressure curves.

compliance model in which the lobar vascular bed was represented by upstream and downstream series resistances with a compliance in parallel with the downstream resistance (Figure 2). In this model, the venous pressure rises immediately to the pressure in the middle compliance when flow through the downstream resistance (R_v) stops. Subsequently, P_a and P_v rise in parallel as flow into the compliance continues. This model provided a simple objective means for identifying a pressure, P_{vi}, associated with the compliant region. In practice, the slowly rising portion of the venous pressure curve could be linearly extrapolated back to the instant of venous occlusion to obtain P_{vi} (Figure 1). Several lines of evidence suggested that, in the dog lung lobe, P_{vi} was a useful microvascular pressure. For example, the pressure drops upstream and downstream from P_{vi} could be manipulated by various pulmonary vasomotor stimuli (3) and the changes in the upstream and downstream pressure drops, in response to these stimuli, paralleled the changes defined using the low-vicosity bolus technique (3). This comparison of results suggested that constriction of the lobar arteries increases pressure drop across R_a in Figure 2, while constriction of the lobar veins increases the pressure drop across R_v in Figure 2. The isogravimetric method, as applied to the lungs by Gaar *et al.* (10), has generally been accepted as measuring the effect microvascular pressure [sometimes referred to as the pressure at the filtration midpoint (11)] in isolated lungs. The observation that P_{vi} is close to the isogravimetric pressure (2,12) suggests that the microvascular hydrostatic pressure controlling transvascular fluid movement and the pressure controlling lobar vascular volume (P_{vi} in Figure 2) are nearly the same. The simple model used to explain the arterial and venous pressure curves following venous occlusion also predicts certain results of other occlusion experiments. For example Hakim *et al.* (4) found that sudden occlusion of the arterial inflow was followed by rapid fall in arterial pressure to nearly P_{vi}, and then by a slower exponential decrease to P_v, and simultaneous occlusion of both arterial inflow and venous outflow (double occlusion) results in an equilibrium pressure (referred to subsequently as P_{do}) which was close to P_{vi} (2).

III.   MULTICOMPARTMENT RC MODELS

The simple RC model in Figure 2 appears to be useful for identifying the arterial and venous site of action of pulmonary vasomotor stimuli and for obtaining a reasonable estimate of the microvascular pressure under conditions in which the normal symmetry of the arterial-venous resistance distribution in the lungs has been altered, for example, by arterial or venous constriction. However, the simple model does not account for all of the features of the occlusion data, suggesting that more complex modeling may be appropriate. Adding complexity to the model has at least two goals. One is to put bounds on the quantitative conclusions drawn using the simple model to evaluate the data. The other is to determine whether a model which takes advantage of additional features of the data can be used to gain more insight into the mechanics of the pulmonary circulation. Although the simple model reproduces the most striking features of the occlusion data (*e.g.*, the rapid rise in venous pressure following venous occlusion followed by a slower rise in both arterial and venous pressures) several aspects of the data point to the fact that the resistance and compliance are distributed from lobar artery to lobar vein throughout the vascular bed. For example, there is a short time delay before the arterial pressure begins to rise following venous occlusion. This time delay is not predicted by the simple model in Figure 2. In addition, we found that the double occlusion pressure (P_{do}) is consistently a little higher than P_{vi}, (2) and Hakim *et al.* (4) found that when the arterial inflow was occluded, the rapid fall in arterial pressure ΔP_a, stopped before reaching the P_{vi} obtained during venous occlusion. These discrepancies between the simple model predictions and the data suggested that one might be able to take advantage of the additional information contained in the data to describe the resistance versus compliance distribution in the lung lobe in more detail. In examining this possibility, we found that there were two more distributed RC networks that contained the largest number of symmetrically arranged compartmental resistances and compliances that could be assigned unique values using an additional piece of information obtainable from the venous occlusion data, namely, the time delay in the arterial pressure curve. This time delay can be converted into the intercept pressure, P_{ai}, by extrapolating the arterial pressure curve back to the instant of occlusion (9). These more distributed models are depicted in Figure 3. Venous occlusion is modeled by opening the venous switch.

For model 1 the slope of the slowly rising portion of the venous pressure curve in Figure 1 could be used to calculate a vascular compliance, C_L, according to

$$C_L = C_u + C_d = \dot{Q}/(dP_v/dt) \tag{1}$$

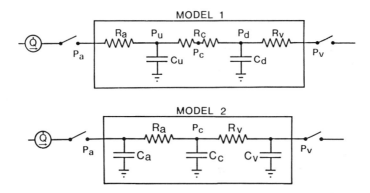

Figure 3. Two multicompartment models with the largest number of symmetrically arranged R's and C's which can be assigned values from the slopes and intercepts of the venous occlusion pressure curves. (Adapted from ref. 9).

Setting $C_u = C_d$, the analysis of model 1 yielded simple algebraic equations that can be used to determine the serial hemodynamic resistance: R_a, R_c, and R_v. Defining the preocclusion arterial venous pressures to be $P_a(0)$ and $P_v(0)$ and noting that P_{ai} and P_{vi} can be obtained by extrapolating the nearly linear portions of the $P_a(t)$ and $P_v(t)$ curves back to the instant of occlusion (Figure 1), the total vascular resistance, R_L, can be subdivided into segmental resistances as follows.

$$R_v = (P_{vi} - P_v(0) - P_a(0) + P_{ai})/\dot{Q} \qquad (2)$$
$$R_c = 4(P_a(0) - P_{ai})/\dot{Q} \qquad (3)$$

and

$$R_a = R_L - R_c - R_v \qquad (4)$$

where

$$R_L = (P_a(0) - P_v(0))/\dot{Q} \qquad (5)$$

The preocclusion pressure at the midpoint of R_c ($P_c(0)$) is theoretically equal to P_{do}, the equilibrium arterial and venous pressure following double occlusion, but it can also be calculated from the venous occlusion data (9) according to

$$P_c(0) = P_a(0) - P_{ai} + P_{vi} \qquad (6)$$

For model 2

$$C_L = C_a + C_c + C_v = \dot{Q}/(dP_v/dt) \qquad (7)$$

assuming that $C_a = C_v$ the central conpliance and upstream and downstream resistances could be calculated from

$$C_c = C_L ((4P_{ai} - 3P_a(0) - P_v(0))/P_a(0) - P_v(0)))^{1/2} \tag{8}$$

$$R_d = R_L (((P_{vi} - P_v(0)/P_a(0) - P_v(0))) - .25(1 - (C_c/C_L))^2) (C_L/C_c) \tag{9}$$

$$R_u = R_L - R_d \tag{10}$$

For model 2 the preocclusion pressure at C_c is

$$P_c = (P_a(0) - P_v(0))(R_d/R_L) + P_v(0) \tag{11}$$

We found that in the dog lung lobe P_c calculated according to equation (11) was close to the measured value of P_{do}. Thus, the two alternative models could represent the key features of the data in the time period shortly after venous occlusion and provide a useful estimate of microvascular pressure.

The arterial occlusion data, such as shown in Figure 4, can theoretically provide an additional piece of information that allows for the individual compartmental compliances to be determined independently. For example, if in model 1, C_u and C_d are allowed to vary independently then for venous occlusion:

$$(R_c/R_L)(C_uC_d/C_L{}^2) = (P_a(0) - P_{ai})/(P_a(0) - P_v(0)) \tag{12}$$

and

$$(R_c/R_L)(C_u{}^2)/C_L{}^2 + (R_v/R_L) = (P_{vi} - P_v(0))/(P_a(0) - P_v(0)) \tag{13}$$

The four measured pressures $P_a(0)$, $P_v(0)$, P_{ai} and P_{vi} are again defined in Figure 1. Equations (1), (4), (12), and (13) are four equations in the five unknowns R_a/R_L, R_c/R_L, R_v/R_L, C_u/C_L and C_d/C_L. To obtain a fifth independent equation P_u and P_d are defined to be the pressures of the compliances C_u and C_d, respectively. The steady state is described by the pressures $P_a(0)$, $P_u(0)$, $P_d(0)$, and $P_v(0)$, and the flow $\dot{Q}$. For arterial occlusion, the arterial switch is opened while P_v is held constant at $P_v(0)$. The governing differential equations which describe the time variation of $P_u(t)$ and $P_d(t)$, respectively, are:

$$C_u dP_u dt = - (P_u - P_d)/R_c \tag{14}$$

and

$$C_d dP_d dt = (P_u - P_d)/R_c - (P_d - P_v(0))/R_v \tag{15}$$

Mathematically, the instant the arterial switch is opened, the arterial pressure, P_a, undergoes a jump discontinuity from $P_a(0)$ to $P_u(0)$, thus

$$P_a(0) = P_u(0) + R_a \dot{Q} \tag{16}$$

for times t>0, in equations (14) and (15), $P_a(t) = P_u(t)$. The solution of equations (14) and (15), in terms of $P_a(t)$, is of the form

$$P_a(t) = a_1 e^{-k_1 t} + a_2 e^{-k_2 t} + P_v(0) \tag{17}$$

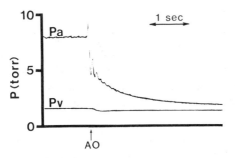

Figure 4. Arterial and venous pressure curves following occlusion of the arterial inflow, AO, to an isolated dog lung lobe.

where:

$$k_1 = ((R_vC_L + R_cC_u) - ((R_vC_L - R_cC_u)^2 + 4R_cR_vC_u^2)^{1/2})/(2R_cR_vC_uC_d) \qquad (18)$$

$$k_2 = ((R_vC_L + R_cC_u) + ((R_vC_L - R_cC_u)^2 + 4R_cR_vC_u^2)^{1/2})/(2R_cR_vC_uC_d) \qquad (19)$$

$$a_1 = ((R_v^2C_L + C_u(R_v + R_c)^2 - R_v(R_cC_d + R_vC_u))\dot{Q})/(2((R_vC_L - R_cC_u)^2 +$$
$$4R_cR_vC_u^2)^{1/2}) + \dot{Q}(R_c + R_v)/2 \qquad (20)$$

and

$$a_2 = (-(R_v^2C_L + C_u(R_v + R_c)^2 - R_v(R_cC_d + R_vC_u))\dot{Q})/(2((R_vC_L - R_cC_u)^2 +$$
$$4R_cR_vC_u^2))^{1/2}) + Q(R_c + R_v)/2 \qquad (21)$$

Thus, equation (17) predicts that $P_a(t)$ is the sum of two decreasing exponentials. This suggests fitting the $P_a(t)$ data with two exponentials using a multiexponential curve fitting technique to determine the zero time intercept, $P_u(0) = (a_1 + a_2 + P_v(0))$. Thus, allowing R_a/R_L to be directly calculated by combining equations (5) and (6) to give

$$R_a/R_L = (P_a(0) - P_u(0))/(P_a(0) - P_v(0)); \qquad (22)$$

using equations (4), (12), (13) and (22), C_u/C_L and R_c/R_L in terms of the measured pressures are:

$$C_u/C_L = (P_a(0) - P_{ai})/(P_u(0) - P_{vi} - P_a(0) + P_{ai}); \qquad (23)$$

$$R_c/R_L = (P_u(0) - P_{vi} - P_a(0) + P_{ai})^2/$$
$$(P_a(0) - P_v(0))(P_u(0) - P_{vi} - 2P_a(0) + 2P_{ai}) \qquad (24)$$

Then C_d/C_L and R_v/R_L can be calculated directly from equations (1) and (4). Since C_L and R_L can be determined from equation (1) and (5), respectively, R_a, R_c, R_v, C_u, and C_d can be calculated from data obtained from two separate occlusion experiments, one being a venous occlusion and the other an arterial occlusion. The use of the arterial occlusion data as described above is, however, subject to the vagaries of multiexponential curve fitting and possibly other considerations which will be discussed below.

These compartmental approaches allow for the calculation of specific compartmental parameters, and suggest that, even though the resistance and compliance are distributed, there is in the normal dog lung lobe, a region between muscular arteries and veins which includes a larger fraction of the vascular compliance than of the vascular resistance, and that advantage can be taken of this characteristic of the intralobar vascular bed to determine the arterial and venous site of vasoconstriction and a useful microvascular pressure P_c (3,9,13).

IV.   THE CONTINUOUS R VERSUS C DISTRIBUTION

One problem with the compartmental approach is that, when used to represent the actually continuous distribution of R and C, the relationships between anatomic and model compartments can be somewhat obscure. As one approach to this problem, we have examined the theoretical bounds that can be placed on the actual continuous distribution by the venous occlusion data (1,7). Figure 5 is an attempt to put the relationship between the serial or longitudinal

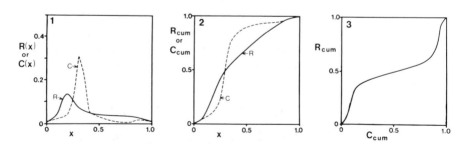

Figure 5. Panel 1: Hypothetical continuous local longitudinal resistance and compliance distributions in a lung lobe. Panel 2: The cumulative resistance and compliance distributions for the local distributions in panel 1. Panel 3: The cumulative R versus C graph obtained by plotting R_{cum} (x) versus C_{cum} (x). (Adapted from ref. 1)

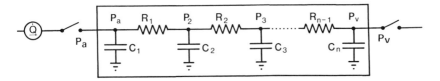

Figure 6. A compartmental representation of a quasi continuous distribution of vascular resistance and compliance.

distributions of R and C into perspective. In panel 1, hypothetical distributions of the local resistance $R(x)$ and compliance $C(x)$ are plotted as a function of a spatial variable (x) from the lobar artery inlet at $x=0$ to the venous outlet at $x=1$. The x variable might be, for example, the fractional distance from the arterial inlet to the venous outlet or fractional cumulative volume from the inlet to the outlet. The local resistance and compliance tend to be distributed differently in relation to the spatial variable as indicated by the structure of the occlusion data previously discussed in regard to the compartmental models. An alternate way of looking at the relationship between R and C is to graph the cumulative functions as in panel 2. If the $R_{cum}(x)$ points are graphed versus the $C_{cum}(x)$ points a cumulative R versus C graph results as depicted in panel 3. The occlusion data contain information about the cumulative R versus C graph. Mathematically, the continuously distributed vascular bed was represented by a large number of serial resistances and parallel compliances as depicted in figure 6. The results of the analysis gave specific boundaries for the continuous distribution compatible with the venous occlusion data as shown in Figure 7. That is, all continuous R_{cum} versus C_{cum} graphs that are compatible with the steady state pressures, $P_a(0)$ and $P_v(0)$, and pressures P_{ai} and P_{vi} are continuously increasing functions within the region W. Thus, if P_c is now defined as the pressure at the midpoint of the cumulative vascular compliance, one important result of this analysis of the continuous model is that the measureable pressure data can be thought of as placing secure bounds on the value of P_c as shown in Figure 8. Figure 9 shows the influence of vasoconstriction in dog lung lobes on the location of P_c along the intravascular pressure drop from lobar artery to lobar vein.

One important result of this analysis and the data presented in Figure 9 is that even though the vascular resistance and compliance are in fact distributed throughout the lobar vascular bed, vasoconstriction occurs in arterial and venous vessels which are upstream and downstream from vessels which are responsible for a major fraction of the lobar vascular compliance. This does not imply that the resistance in these microvessels is insignificant. In fact, in the vasodilated state they may be a substantial fraction of the total vascular resistance (13). However, since the changes in resistance in response to a number of vasomotor stimuli

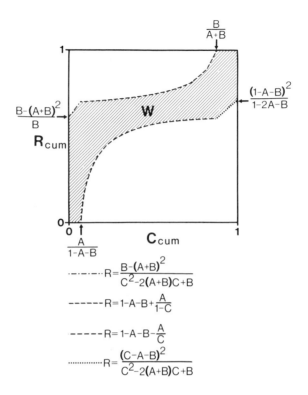

Figure 7. The region W in the cumulative CR plane contains all cumulative R versus C distributions which are compatible with P_{ai} and P_{vi} data. The boundaries of W are in terms of A and B where A = $(P_a(0) - P_{ai})/(P_a(0) - P_v(0))$ and B = $(P_{vi} - P_v(0))/(P_a(0) - P_v(0))$. In the equations for the boundaries of W, R_{cum} and C_{cum} are abbreviated by R and C, respectively. (Adapted from ref. 1).

appear to occur either upstream or downstream from this compliant region the arterial or venous site of vasoconstriction can be readily determined, and a useful estimate of microvascular pressure obtained.

V.   VARIABLE RC AND VISCOELASTIC MODELS

Up to this point, we have considered the vessel walls to be purely elastic and the R's and C's to be constant regardless of vascular volume. However, there are several observations that suggest that more complex viscoelastic vessel wall properties are important in determining the rates of change in the pressures during

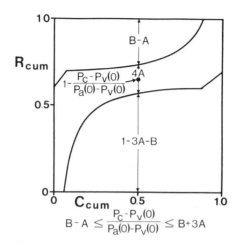

Figure 8. The region W defined according to figure 7 with P_c located at $C_{cum} = 0.5$. P_c is bounded such that $B - A \leq (P_c - P_v(0))/(P_a(0) - P_v(0)) \leq B + 3A$. (Adapted from ref. 7).

the slowly rising phase following arterial or venous occlusion. First, it was observed that the compliance calculated from the slope of the slowly rising pressure following venous occlusion (equation 1) is always less than that obtained from static measurements of vascular compliance (8). In addition, once the R's and C's have been established in the previous RC models by venous occlusion, the rate of fall in arterial pressure following arterial occlusion is slower than predicted by these models. In other words, for a given set of R values a larger vascular compliance is needed to fit the arterial occlusion pressure curves than the venous occlusion pressure curves (*i.e.*, there is hysteresis in the dynamic pressure volume curve). The viscoelastic nature of the vessel walls is further suggested by data from an occlusion experiment in which the venous outflow is occluded and then within a second or two the arterial inflow is occluded. Following the arterial occlusion, both arterial and venous pressures fall below the venous pressure extant at the instant before the arterial occlusion, indicative of relaxation of the vessels walls during this isovolumic state (Figure 10). The previously described models do not predict this behavior. In addition, if the venous occlusion is continued for more than about one second, it becomes evident that the arterial and venous pressure curves are not actually linear and parallel. As time progresses, the curves converge due to the decrease in vascular resistance as the vessels distend and an upward concavity can be seen in both pressure curves as the vascular compliance

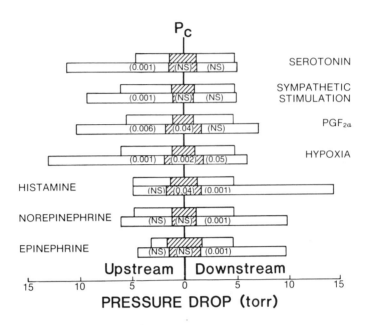

Figure 9. The results obtained with several vasoconstrictor stimuli in isolated dog lung lobes using venous occlusion with data analyzed according to figure 8. The upper bar for each pair of bars was obtained during control conditions, and the lower bar was obtained during vasoconstriction with the indicated stimulus. The length of the unshaded portion of the bar to the left, or upstream side, of P_c is a lower bound on the pressure drop from lobar artery to P_c and the unshaded portion to the right, or downstream side, of P_c is the lower bound on the pressure drop from P_c to the exit from the lobar vein. The shaded portion of each bar indicates the bounds on P_c under these conditions. In other words, the pressure at the cumulative compliance midpoint, P_c, is somewhere within the shaded portion. The numbers in parentheses are numbers larger than the probability that the change in each individual pressure drop is not different from control. NS means $P > 0.05$). Serotonin infusion, electrical stimulation of the stellate ganglion (sympathetic stimulation), $PGF_{2\alpha}$ infusion and hypoxia mainly increased the pressure drop upstream from P_c while histamine, norepinephrine and epinephrine infusion mainly increased the pressure drops downstream from P_c. (Adapted from ref. 13).

decreases with vessel distension. A compartmental model that can account for the additional features of the data is shown in Figure 10.

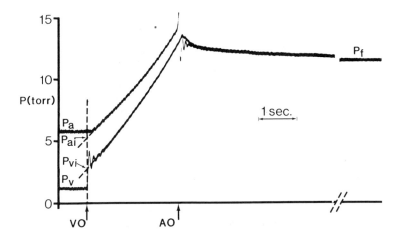

Figure 10. The P_a and P_v curves obtained when the inflow to an isolated lung was occluded (AO) shortly after the outflow was occluded (VO). P_f is the final equilibrium pressure. (from Ref. 8).

This model consists of three serial hemodynamic resistances: R_a, R_c, and R_v as in model 1, Figure 3. However, the resistances are separated by parallel viscoelastic elements, arranged as St. Venant elements (14), instead of the simple elastic elements. The arrows drawn through the circuit elements signify those elements which are volume dependent, *i.e.*, decreasing R and C with increasing volume.

In the preocclusion steady state (*i.e.*, when both switches s_1 and s_2 in Figure 11 are closed), the governing equations are:

$$\dot{Q} = (P_a(0) - P_1(0))/R_a = (P_1(0) - P_2(0))/R_c = (P_2(0) - P_v(0))/R_v \qquad (25)$$

and

$$P_1(0) = P_3(0); \quad P_2(0) = P_4(0) \qquad (26)$$

and the total vascular resistance, R_L, is given by eq. 4.

For the venous occlusion part of the experiment (modeled by opening switch s_2), the flow out of the lung lobe is equal to zero while the flow into the lung remains constant. The venous pressure, P_v, instantaneously becomes equal to P_2 according to

$$P_v(0^+) = P_v(0^-) + R_v\dot{Q} = P_2(0) = P_4(0) \qquad (27)$$

where $P_v(0^+)$ and $P_v(0^-)$ are values of $P_v(t)$ on either side of the jump discontinuity at t=0. For the analog circuit of Figure 11, the governing differential

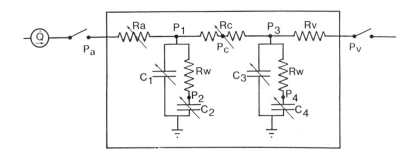

Figure 11. A compartmental model in which the values of some of the R's and C's vary with vascular volume (i.e., with the pressures across the C's) and the vessel walls are viscoelastic. The diagonal arrows designate the volume dependent elements. Occlusion occurs when switches s_1 and/or s_2 are opened. $\dot{Q}$ is the flow into the artery and is constant as long as s_1 is closed. (from ref. 8).

equations for venous occlusion are:

$$C_1 dP_1/dt = \dot{Q} - (P_1 - P_v)/R_c - (P_1 - P_3)/Rw_1 \tag{28}$$

$$C_2 dP_v/dt = (P_1 - P_v)/R_c - (P_v - P_4)/Rw_2 \tag{29}$$

$$C_3 dP_3/dt = (P_1 - P_3)/Rw_1 \tag{30}$$

$$C_4 dP_4/dt = (P_v - P_4)/Rw_2 \tag{31}$$

where C_1 and C_2 along with Rw_1, Rw_2, C_3, and C_4 represent the viscoelasticity of the vessel walls. The arterial pressure, P_a, is related to P_1 by

$$P_a = P_1 + R_a \dot{Q} \tag{32}$$

The initial conditions for equations (28)-(32) are given by equations (25), (26), and (27).

From the solution of model 1, it can be shown that the difference between the $P_a(t)$ and $P_v(t)$ curves at any time following venous occlusion is directly proportional to a linear combineation of R_a and R_c (9). In recognition that, for Poiseuille flow, the hemodynamic resistance is inversely proportional to the fourth power of the vessel diameter, one might assume that the lumped hemodynamic resistances, R_a and R_c, and inversely proportional to the square of the blood volume in those vessels contributing to these resistances, Q_a and Q_c respectively, *i.e.*

$$R_a = K_a/Q_a^2; \quad R_c = K_c/Q_c^2 \tag{33a,b}$$

where K is a proportionality constant which may include blood viscosity, the number of parallel interconnecting vessels, etc. The volumes Q_a and Q_c are then assumed to increase in proportion to the blood volume accumulated during venous occlusion according to

$$Q_a = Q_a(0) + \varepsilon_a \dot{Q}t; \quad Q_c = Q_c(0) + \varepsilon_c \dot{Q}t \tag{34a,b}$$

where $Q_a(0)$ and $Q_c(0)$ are the respective blood volumes prior to venous occlusion and ε_a and ε_c represent the fractions of the accumulated blood volume, $\dot{Q}t$, which contribute to Q_a and Q_c, respectively. Denoting the preocclusion values of the resistances by $R_a(0)$ and $R_c(0)$, the combination of equations (33) and (34) yields after algebraic rearrangement,

$$R_a(t) = R_a(0)/(1 + \varepsilon_a \dot{Q}t/Q_a(0))^2; \quad Rc(t) = R_c(0)/(1 + \varepsilon_c \dot{Q}t/Q_c(0))^2 \tag{35a,b}$$

Equations (35a and b) were used in equations (28), (29), and (32) to simulate the volume dependency of hemodynamic resistance.

To account for the volume dependency of compliance we assume that the compliance is a decreasing linear function of volume; namely,

$$C_i(t) = C_i(0) - \alpha(Q_i(t) - Q_i(0)); \quad i = 1\text{-}4 \tag{36}$$

where $C_i(t)$ and $Q_i(t)$ represent the time-varying compliance and volume of the individual compliance elements after VO, respectively; $C_i(0)$ and $Q_i(0)$ are the respective values before occlusion. The $\alpha = - dC_i/dQ_i$ is a constant parameter independent of i. Thus, since $C_i = dQ_i/dP_i$, we can integrate to obtain:

$$C_i(t) = C_i(0) \exp(- \alpha(P_i(t) - P_i(0)) \tag{37}$$

Equation (37) was used in equations (28)-(31) to simulate the volume dependence of compliance.

One can show how the various model elements contribute to the characteristic shapes of the experimental VO-AO curves via simulation. Since the interactions between the model elements are complex, it is instructive to examine the individual effects of each model element separately. As a starting point, Figure 11 shows a VO-AO simulation using model 1 from Figure 3 in which all the model elements are assumed to be constant, that is, independent of lobar volume (and pressure). The results are shown in Figure 11 as the dashed line in each panel. After a short initial transient period, $P_a(t)$ and $P_v(t)$ become parallel, lineal functions of time, and

$$P_a(t) - P_v(t) = (R_a(0) + R_c(0)/2)\dot{Q} \tag{38}$$

At the time of arterial occlusion, P_a falls and P_v rises such that the asymptotic value of vascular pressure, P_f, is between the values of $P_a(t)$ and $P_v(t)$ which obtain at the instant before arterial occlusion.

The influence of volume dependence of hemodynamic resistance can be shown by setting α, Rw_1, and $Rw_2 = 0$ and $\varepsilon_a/Q_a(0) = \varepsilon_c/Q_c(0) > 0$ in the model in Figure 11. (In this and subsequent simulations setting Rw's equal to zero was accomplished by adding equation (28) to equation (30) and adding equation (29) to equation (31) and setting $P_1 = P_3$ and $P_v = P_4$). The effect of the volume dependence of resistance (equation 35) on the model results is shown as the solid lines in Figure 12A. In contrast to the results obtained when R_a and R_c are constant (dashed lines), the $P_a(t)$ curve has a smaller slope than the $P_v(t)$ curve. Thus, convergence of $P_a(t)$ and $P_v(t)$ results from the decrease of R_a and R_c with volume accumulation following VO.

The most obvious manifestation of the viscous behaviour of the vessel walls is the decrease in both P_a and P_v following AO. To show the effect of adding wall viscosity alone, the values of the elements of the model of Figure 11 can be kept constant (*i.e.*, $\varepsilon/Q(0)$ and $\alpha = 0$), while Rw_1 and Rw_2 are given finite values. This results in the solid lines shown in Figure 12B and demonstrates that the impact of the viscoelastic elements is to increase the initial slopes of $P_a(t)$ and $P_v(t)$. This is because the compliances C_3 and C_4 fill relatively slowly at first due to the effect of Rw_1 and Rw_2. Later, as the pressure drop across Rw_1 and Rw_2 are established, compliances C_2 and C_4 begin to fill in proportion to their contribution to the total compliance, and the slopes approach $\dot{Q}/C_L$. Following AO there is an initial rapid fall in P_a to meet a rising value of P_v. Then both pressures fall slowly in an exponential fashion to an equilibrium pressure below the values of both P_a and P_v just prior to AO. This is the model equivalent of stress relaxation as the pressure drops across the Rw's are dissipated and the volume is shared by the C's.

To demonstrate the impact of the volume dependence of the lobar vascular compliance on the model results, the hemodynamic resistances can be held constant (*i.e.*, $\varepsilon/Q(0) = 0$); and Rw_1 and Rw_2 set equal to zero; and the compliances allowed to vary according to equation (37) with a finite value for α. The simulation results are shown as solid lines in Figure 12C. Now, after the initial transient period, the slopes of $P_a(t)$ and $P_v(t)$ increase. Since the slopes of $P_a(t)$ and $P_v(t)$ are inversely proportional to compliance, the impact of decreasing the compliance is to produce a concave upward trend in the $P_a(t)$ and $P_v(t)$ curves following VO.

The combined effects of viscoelasticity and of volume dependence on resistance and compliance and are all included to give the solid lines in Figure 12D). The convergence of the $P_a(t)$ and $P_v(t)$ curves following VO due to the

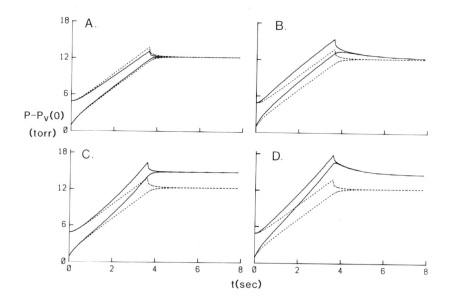

Figure 12. A simulated VO-AO experiment for the model in fig. 11 compared to model 1 in fig. 3 (dashed lines).A. With no wall viscosity (i.e., Rw_1 and Rw_2 = 0) and with C's constant (solid lines). Shows the effects of volume dependence of vascular resistance. B. With the R's and C's constant showing the effects of wall viscosity (solid lines). C. With no wall viscosity and the hemo-dynamic R's constant showing the effects of volume dependent compliance (solid lines). D. With variable R's and C's and with wall viscosity (solid lines). (From ref. 8).

volume dependence of hemodynamic resistance, the upward concavity of the $P_a(t)$ and $P_v(t)$ following VO due to the volume dependence of compliance, and the decrease in $P_v(t)$ and $P_a(t)$ following AO due to viscoelasticity can be seen.

This more complicated compartmental model appears to include the important elements and flexibility necessary to reproduce the key features of the experimental data, but due to the mathematical nonlinearity of the model and the fact that the number of model parameters appears to exceed the number of independent and/or readily quantifiable data obtainable from a set of occlusion curves, it is not clear that the data can provide unique estimates of each model parameter. However, approximations can be made which allow calculation of certain parameters for purposes of characterizing the experimental data and for quantitative comparisons between experimental conditions. This again includes P_c calculated using P_{ai} and P_{vi} as indicated in Figure 8. Examples of additional

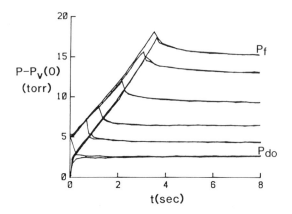

Figure 13. A composite of several VO-AO experiments from one lung with each AO carried out at a different time following VO. The final equilibrium pressure is P_f. P_{do} is the equilibrium pressure obtained when VO and AO are carried out simultaneously. (Adapted from ref. 8).

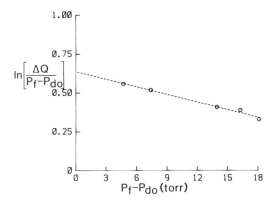

Figure 14. $\ln(\Delta Q/(P_f - P_{do})$ versus $P_f - P_{do}$ from five VO-AO on one lung. The dashed line is the linear regression line having slope $-\alpha/2$ and intercept $\ln(CL(0))$ according to equation (41). (Adapted from ref. 8).

parameters are the static vascular compliance C_L and the fractional decreases in compliance with increasing Q, namely, α/C_L. These can be calculated as follows. A few seconds after AO, the pressure across the compliance elements accomodating the stored blood volume approach P_f. Then equation (31) can be considered to represent the total vascular compliance, C_L.

$$C_L = C_L (0) \exp(- \alpha(P_f - P_{do})) \tag{39}$$

A series of VO-AO experiments with a variation in the time between VO and AO provides a range of values for $P_f - P_{do}$ as in Figure 13. Since the static vascular compliance is defined as $C_L = dQ_L/dP_f$, integration of equation (39) expresses the blood volume stored in the lung as

$$\Delta Q = (C_L(0)/\alpha)(1 - (- \alpha(P_f - P_{do})) \tag{40}$$

Since graphs of $\ln(\Delta Q/(P_f - P_{do}))$ versus $P_f - P_{do}$ for the data are reasonably linear (e.g., in Figure 14), we can take advantage of this result by expanding equation (40) in a Maclaurin series (8), the result being that, since $\alpha(P_f - P_{do})/2$ is small, both $C_L(0)$ and α can be obtained from a linear regression analysis of the $\ln(\Delta Q/(P_f - P_{do}))$ versus $(P_f - P_{do})$ data obtained from a series of VO-AO experiments according to

$$\ln(\Delta Q/P_f - P_{do})) = \ln C_L(0) - \alpha(P_f - P_{do})/2 \tag{41}$$

VI.   OTHER FACTORS WHICH MAY INFLUENCE THE OCCLUSION DATA

An additional factor contributing to the shapes of the pressure curves is the effect of inertia of the flowing blood at the time of occlusion. The rapid deceleration of the blood upstream (venous occlusion) or downstream (arterial occlusion) contributes to the immediate changes in venous and arterial pressures, respectively. Oscillations can commonly be seen in the time period immediately following occlusion. These oscillations die out rather quickly. In the venous and double occlusion experiment a quasi steady state ensues in which the inertance of the blood is not important (1,9). Thus, extrapolation of the longer time data back to the instant of occlusion appears justified. The slow portion of the arterial pressure drop following arterial occlusion is not a steady state because the blood continues to decelerate during the entire period of the arterial pressure decay. The rate of change in flow is much slower than at the instant of occlusion, and it may be justifiable to ignore blood inertance during this period, thus, allowing for extrapolation back to zero time as indicated above. However, in the case of arterial occlusion the extrapolation is nonlinear, and the absence of early time data due to the oscillatory pressure behavior tends to be a more significant problem. This aspect of the effect of inertia is not particularly welcome when the data are to be

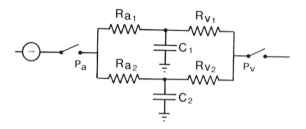

Figure 15. A simple parallel T section model.

evaluated using the compartmental RC models, and accurate early time data in which the inertial effects dominate are difficult to obtain.

In the models discussed above the vascular bed is considered to be a series of compartments, or, as if all of the parallel pathways through the lungs had identical relative distributions of R versus C. In such an organ there would be no information about the parallel nature of the bed in the occlusion data. On the other hand, if parallel heterogeneity of R versus C distributions of sufficient magnitude existed, it could add complexity to the interpretation of the data. Given the well documented heterogeneity in local blood flow in the lungs (15,16) it would not be surprising, and perhaps even likely, that heterogeneity in the RC distribution among parallel pathways exists as well. Examination of the simplest model representation of the effects of this kind of parallel heterogeneity may serve to put some of the complexity into perspective. Such a model is shown in Figure 15. Note that this model is identical to that in Figure 2 when $Ra_1 = Ra_2$, $Rc_1 = Rv_2$, and $C_1 = C_2$. However, in general the parallel model for venous occlusion gives

$$P_{vi} + P_v(0) = \dot{Q}Rv_1Rv_2/(Rv_1 + Rv_2)$$

and the rapid fall in P_a at the instant of arterial occlusion is

$$\Delta P_a = \dot{Q}Ra_1Ra_2/(Ra_1+Ra_2),$$

but $\quad P_a(0)-P_v(0) = \dot{Q}(Ra_1 + Rv_1)(Ra_2 + Rv_2)/(Ra_1 + Rv_1 + Ra_2 + Rv_2).$

Thus, if the Ra's and/or the Rv's are not equal, P_{vi} will not equal $P_a(0) = \Delta P_a$ even though the compliance in each individual pathway is not distributed. Thus, it is conceivable that the arterial and venous occlusion data contain information about the parallel heterogeneity in the resistance versus compliance distribution as well as the longitudinal distribution.

Holloway *et al.* (5) have investigated the use of the arterial occlusion approach for evaluating capillary pressure *in vivo*. If a balloon tipped catheter is placed in a lobar artery and then inflated to obtain a wedge pressure the time course of the fall in pressure at the catheter tip contains information about the resistance versus compliance distribution between the catheter tip and the left atrium. A fairly rapid fall followed by slower decay, reminiscent of the response of the simple RC model, was observed (5). This approach has the promise of being useful for estimating pulmonary capillary pressure *in vivo*. However, it can be difficult to identify a clear break in the decay curve, and back extrapolation of the exponential decay can be equivocal. On the other hand, pulmonary vaso-constriction with arterial or venous constrictors show clear differences in the exponential decay of the catheter tip pressure to the steady wedge pressure. When pulmonary artery diastolic pressure is close to the left atrial pressure, the post balloon-inflation pressure curve may not be of sufficient quality for the purposes of detailed analysis. Under these conditions pulmonary capillary pressure is close to the diastolic pressure anyway. However, when diastolic pressure is high relative to left arterial pressure, the quality of the data tends to be better, and this is the situation when it is of clinical significance to know whether the capillary pressure is closer to arterial pressure or to left atrial pressure. A rapid fall in the catheter tip pressure to the steady wedge pressure suggests that capillary pressure is close to left atrial pressure, whereas a slow fall in pressure suggests that capillary pressure is closer to arterial pressure. Thus, alternative methods for objectively and quantitatively evaluating these pressure curves might prove useful.

VII.   SUMMARY

In conclusion, the occlusion data contain information about the longitudinal distribution of resistance versus compliance in the pulmonary vascular bed. The venous occlusion data allow one to determine the value of an intravascular pressure, Pc, which can be thought of as a pressure at a point located along the arterial to venous distribution of cumulative vascular compliance where half the compliance is upstream and half is downstream. Pc can be found in the sense that an upper and lower bound on its value can be calculated in a simple manner using the data. If the upper and lower bounds are narrow, then the vascular compliance is concentrated near Pc. In general, the compliance appears to be concentrated at the microvascular level within the intra-lobar vascular bed, and vasoconstriction within a lung lobe tends to occur upstream and downstream from this concentrated compliance. This conclusion is based on the observation that the width of the bounds on Pc are minimally influenced by vasoconstriction (Figure 9; 13). This configuration of the resistance versus compliance in the lung lobe results in a situation wherein Pc and the double occlusion pressure, Pdo, are essentially equal. Although the double occlusion procedure alone does not allow bounds to be determined, it is particularly useful for obtaining microvascular pressure in studies of lung fluid balance (17,18) because it can be obtained without the transient increase or decrease in microvascular pressure produced during arterial or venous occlusion. It is also useful for studying the lung in situ (2). The addition of the other occlusion maneuvers such as arterial occlusion may provide aditional information which can specify parameters in more complex models, and thus provide a more detailed analysis of the mechanics of the pulmonary circulation. More complete understanding of the relationships between the hemodynamic resistance versus compliance distributions obtained from such analyses, and the functional and anatomical compartmentalization of the lung vasculature remains a challenge for future studies.

REFERENCES

1. Bronikowski TA, Linehan JH, and Dawson CA. (1984) *Microvasc Res* 28:289.
2. Dawson CA, Linehan JH and Rickaby DA. (1982) *Ann NY Acad Sci* 384:80.
3. Hakim TS, Dawson CA and Linehan JH. (1979) *J Appl Physiol* **47**:142.
4. Hakim TS, Michel RP and Chang HK. (1982) *J Appl Physiol* **52**:710.
5. Holloway H, Perry M, Downey J, Parker J and Taylor A. (1983) *J Appl Physiol* **54**:846.
6. Rock P, Patterson GA, Permutt S and Sylvester JT. (1985) *J Appl Physiol* **59**:1891.
7. Bronikowski TA, Dawson CA and Linehan JH. (1985) *Microvasc Res* 30:306.
8. Linehan JH, Dawson CA and Rickaby DA. (In press) *J Appl Physiol*.
9. Linehan JH, Dawson CA and Rickaby DA. (1982) *J Appl Physiol* 53:158.
10. Gaar KA, Taylor AE, Owens LJ and Guyton AC. (1967) *Am J Physiol* 213:910.
11. Taylor AE and Parker JC. (1985) *In* **Handbook of Physiology. Section 3: The Respiratory System. Vol. I, Circulation and nonrespiratory functions.** Amer Physiol Soc:Bethesda.
12. Parker JC, Kvietys PR, Ryan KP and Taylor AE. (1983) *J Appl Physiol* 55:964.
13. Linehan JH and Dawson CA. (1983) *J Appl Physiol* 55:923.
14. McDonald DA. (1974) **Blood Flow in Arteries.** Williams and Wilkins:Baltimore.
15. Hakim TS. (1986) *In* **Pulmonary Circulation in Health and Disease.** (JA Will, CA Dawson, EK Weir, CK Buckner, eds). Academic Press:Orlando.

16. Hughes JMB, Glazier JB, Maloney JE and West JB. (1968) *Resp Physiol* **4**:58.
17. Selig WM, Noonan TC, Kern DF and Malik AB. (1986) *J Appl Physiol* **60**:1972.
18. Townsley MI, Korthuis RJ, Rippe B, Parker JC and Taylor AE. (1986) *J Appl Physiol* **61**:127.

Models of the Pulmonary Hemodynamics Based on Anatomic and Functional Data[1]

YUAN-CHENG B. FUNG
MICHAEL R.T. YEN
SIDNEY S. SOBIN
Department of AMES/Bioengineering
University of California, San Diego
La Jolla, CA 92093

I.   INTRODUCTION

Blood flow in the lung is characterized by many variables, including

1) Dynamic variables such as the velocity and pressure at every point as functions of time, the flow rate in every vessel, the amplitude and frequency of flow pulsation, the distribution of the airway pressure, pleural pressure, parenchymal tissue stresses, the pressure and flow in the right ventricle through the pulmonary valves, and those in the left atrium through the mitral valves;

2) Anatomical variables such as the diameter and length of every branch of blood vessels, the branching pattern of the vessels from generation to generation

3) Rheological variables such as the compliance and visco-elasticity of every vessel (which varies from generation to generation), the hematocrit and hence the apparent viscosity of the blood (which is smaller in small blood vessels of diameter less than 1 mm);

4) Neuro and endocrine variables;

5) Idiosyncratic and pathological variables.

[1]*Various parts of this work were supported by grants from USHSS, NIH, NHLBI and National Science Foundation over the past fifteen years.*

To comprehend a phenomenon governed by so many variables requires a theory which helps a) To formulate problems definitively, b) To recognize all the ad hoc hypotheses and axioms, c) To deduce various relationships among variables, d) To obtain solutions that can be validated.

A theory is often called a mathematical model. A theory is wrong if the deductive process is faulty. One theory can be less accurate than another. When two theories arrive at the same conclusions, scientists generally prefer the one with fewer ad hoc hypotheses.

In the following I shall present a model for steady blood flow in the lung, connecting dynamic variables with anatomical and rheological variables on the basis of the laws of conservation of mass and momentum, without other ad hoc hypotheses. The neuro and endocrine variables as well as the idiosyncratic and pathological variables are ignored. If we assume that the neuro, endocrine, idiosyncratic, and pathological factors affect pulmonary hemodynamics through their effects on anatomical and rheological variables, then the present theory can form a basis to investigate the influence of these variables on hemodynamics. If the inertial effects are added, then the theory can be extended to cover nonstationary flows.

II.   BASIC CONCEPTS

Consider the pressure-flow relationship in pulmonary circulation. It is well known that if an incompressible Newtonian fluid flows in a rigid tube of uniform diameter D the volume flow rate, Q, is linearly proportional to the difference of pressures at the two ends of the tube:

$$\frac{128\mu L}{\pi} Q = D^4 (P_{entry} - P_{exit}) \tag{1}$$

This is known as the Poiseuille's law, see Fig. 1, top row, and Ref (1), p. 84. Here μ is the coefficient of viscosity of the fluid, L is the length of the tube, and the subscripts "entry" and "exit" refer to the ends of the tube.

If the tube is elastic, however, the result is different. Refer to the illustration at the bottom of Fig. 1. As the fluid flows down the tube, pressure drops because of viscous dissipation of energy. As the pressure is reduced, the diameter of the tube decreases. The velocity increases when the cross sectional area of the tube is decreased. The increased velocity of flow accelerates the decreasef pressure. Decreasing pressure decreases diameter, and so forth. Thus a feedback mechanism exists which causes the tube wall to converge more and rapidly toward

the exit end. If the diameter (D) of the elastic tube changes with the pressure p
according to a linear law:

$$D = D_0 + \alpha p = D_0 (1 + \beta p) \tag{2}$$

which has been found to be valid for pulmonary arteries and veins (Ref. 1, pp.
212-214, 302-306), then for a steady flow of a Newtonian viscous incompressible
fluid in such a tube we have (see Ref 1, pp.4 and 334):

$$\frac{640\mu\alpha L}{\pi} \quad Q = [D(o)]^5 - [D(L)]^5 \quad =[D_0 + \alpha p_{entry}]^5 - [D_0 + \alpha p_{exit}]^5 \tag{3}$$

Here D_0 is the tube diameter when p is zero, p is the transmural pressure, α is the
compliance constant. This is called the fifth power law for flow in an elastic tube.
Equation [3] may be corrected for loss due to turbulence and bifurcation by
replacing μ with the "apparent" viscosity which depends on the Reynolds number.
To account for the effect of change of kinetic energy along the stream, at each
junction of a vessel of order n to one of order n+1 a static pressure drop equal to

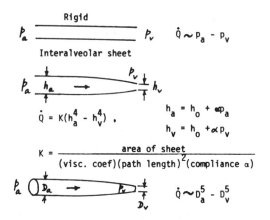

Figure 1. Formulas related to flow in a rigid tube, an elastic sheet, and
an elastic tube.

$$\frac{1}{2} \rho \, v_{n+1}^2 - \frac{1}{2} \rho \, v_n^2 \qquad\qquad [4]$$

should be added according to the well known Bernoulli's equation (see Ref. 1, p.18). Here v_n is the mean velocity of flow in the vessel of order n.

The pulmonary capillary blood vessels are rigid (with respect to blood pressure) in the plane of the interalveolar septum, and elastic in the direction perpendicular to the plane of the interalveolar septum (see Ref. 1, pp. 306-309). Hence its flow-pressure relation-ship is somewhere between Eqs. [1] and [3]. If the local average height of the lumen of the pulmonary capillaries in an interalveolar septum is denoted by h and called the "thickness" of the alveolar sheet, then experimentally it has been found that

$$h = h_o + \alpha \, (p - p_A) \qquad\qquad [5]$$

for $0 < (p - p_A) <$ an upper limit of about 25 cmH_2O (for cat) or 15 cmH_2O (for man). Here p is the local blood pressure in the capillary, p_A is the alveolar gas pressure, h_o is the sheet thickness when $p = p_A$, and c is the compliance constant of the capillary sheet. Using Eq. [1], together with the equations of continuity and motion, and an experimentally verified linear relationship between local velocity of flow and pressure gradient, we obtain the result (see Ref. (1), p. 331)

$$\frac{4\mu k f L^2 \alpha}{SA} \, Q = [h(o)]^4 - [h(L)]^4$$

$$= [h_o + \alpha(p_{art} - p_A)]^4 - [h_o + \alpha(p_{ven} - p_A)]^4 \qquad [6]$$

Here p_{art}, p_{ven} are the pressures at the arteriolar and venular ends of the capillary sheet, A is the capillary sheet area, S is the vascular space-tissue ratio, [see (1), p. 298-300], k and f are dimensionless factors relating to sheet geometry [see (1), pp. 312, 313], L is the average length of blood pathway between the inlet and outlet of the sheet.

Since the vascular space is an assemblage of elastic vessels it is clear that the pressure-flow relation of the whole lung can be obtained by a systematic application of the six equations [1] - [6]. It is then evident from these equations that the morphological and rheological data needed are the values of D_o, α, L, μ, for every branch of pulmonary arteries and veins, and h_o, a, L, S, A, μ, k, and f of the pulmonary capillaries.

III.   COLLECTION OF THE MORPHOLOGICAL AND RHEOLOGICAL
        DATA

Many authors have published morphological and rheological data on pulmonary arteries, veins, and capillaries of various animals, but the data were fragmentary. Our collection of the first complete set of the desired data on the cat took several years. Our results are summarized in Ref. (1), pp. 336-339. Table I shows such a set of data of the pulmonary arteries of the cat's right lung [see (1), p. 337]. Similar data have been obtained for the veins [see (1), p. 338, 33]. Data on the pulmonary capillaries, arterioles, and venules were obtained earlier [see summary in (1), pp. 295-313]. Additional data obtained since 1984 are given in (2)-(6).

The rheological properties of the pulmonary blood vessels are very different from those of peripheral vessels. Figure 2 shows the diameter *vs.* blood pressure relationship of pulmonary veins, [see (1), pp. 209-218 for details]. The relationship is linear! It is remarkable that the **pressure-diameter relationship does not change its slope when the transmural pressure, expressed either as p - p_A, or as p - p_{PL}, changes from positive to negative values.** From a mechanics point of view, this implies that the pulmonary veins do not buckle, or collapse, when the

TABLE I. Morphometric data of pulmonary arteries of the cat measured at transpulmonary pressure $P_A - Ppl = 10$ cmH$_2$O.

| Order | | $D_{on},$ | $L_n,$ | $\mu_n,$ | Compliance | |
n	N_n	cm	cm	cP	$\alpha, 10^{-4}$ cm P_a^{-1}	$\beta, 10^{-4}$ P_a^{-1}
1	300,358	0.0024	0.0116	2.5	0.00463	1.928
2	97,519	0.0044	0.0262	3.0	0.00848	1.928
3	31,662	0.0073	0.0433	3.5	0.01407	1.928
4	9,736	0.0122	0.0810	4.0	0.02352	1.928
5	2,925	0.0192	0.1510	4.0	0.02154	1.122
6	774	0.0352	0.2720	4.0	0.02802	0.7959
7	202	0.0533	0.4600	4.0	0.03807	0.7143
8	49	0.0875	0.8190	4.0	0.09818	1.122
9	12	0.1519	1.5260	4.0	0.40451	2.663
10	4	0.2486	1.1870	4.0	0.66202	2.663
11	1	0.5080	2.5000	4.0	1.35280	2.663

Ppl, pleural pressure; PA, airway pressure; Nn, no. of branches in right lung; Don, diameters at zero transmural pressure; Ln, length, μn, apparent viscosity coefficient; Pa, arterial pressure.

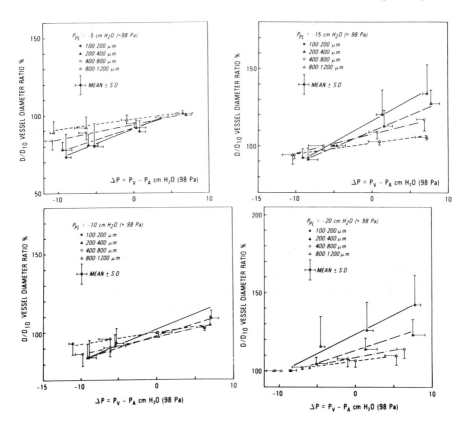

Figure 2. Distensibility of pulmonary veins of the cat subjected to positive and negative p_v - p_A. Vessel diameter is normalized against its value at p_v $-p_A = 10$ cmH₂O. Reproduced by permission of American Physiological Society, J Appl Physiol 54:1543, 1983.

transmural pressure becomes negative, (*i.e.*, when the circumferential stress in the vessel wall becomes compressive). This important feature is examined further and confirmed by other evidences [see (1), pp. 209-213]. In contrast, peripheral veins have nonlinear pressure-diameter relationship [see (7), Chap.8, pp. 290-295] and collapse readily under negative transmural pressure [see (1), pp. 168-186]. When the diameter of a peripheral vein is plotted against transmural pressure, the curve is exponential when the transmural pressure is positive, and a sudden and large change of slope occurs when the transmural pressure changes sign.

The pulmonary capillaries also behave very differently than the peripheral capillaries. The later are known to be very rigid and noncollapsible, except in very thin membranes such as bat's wing and rat's salivary gland. The pulmonary capillaries are very compliant. Their properties can be expressed in terms of the average thickness, h, of the capillary vascular space in the interalveolar septum. The experimental results [see (1), p. 306-309] may be summarized as follows:

h = 0 if Δp is negative, and smaller than $-\varepsilon$,
where ε is a small number about 1 cm H_2O.   [7a]

$h = h_o + \alpha\Delta p$ if Δp is positive and smaller than
    a certain limiting value.   [7b]

h tends to be a limiting value h_α if Δp increases
    beyond the limiting value.   [7c]

In the small range $-e < \Delta p < 0$, h increases from
    0 to h_o. A rough approximation is
      $h = h_o + (h_o/\varepsilon)\, \Delta p.$ [7d]

The area of the interalveolar septum depends on
    $p_A - p_{PL}$, but not on Δp.   [7e]

Here $\Delta p = p - p_A$, p being the local blood pressure, p_A being the alveolar gas pressure. The constants α, h_o, ε, vary with the trans-pulmonary pressure, $p_A - p_{PL}$, to some extent.

Of great importance to the mathematical model are Eqs [7a] and [7b]. [7a] describes the collapse of capillaries when Δp is negative. [7b] defines the region in which Eqs. [5] and [6] are valid.

IV.   MODELING THE WHOLE LUNG

To analyze blood flow in the whole lung, it is necessary to specify a vascular circuit which is consistent with the statistical data on branching pattern. Inasmuch as such a specification is nonunique, the result is stochastic.

A detailed analysis based on the data and formulas outlined above and two specific patterns of circuits is presented in Ref. (5), in which the results are given in various curves: (1), the flow Q as a function of p_a for fixed p_v but variable p_{PL}, (2), the variation of Q *vs.* p_a for the different circuits that are both consistent with the statistical data on branching pattern, (3), flow Q *vs.* p_v fixed p_a, p_A, and p_{PL}, (4), the distribution of pressure *vs.* the order number of the blood vessels, (5), the transit time of blood *vs.* flow rate Q. These results are compared with data published in the literature and the agreements are found to be reasonable. These comparisons are, however, not definitive because the physiological measurements were obtained from dogs, but a complete set of morphological and rheological data for the dog does not exist; so data of the cat were used with a reasoned but arbitrary scaling.

To obtain a definitive validation, perfusion experiments were done on cat lung (4), and the results are compared with the model outlined above. This comparison shows good agreement between theory and experiment in zone 3 condition, but it also shows that additional consideration is needed in order to model pulmonary blood flow in zone 2 condition. The good agreement in zone 3 condition is illustrated in Fig. 3. One parameter was used to adjust the theoretical curve to obtain a good fit. This is the area, A, of the alveolar wall in which there

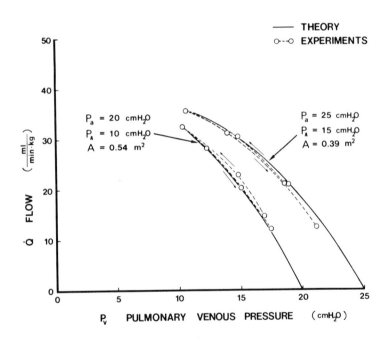

Figure 3. Pressure-flow relationship in two right lungs of cat in zone 3 condition. In the case in which $p_A = 15$ cmH$_2$O, it was found that $p_v = 8.0$ cm H$_2$O when flow (Q) reached the peak value of 38 ml/min/kg. Hence, when p_v was cycled between 22 and 10 cmH$_2$O, flow condition was in zone 3; i.e., $p_{ven} > p_A$ throughout, although $p_v < p_A$ in part of cycle. Test correspond to the lower curve has a Q_{max} of 44 ml/min/kg when p_v was 2.4 cmH$_2$O. Theoretical curves were drawn with alveolar wall surface area A (half lung) indicated in figure. Good fit is obtained by adjusting the values of A. p_a is arterial pressure. From Ref. (3) reproduced by permission.

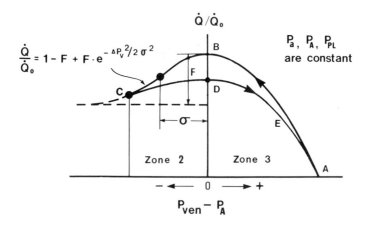

Figure 4. Reduction of area of perfused alveolar sheets due to collapse of capillary blood vessels and adhesion of endothelial cells in zone 2 condition is directly related to reduction of flow through lung. A mathematical expression for reduced flow and reduced alveolar area in region BC (zone 2) is given in Eq. [9]. From Ref. (3), reproduced by permission.

is flow, (area of the "open" part of the interalveolar septa, equal to one-half of the gas exchange area). In Fig. 3, A is that of the right half lung. When everything else is fixed the flow is proportional to A, (see Eq. [6]); hence roughly speaking the theoretical curve is raised upward if A is increased. Experimental determination of A by stereological methods is subjected to considerable uncertainty; the value of A depends on the geometric hypothesis used, and different authors published diverse values; see detailed discussion in (3,6). Furthermore, according to the theory presented below, a fraction of the interalveolar septa may be collapsed, and the collapse reduces the value of A. These factors, in addition to the individual variation of one animal from another, justify our use of A as a floating parameter. That the value of A so determined lies in the ball park of the areas obtained by stereological methods is in itself a validation suggesting the correctness of the mathematical model.

For pulmonary blood flow in zone 2 condition there exists a new feature which is illustrated in Figs. 4 and 7. When the airway, pleural, and arterial pressure are fixed and the venous pressure is decreased continuously, the flow first increases, reaches a peak, then decreases with further decrease of the venous pressure. This is the "waterfall" or "sluicing" phenomenon. If p_v were increased again the flow at the same p_v is smaller than the value achieved earlier while p_v was decreasing. A hysteresis loop is obtained. These features are analyzed below.

V.   A NEW THEORY OF ZONE 2 FLOW

To analyze the zone 2 flow, we first pin down the exact location of the sluicing gates. We conclude that the sluicing gates are located at the end of the capillary blood vessels, where the alveolar sheet is connected to a draining venule. The first evidence was obtained by catalyzed silicone rubber castings of 3 cats' lungs perfused when the polymer fluid was at a low viscosity of 20 centipose, equilibrated (flow stopped) at negative transmural pressures ($p - p_A$) of -23, -17, and -2 cmH_2O while $p_{PL} = 0$, solidified in one hour, hardened for 2 or more weeks, tissue corroded with 10% KOH. These castings show that the capillaries were readily corroded away, whereas the smallest veins that remained on the venous tree have mean diameters of about 22 μm, which is close to what we have measured earlier of the diameters of the smallest pulmonary venules subjected to positive transmural pressure (see Ref.1, pp. 209-213). Hence the venules do not collapse under negative transmural pressure although the capillaries do. The second evidence was provided by the compliance measurements mentioned earlier: The compliance of veins of all sizes does not change when $p - p_A$ or $p - p_{PL}$ changes sign; whereas the capillaries do become very compliant in the range
$-e < p - p_A < 0$ (see Eq. [7d], in which the compliance constant is h_o/e). A third evidence is provided by a detailed theoretical analysis of the sluicing gate presented in Ref. (2). These evidences all confirm our conclusion that the sluicing gates are located at the ends of the capillaries.

Next, we show that the partial differential equations describing sheet flow can admit the solution $h = 0$ without violating any boundary conditions, (3). But $h = 0$ means collapse of capillary sheet. For such collapse to occur the sheet must be attached directly to a venule in which the transmural pressure $p_{ven} - p_A$ is negative.

Thirdly, in the waterfall region, $p_{ven} - p_A < 0$, the flow is essentially constant. Hence the pressure distribution in the arteries and veins (noncapillary vessels) is essentially independent of $p_{ven} - p_A$. Hence the right hand side of Eq. [6] is essentially independent of $p_{ven} - p_A$, and Eq. [6] shows that the flow Q is directly proportional to the area of the capillary sheet in which blood flows. It follows that in this region, the percentage decrease in flow is approximately equal to the percentage of the area of the collapsed capillary sheets in the total alveolar area:

$$\frac{Q_o - Q}{Q_o} = \frac{A_c}{A}$$

                                                                                    [8]

where Q is the total flow, Q_o is the flow computed from Eq. [6] (flow at point B in Fig. 4) with A representing the total area of the alveolar sheets in which flow exists when $p_{ven} = p_A$, while A_c is the area of the sheets collapsed (where h = 0) when p_{ven} is reduced to a value below p_A.

Thus, theoretically, the flow reaches a maximum when $p_{ven} - p_A = 0$. We may take the condition $p_{ven} - p_A = 0$ as the dividing line between zone 2 and zone 3, as is shown in Fig. 4.

Now, A_c is zero when $p_{ven} - p_A = 0$. For further decrease of p_{ven} let us designate $p_{ven} - p_A$ by Δp. If the maximum fraction of A_c/A is F when $\Delta p -> \infty$, we propose a relationship (see Fig. 4):

$$\frac{Q}{Q_0} = 1 - F(1 - e^{-\Delta p^2/2\sigma^2}) \qquad [9]$$

which seems to fit experimental data very well.

VII. ESTIMATION OF COLLAPSED AREA

A fundamental question about the collapse of an interalveolar septum may be formulated as follows. Consider a sheet open to the left to an arteriole with $p_{art} > p_A$ and to the right to a venule with $p_{ven} < p_A$, as is shown at the top of Fig. 5. A segment of length ξ next to the venule is collapsed. Determine ξ according to the principles of mechanics.

The answer can be obtained according to the principle of virtual work. When an alveolar sheet collapses (h = 0), the endothelial surfaces of the capillary blood vessels may adhere, thus reducing the free energy of the membrane. Reseparation needs additional energy. Further, as the area of contact increases work is done by the external forces, and strain energy is stored in the membrane. When the sum of these work and energy, W, is carefully computed as a function ξ, a curve of W vs. ξ is obtained. According to the principle of virtual work, the condition of equilibrium is obtained at that value of ξ where $\partial W/\partial \xi = 0$. According to the principle of dynamic stability, the equilibrium is stable if the curve concaves upward, i.e., if the second derivative is positive, $\partial^2 W/\partial \xi^2 > 0$; whereas it is unstable if $\partial^2 W/\partial \xi^2 < 0$.

The computation of W as a function of ξ is presented in (3). A curve which concaves downward was obtained. Hence any equilibrium is unstable, implying that the collapse of an interalveolar septum, once started, will continue until it is arrested by other means, such as the case shown in Fig. 6.

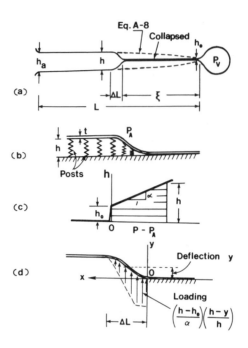

Figure 5. Schematic drawings for analysis of deflection pattern of collapsed interalveolar septa A: <u>dotted lines</u>, walls of sheet before collapsing; <u>solid lines</u>, walls of collapsed sheet; h is sheet hickness; E is collapsed region; L is length of sheet; ΔL is length of transition zone. Posts are drawn as springs, which balance the transmural pressure, p - p_A. C: elastic characteristics of sheet described by Eq. [7b]. a is compliance constant. D: out-of-balance spring forces causing deflection of wall when right-hand side of sheet is collapsed. Wall deflection measured from middle line of sheet is denoted by y. From Ref. (3), reproduced by permission.

Warrell *et al.* (8) have obtained micrographs of quick-frozen dog lung perfused under zone 2 condition. Figure 3 of Ref (8) shows a number of collapsed septa typical of our Fig. 6. Warrell *et al.* called the phenomenon "patchy filling".

With this result we can compute the limiting size of the collapsed sheet, the factor F in Eq. [9]. We have found (6) that each terminal venule in the cat lung drains on the average 18 alveoli. Assuming the alveoli to be dodecahedrons we obtain F = 0.156. Experimental value of F is 0.104 ± 0.016 (S.E.)

With these results the comparison between theory and experiment is illustrated in Fig. 7.

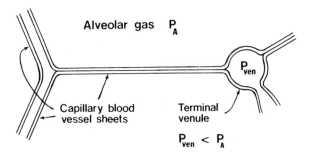

Figure 6. A pulmonary capillary sheet is collapsed and the collapse is arrested by two open septa at the left end. From Ref. (3), reproduced by permission.

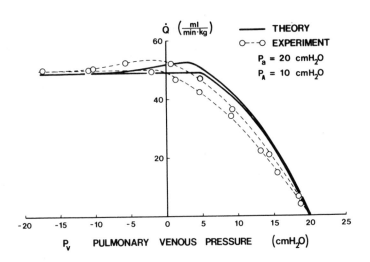

Figure 7. Comparison of theoretical and experimental results. Theoretical curves were based on data given in (1), and $A = 0.84$ m^2 for half lung. In zone 2 condition, Eq. [9] was used. Curve fitting yields $o = 5.3$ and $F = 0.093$. In return stroke, it is assumed that the collapsed alveolar sheets are not reopened, unless the pulmonary arterial pressure is increased under zone 3 condition. From Ref. (3), reproduced by permission.

VII.   CONCLUSIONS

The model presented here is based on the laws of conservation of mass and momentum and the measured morphological and rheological data. It yields results which are in reasonable agreement with those obtained by perfusion experiments. In zone 2 condition, defined by $p_{ven} - p_A < 0$, some interalveolar septa connected with venules may be collapsed. On increasing the venous pressure again after it reached a minimum, the collapsed capillary sheets may not reopen until a large flow is imposed in zone 3 condition. It follows that the total area of open interalveolar septa depends on the perfusion history of the lung. In order to obtain repeatable results independent of history, it is advised that the lung be "preconditioned" by perfusing it with a large flow in zone 3 condition to open up all capillaries before any experiments are performed.

Further developement of the model should include the addition of inertial, neurological, endocrinological, and pathological variables to the model. The addition of inertial variables can be handled by numerical simulation. Our formulation is presented in Ref (9), but it has not yet been tested extensively. The large existing literature will help, of course. On the other hand, we believe that the influence of neurological, endocrine, and pathological variables can be revealed through their effects on the geometry and elasticity of the blood vessels, airways, parenchyma, pleura, chest wall, and muscle. Compared with what lies in the future, the existing models are merely a beginning. They do contribute to reinforce our conviction that a rational approach accompanied by patient collection of the needed anatomical and rheological data will deepen and simplify our understanding of the lung.

ACKNOWLEDGMENTS

Most of the anatomical, rheological and pressure-flow data of the cat lung presented above were obtained with the collaboration of our colleagues Herta Tremer, Tom Rosenquist, Roberta Lindal, Linda Foppiano, Nancy Bingham, Feng Yuan Zhuang, and H.H. Ho. We are deeply indebted to them, as well as to Sol Permutt, John West, and others who have contributed much to the clarification of pulmonary blood flow. References to original publications are given in Ref. (1), pp. 365-369.

REFERENCES

1. Fung YC. (1984) **Biodynamics: Circulation.** Springer-Verlag:New York.
2. Fung YC and Zhuang FY. (1986) *J Biomech Eng* **108**:175.
3. Fung YC and Yen RT. (1986) *J Appl Physiol* **60**:1638.
4. Yen RT and Sobin SS. (1986) *In* **Frontiers in Biomechanics.** (GW Schmid-Schönbein, SL-Y Woo and BW Zweifach, eds), Springer-Verlag:New York.
5. Zhuang FY, Fung YC and Yen RT. (1983) *J Appl Physiol* **55**:1341.
6. Zhuang FY, Yen MRT, Fung YC and Sobin SS. (1985) *Microvasc Res* **29**:18.
7. Fung YC. (1981) **Biomechanics: Mechanical Properties of Living Tissues.** Springer-Verlag:New York.
8. Warrell DA, Evans JW, Clarke RO, Kingaby GP and West JB. (1972) *J Appl Physiol* **32**:346.
9. Seguchi Y, Fung YC and Ishida T. (1986) *In* **Frontiers in Biomechanics.** (GW Schmid-Schönbein, SL-Y Woo and BW Zweifach, eds) Springer-Verlag:New York.

Interpretation of Pressure-Flow Curves in the Pulmonary Vascular Bed

W. MITZNER
I. HUANG
Environmental Health Sciences
Johns Hopkins University
School of Hygiene and Public Health
Baltimore, Maryland 21205

I.   INTRODUCTION

In this presentation, we will consider two different models of the pulmonary circulation as they are applied to the understanding and analysis of pressure-flow curves. Knowledge of the pressure-flow curve in different conditions provides a dimensional improvement in our understanding of the hemodynamic changes in these different conditions, compared to a single measurement of pressure and flow. Although it may not always be possible to obtain sufficient data to generate a pressure-flow curve, if one has an understanding of the nature of this curve, in some situations it may be helpful in interpreting observed changes in total vascular resistance through the lung in other situations.

For example consider the hypothetical curve shown in Figure 1A. Such a curve is typical of the kind of pressure-flow relationships seen in lungs from several different species (1). There is usually some curvilinearity, with the convexity toward the pressure axis. In situations where the perfusion is controlled with a pump, one can obtain the whole curve, including a measured pressure at zero flow. More commonly, for a variety of reasons a direct measure of this zero flow pressure is not obtained, and one must analyze a piece of the curve as shown here by the solid line. It is also quite common for the extrapolated lower tail of this curve to intersect the pressure axis at a pressure in excess of the outflow

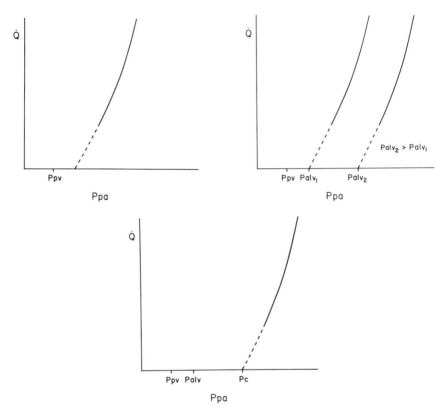

Figure 1: A(left): Hypothetical pulmonary pressure-flow curve. The extrapolated tail of the curve intersects the pressure axis above pulmonary venous pressure (Ppv). $\dot{Q}$ = blood flow, Ppa = pulmonary artery pressure. B(right): Effect of changes in alveolar pressure (Palv) in a zone 2 lung. Increasing Palv shifts the curve to the right. C(below): Effect of vascular tone in causing a critical pressure (Pc). When Pc exceeds Palv the extrapolated intercept exceeds Palv.

pressure, i.e., the pulmonary venous pressure. There are a variety of reasons why this might occur and these will be schematically illustrated in the next several figures. The fact that the curve is non-linear and the extrapolation does not intersect the pressure axis at the venous outflow pressure may lead to an incorrect conclusion regarding changes in the pulmonary vasculature if only single pressure-flow points are obtained (1,2). For example, if an intervention caused the cardiac output to fall, there would be a measured increase in total pulmonary resistance even though there was no effect of the intervention on the pulmonary vasculature. Furthermore, even if there were a change on the pulmonary vessels such that there were a shift of the curve left or right, if the cardiac output also changed, it would be possible to measure the same total pulmonary resistance. In both of these situations, if only a piece of the total pressure-flow curve were known, these incorrect conclusions might be avoided.

The least controversial reason for a zero flow intercept in excess of outflow pressure is the zone 2 situation where alveolar pressure exceeds pressure at the capillary outflow. This situation is illustrated in Figure 1B. Here, because the capillaries cannot sustain a negative transmural pressure, the alveolar pressure becomes the effective downstream pressure seen from the pulmonary artery. It has been shown that when alveolar pressure is increased the pressure-flow curves shift to the right by an amount roughly equal to the increase in P_{alv} (3).

Another reason why the zero flow pressure intercept might exceed the the outflow pressures is that vascular tone may itself create an effective outflow pressure at some active locus in the vasculature. This situation has been analyzed in detail (4), and the hemodynamics established are considered similar to the effect of alveolar pressure on the capillaries. That is, a Starling resistor may be established at a vascular locus where the vascular tone is increased sufficiently. The Starling resistor analogy in the pulmonary capillaries has been criticized as being inappropriate because the Reynolds number is too low to support any degree of flutter (5), and this criticism may also apply to other regions of the vasculature. However, an effective downstream pressure will be established by the surrounding tone or pressure even where viscous forces predominate, as long as the vessel is collapsible and the effective surrounding pressure exceeds the intravascular pressure. A theoretical analysis of such viscous flow limitation is well described (6). Although most experimental uses of Starling resistors occur with high Reynolds number conditions, in the present discussion we use the term Starling resistor for convenience in referring to any flow conditions where an effective downstream pressure is generated.

Figure 1C illustrates the situation where vascular tone is sufficient to increase the effective downstream pressure to a level above the alveolar pressure. One might reasonably ask whether such a situation ever occurs in a real lung. A complete answer to this question, however, depends on data which are not yet available. What is clear is that pressure-flow curves as shown in Figure 1C have been observed (7), but what is not clear is the mechanism responsible for their shape. That is, this type of non-linear pressure-flow curve might result from a Starling resistor in the vasculature, or it might result from vascular distensibility which would serve to decrease vascular resistance as the pressure across the vessel walls increases. In the following discussion, we will consider in some detail how these two possibilities can be applied to explain the effect of hypoxia on the pulmonary pressure-flow curves in pig lungs.

II.   PULMONARY PRESSURE-FLOW DATA AND MODEL ANALYSIS

A.   Starling Resistor Model

Figure 2 shows the results of a previous study where the pressure-flow curves were measured in isolated perfused pig lungs (7) (the pressure and flow axes are transposed in this original figure). The venous outflow pressure was zero (atmospheric) and a PEEP of 5 cmH$_2$O was used. In this study we did not measure the mean transpulmonary pressure, but we estimate it to be about 10 cmH$_2$O. In our original explanation of the mechanism responsible for these curves, we used a Starling resistor model. The basic features of this model are outlined as follows. As a first approximation we ignored vessel distensibility, and there were two reasons for so doing. First, there were no data available on the distensibility of the pig pulmonary vasculature, so any inclusion of vascular distension would have been entirely arbitrary. Second, the pulmonary artery pressure in the pig tends to be considerably higher than most other species, and we considered the possibility that either the vessels were very stiff to accommodate high pressure, or that in control conditions they were already distended to their elastic limits so that vessel size would remain relatively constant.

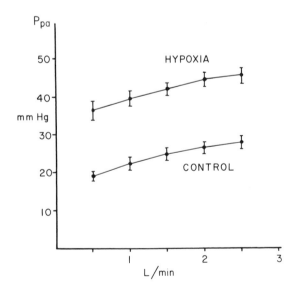

Figure 2: Effect of hypoxia on pulmonary pressure-flow curves in pig lung. Data from reference 7.

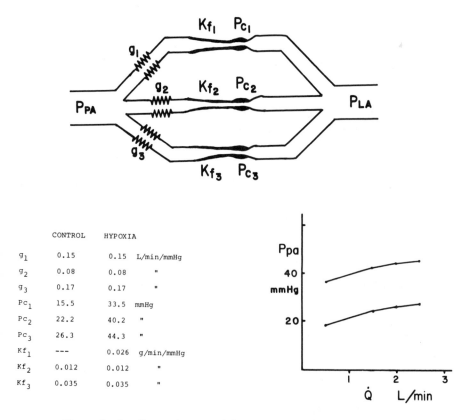

	CONTROL	HYPOXIA	
g_1	0.15	0.15	L/min/mmHg
g_2	0.08	0.08	"
g_3	0.17	0.17	"
Pc_1	15.5	33.5	mmHg
Pc_2	22.2	40.2	"
Pc_3	26.3	44.3	"
Kf_1	---	0.026	g/min/mmHg
Kf_2	0.012	0.012	"
Kf_3	0.035	0.035	"

Figure 3: Starling resistor model consisting of 3 parallel branches used to model the data of Figure 2. Curves shown here are generated from the model variables on left (from reference 7— Kf data refers to local filtration coefficients not being considered here).

Given this assumption of non-distensible vessels, we then accounted for the curvilinearity of the pressure-flow curve by assuming a parallel distribution of critical pressures. That is, we considered the vasculature to consist of Starling resistors in parallel where the effective downstream pressures of each branch were not equal. If one accepts that such Starling resistors can exist in the pulmonary circulation, then it is quite reasonable to assume that the critical pressures of every parallel channel are not equal. Using this model, we could fit our data quite well using 3 parallel branches, and this model is shown in Figure 3. The respective conductances (g_1 - g_3) of each branch were determined from the original data.

B.   Distensibility Model

About two years after these data and model were published, the model of
the pulmonary circulation based on detailed morphometric and elasticity data in the
cat was described by Zhuang *et al.* (8). In this model they described the shape of
the pressure-flow curve as resulting from distension of the pulmonary vessels with
increasing pressure. In their model they included Starling resistors, but only in the
capillary sheet in the zone 2 situation where the effective downstream pressure was
equal to the alveolar pressure. This model has several pleasing features, not the
least of which is the fact that it attempts to consider the true structure of the
circulation based on measurements of that structure. For this reason, it has the
potential for helping understand the mechanisms of a variety of observed changes
in the pulmonary pressure-flow curve.

We therefore attempted to apply the principles of the model of Zhuang *et
al.* to the above results with hypoxia. In order to do this we were required to make
several somewhat arbitrary assumptions to allow us to scale the data from the cat
to that of the pig. This scaling posed a considerable problem since there are no
similar morphometric data available for the pig circulation. As a first
approximation we have scaled vessel diameter and length by the cube root of lung
volume. The relative lung volumes of pig and cat as functions of body weight
were determined from published data (9). Assuming a nominal cat weight of 3 kg
for the data used by Zhuang *et al.*[1] and the 27 kg weight of young pigs we used,
we get a body weight ratio of 9. Since the ratio of lung volumes at TLC between
pig and cat is only about half the body weight ratio, we used a linear scaling factor
of 1.6 (*i.e.*, $4.5^{1/3}$). The capillary sheet area was also initially scaled as the $2/3$
power of 4.5, or 2.7, but the capillary thickness and length were left unchanged.
Because our data were from whole lungs and the data of Zhuang *et al.* were from
$1/2$ the lung, we multiplied the number of branches of each order by 2. The
compliance of all orders of branches was initially left at the same values used for
the cat, that is, a diameter change of between 1 and 2% per cmH_2O transmural
pressure. Because the veins of the dog have been shown to have an elastic limit at
relatively low pressure (10-15 cmH_2O; 12), we also included an elastic limit in the
pig at a slightly higher pressure of 25 cmH_2O. Pressure flow curves were
constructed assuming a dichotomous branching network (model l; 8). For fixed
alveolar and venous outflow pressures, we calculated the pressure gradient through
each order for a sequence of fixed flow rates using the formulas described by
Zhuang *et al.* (8).

---

[1]*Actually, the arterial morphometry data was from cats with a body
weight range of 3.1 - 5.9 kg (10) and the arterial elasticity data from cats with a
range of 1.8 - 3.5 kg (11).*

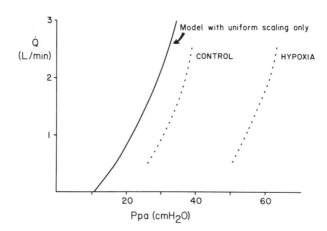

Figure 4: Fit of model of Zhuang et al. (8) to data of Figure 2. Scaling from cat to pig was with a fixed proportion of linear dimensions. See text. The dashed curves are data from Figure 2.

Figure 4 shows the results of this model with the above direct proportional scaling to the pig. As the figure shows, the fit of the control data is not perfect, but considering all the assumptions is really not all that bad. Part of the problem with the actual pig lung data is that the curves are quite steep at high pressure, so that in order to have zero flow at 10 cmH_2O the curves must make a rather sharp bend. We experimented with the model variables to determine what kind of changes would be needed to account for such a pressure-flow shape. This was also done with the anticipation of also being able to account for the kind of parallel shift seen with hypoxia. We found that to achieve a sharp bend in the pressure-flow curve, one needs to place a constriction downstream and also increase the compliance of the orders where the constriction has occurred. To implement vascular constriction in the model, we simply decreased the resting vessel diameter at zero transmural pressure (d_o). To match the control curve shown in Figure 3, we reduced the d_o of arterial and venous orders 1-4 by 37%. This reduction makes the smallest order vessels of the pig about the same size as that of the cat. This assumption may not be as bad as it first might seem, since the capillary sheet thickness across species would not be expected to vary much in proportion to body weight or lung volume. Thus the lowest order vessel entering into the sheet might also be expected to be of similar diameter across species. The large species would also have more than 11 orders of branches and thus a greater number of vessels in tbe smaller orders. We have chosen not to scale the number of orders and the branching order ratio because this would include additional arbitrary assumptions. As it turns out, however, without these additional assumptions one can fit the data quite nicely, and we would not expect the qualitative effects on the pressure-flow curves which we studied to be altered by simply increasing the number of branching orders.

To fit the control curve we also needed to increase the vessel compliance in orders 1-4. Whether it is reasonable to increase compliance in a constricted vessel will be discussed later, but one can appreciate the effect of a decrease in diameter in the small arteries at the same time as the compliance is increased in the curves shown in Figure 5. As can be seen one can obtain a nearly perfect fit to the control data with the specific changes shown.

Since most investigators agree that a major site of constriction during hypoxia is in the small pulmonary arterioles, to model the changes during hypoxia, we simply increased the degree of constriction of the small arterioles. Figure 6 shows the effect of simply decreasing the control d_0 by 75% in orders 1-4 and increasing the compliance of these orders, by a factor of 2.7. This figure makes it clear that one can simulate parallel shifts of the pressure-flow curves by imposing both a decreased diameter and an increased compliance in small order arterioles. Intuitively, that this will work makes some sense since, at low pressures the resistance is greatly increased and the curve is relatively flat. But when the pressure in the constricted vessels begins to increase, because of the increased compliance, these vessels dilate rapidly thereby decreasing vascular

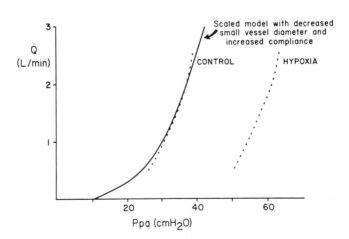

Figure 5: Improved fit of control curve of Figure 2 data (dashed lines). Scaling was the same as used in Figure 4, except that arterial and venous orders 1-4 had d_0 reduced by 37% and compliance increased 20%. See Text.

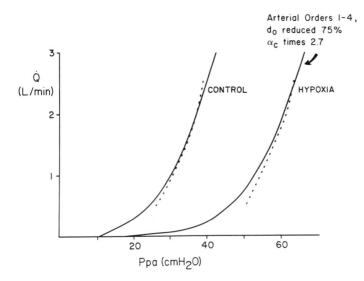

Arterial Orders 1-4,
d_0 reduced 75%
α_c times 2.7

Figure 6: Fit of hypoxia curve to Figure 3 data (dashed lines). The parallel shift could be modeled by decreasing d_o of arterial orders 1-4 by 75% and multiplying the compliance of the control curve (α_c) by 2.7.

resistance, and the pressure-flow curve then turns sharply upward. It turns out that the pressure flow curves are exquisitely sensitive to the local compliance at the site of constriction. As an illustration, the curve in Figure 7 shows the effect of a 10% increase and decrease in compliance. These 10% changes in compliance cause significant parallel shifts of the hypoxia curve.

III.   DISCUSSION

Although the above analysis shows that it is quite simple to model a parallel shift of the pressure-flow curve with a resistance-compliance type of model based on morphometric data, we still need to consider whether the changes required for such a shift are physiologically meaningful. That is, is it reasonable to expect that a constricted vessel is more compliant. This possibility seems to be counter-intuitive, since we normally think of a constricted vessel as being stiffer. Indeed, measurements of total lung vascular compliance in the pig during hypoxia do show a decrease (13). But since the contribution of the smallest order arterioles to the total compliance is relatively little, it is still possible that these small

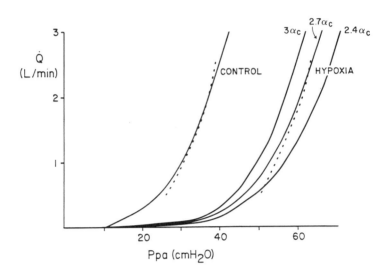

Figure 7: Curves showing the sensitivity of the location of the pressure-flow curves to the vascular compliance of the constricted vessel. A 10% increase or decrease in compliance results in a significant shift of the hypoxia curve.

constricted vessels have increased distensibility. Depending on how the constriction occurs and how the smooth muscle is linked up with the elastin and collagen matrix it may not be unreasonable to expect that an increased compliance could occur in a limited region and pressure range. Furthermore, in a constricted state the muscle itself might become the most compliant part of the wall, with increasing pressure acting to pull apart the constriction.

Such observations of vascular constriction with increased compliance were made in both arteries and veins by Alexander (14). Figure 8 shows the effect of epinephrine on the circumference-tension relationship of an aortic segment *in vivo* (Figure 3 from ref. 14). As the figure clearly shows, there is a substantial increase in vessel compliance at the same time as the d_o or unstressed circumference is decreased. He attributed this increased compliance to the properties of smooth muscle, which he considered to be the most distensible of the elements comprising the aortic wall. In other studies he also showed that this phenomenon of constriction with increased compliance was not limited to high pressure vessels such as the aorta, but could also be seen in systemic and splanchnic veins. We are not aware of any similar measurements on small pulmonary arteries, but, certainly on the basis of Alexander's work, the possibility of finding pulmonary vascular constriction with increased compliance has to be seriously considered.

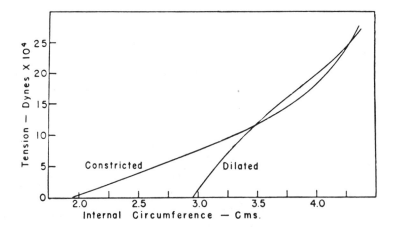

Figure 8: Results of Alexander (14) showing increased compliance in a constricted canine aorta.

Finally, we would like to consider the advantages and disadvantages of the two models presented. At the present time there are not enough data available to claim with any degree of certainty that one model is better than the other. Operationally, the Starling resistor model is simpler and it can be easily used to fit the steep pressure-flow curves shown in Figure 3 very well, and readily allows for regional flow differences. It also provides a convenient and useful interpretation of the zero-flow pressure intercept. Although the pressure at zero-flow was not measured in the above hypoxia study, in other situations where the Starling resistor model has been applied, the measured pressure at zero flow does indeed exceed the outflow pressure (3). However, since the actual pressure at zero-flow only represents the lowest critical pressure of the various parallel branches (2), a measure of the actual arterial pressure at zero flow may not always be a very useful measure. Rather, it is the mean critical pressure which provides the effective downstream pressure when all parallel branches are open.

One of the best tests for the existence of a Starling resistor is to raise the true outflow pressure at constant flow. In an ideal Starling resistor model, there will be no change in inflow pressure until outflow pressure rises sufficiently to increase pressures at the critical locus to a level which exceeds the collapse pressure. This test will obviously not work in vascular beds where there is a local venous-arterial reflex (15), but such a local reflex has not been demonstrated n the pulmonary vasculature. Indeed, in a canine zone 2 lung perfused with constant flow, raising pulmonary venous pressure has no effect on the pulmonary arterial pressure until Ppv approaches the alveolar pressure (unpublished observations). We did not do this test in the pig hypoxia studies described above, but such experiments were done by Rock *et al.* (16). They were able to show that during normoxia with a PEEP of 5 cmH$_2$O, increases in left atrial pressure (Pla) did not increase pulmonary artery pressure until Pla exceeded about 7 cmH$_2$O. During hypoxia, however, pulmonary artery pressure was not increased by increases in Pla up to 20 cmH$_2$O. This result was interpreted by them as strong support for muscle tone acting at a Starling resistor locus.

Further support for the Starling resistor model in the pig came from later studies where we studied the interaction of hypoxia with increases in alveolar pressure (17). These results showed that hypoxia and lung inflation acted in an additive fashion on the extrapolated critical pressure. That is, hypoxia caused a parallel shift in the pressure-flow curve and this shift was increased by increases in alveolar pressure. Since in a Starling resistor, vascular tone and surrounding pressure at the critical locus are additive (4,17), we could account for this experimental finding simply by assuming that the Starling resistor or critical locus was within alveolar vessels. As will be discussed subsequently, the morphometric distensible model also demonstrates this additive parallel shift property, so that these tests cannot be used to distinguish between the models.

In considering the morphometric model of Zhuang *et al.* (8) extrapolated to the pig, there are several very desirable features. It is based on physical elements of the structure of the pulmonary vasculature. It also includes quantification of the fact that pulmonary vessels are not rigid tubes. One already mentioned limitation of the present model scaled for the pig is that the scaling is rather arbitrary. Our original goal was to see if we could simulate the change in the observed curves with hypoxia, and to this end we adjusted the variables to first get a good match for the control curve. Clearly, the pig lung is quite different from the cat, but there are no comparable pig data on which to do much better. Among questions which need answers are the following:

1) How many orders of branching are there?
2) How many numbers of branches per order are there?
3) What is the distensibility of the individual orders? and
4) What are the physical properties of the capillary sheet?

Although in the extrapolation of the published cat data to the pig we used several questionable assumptions, this problem could be eliminated with direct morphometric and elasticity measurements in the pig. We also used a symmetric branching model (Model 1 of Zhuang *et al.*) for simplicity in calculating the pressure drop of each order. In the cat, using the slightly asymmetric branching pattern (Model 2) reduced the total pulmonary vascular resistance by about 25%, but even this pattern greatly oversimplifies the actual branching pattern in the real lung. It must be that as one approaches the actual branching pattern, the total resistance would decrease even more, but it is not clear at the preset time how to approach mathematically this limit. This problem remains a significant one in using the morphologic model of Zhuang *et al.* (8).

As already mentioned, the Starling resistor model can easily incorporate parallel shifts due to lung inflation. In the distensibility model, it was possible to account for a parallel shift of the pressure flow curves with hypoxia by constricting vessels and increasing their compliance. If we now consider the effect of increasing alveolar pressure, we have the following situation. Since the hypoxic constriction was in orders 1-4, and since these orders were considered to be alveolar vessels by Zhuang *et al.* (8), the increased Palv will act to decrease their diameter even further. Downstream from the arterial constriction we now have a zone 2 Starling resistor at the capillary sheet outflow, so that increases in alveolar pressure cause one-for-one increases in intravascular capillary pressure. Although it is not intuitively obvious how these two non-linear series resistance changes will affect the pressure-flow curves, it turns out that the interaction of hypoxia and lung inflation act additively to cause parallel shifts of the curve. This result is shown in Figure 9. It is worth emphasizing that if orders 1-4 were considered to

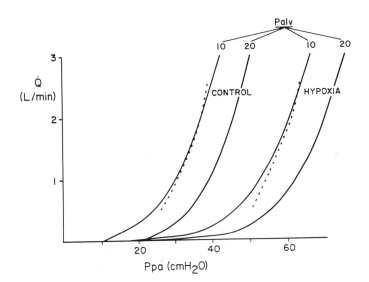

Figure 9: Effect of hypoxia and increased alveolar pressure (Palv) on the pressure-flow curves generated by the model of Zhuang et al. (8). Hypoxia and Palv are seen to act additively. Dashed curves are data from Figure 2.

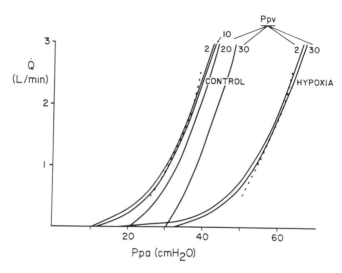

Figure 10: Effect of hypoxia and increased pulmonary venous pressure
(Ppv) on the pressure-flow curves generated by the model of Zhuang et al. (8).
When Ppv is below the extrapolated tail of the curve at normal flow, it has little
effect on the curve. See text. Dashed curves are data from Figure 2.

be extra-alveolar vessels with extravascular pressure equal to pleural pressure, then
with increased Palv the curves would still shift to the right, but the magnitude of
the shift would be considerably less than the increase in Palv.

It is also of interest to consider the effect of increases in venous outflow
pressure (Ppv) in the model of Zhuang et al. (8), since this has been considered to
be a test of the Starling resistor model. It turns out, however, that the Zhuang
model also demonstrates little effect of venous pressure increases until the venous
pressure roughly exceeds the extrapolated zero-flow pressure intercept. Figure 10
shows the effect of increasing venous pressure from 2 to 30 cmH$_2$O, with alveolar
pressure at 10 cmH$_2$O. As can be seen, in the control condition the two curves
with venous pressure of 2 and 10 are nearly identical, but the curves with Ppv of
20 and 30 are shifted to the right. During hypoxia, increases in Ppv from 2 to 30
cmH$_2$O have little effect. The reason why increases in Ppv have little effect when
Ppv is less than the extrapolated zero-flow pressures is related to the fact that these
increases contribute to the distension of the pulmonary veins. As Ppv increases,
the venous diameters increase and their resistances decrease accordingly. It was
initially quite surprising to find that this distension almost completely balanced
the increased Ppv, to the degree where it behaved operationally like a Starling

resistor. Note also that the shift of the curves in the normal flow range is less than the increase in venous pressure. That is, at high venous pressure much of the effect is on the lower tail of the curve and not on the steep portion. Thus the ratio of the change in P_{pa} to the change in P_{pv} at fixed flow in the normal range is less than 1 (about 0.5 in this example when P_{pv} increases from 20-30). The fact that this ratio is less than unity results partially from the fact that the model as presently used places no limit on the maximal diameter of the arteries or capillary sheet. If we were to include elastic limits in these vascular compartments, then the P_{pa}/P_{pv} ratio should approach unity.

In summary, we have analyzed experimental data on pulmonary vascular pressure-flow curves within the context of two distinct models. The data which show parallel shifts of the curves can be described quite well using a Starling resistor model. The model described by Zhuang et al. (8) based on vascular morphometry and elasticity can account equally well for such parallel shifts if the compliance of the constricted vessels is allowed to increase. Increased compliance of the constricted vessels is the only manipulation we could make in the model to account for parallel shifts. However, whether such a change actually occurs in the small vessels with hypoxia remains to be determined.

REFERENCES

1.   Mitzner W. (1983) *In* **Clinics in Chest Medicine.** (RA Matthay, ed) W.B. Saunders Co: Philadelphia, 4(2):127.
2.   Mitzner W. (1974) *Am J Physiol* **227**: 513.
3.   Graham R, Skoog C and Oppenheimer L. (1982) *Circulation Res* **50**:566.
4.   Permutt S and Riley RL. (1963) *J Appl Physiol* **18**:924.
5.   Fung YC and Yen RT. (1986) *J Appl Physiol* **60**:1638.
6.   Wilson TA, Rodarte J and J Butler. (1986) *In* **Handbook of Physiology III: The Respiratory System.** Amer Physiol Soc: Bethesda, Maryland.
7.   Mitzner W and Sylvester JT. (1981) *J Appl Physiol* **51**:1065.
8.   Zhuang FY, Fung YC and Yen RT. (1983) *J Appl Physiol* **55**:1341.
9.   Lum H and Mitzner W. (1985) *Amer Rev Resp Dis* **132**:1078.
10. Yen, RT, Zhuang FY, Fung YC, Ho HH, Tremer T and Sobin S. (1984) *J Biomechanical Eng* **106**:131.
11. Yen RT, Fung YC and Bingham N. (1980) *J Biomechanical Eng* **102**:170.
12. Smith JC and Mitzner W. (1980) *J Appl Physiol* **48**:450.

13.   Rock P, Permutt S and Sylvester JT. (1984) *Amer Rev Resp Dis* **129**:A341.

14.   Alexander RS. (1954) *Circulation Res* **2**:140.

15.   Mitzner W. (1974) *J Appl Physiol* **37**:706.

16.   Rock P, Patterson G, Permutt S and Sylvester JT. (1985) *J Appl Physiol* **59**:1891.

17.   Sylvester JT, Mitzner W, Ngeow Y and Permutt S. (1983) *J Appl Physiol* **54**:1660.

Gravity Nondependent Distribution of Pulmonary Blood Flow[1]

TAWFIC S. HAKIM[2]
ROBERT LISBONA
GEOFFREY W. DEAN
Department of Physiology
McGill University
Montreal, Quebec H3G 1Y6

I.   INTRODUCTION

The role of gravity in the distribution of pulmonary perfusion was first suggested by Orth (1). The introduction of radioactive gases led to the confirmation of such a role (2; chapters 3,8,9). In the upright man, the apical regions of the lungs receive less blood flow than the basal regions, and it is generally accepted that this phenomenon is due to gravity. Permutt *et al.* (3) pointed out that because alveolar pressure (P_{alv}) is uniform throughout the lung, whereas pulmonary vascular pressure increases 1 cm H_2O per 1 cm distance down the lung, the driving pressure which determines blood flow to a given region will depend upon the vertical height of the region. West *et al* . (4) thus divided the lung into three zones according to the relative magnitude of the alveolar pressure to pulmonary arterial pressure (P_a) and pulmonary venous pressure (P_v). There are, however, a number of findings which cannot be readily explained on the basis of this concept. These have received relatively little attention because they downplayed the effect of gravity.

[1]*This work is supported by a grant from the Medical Research Council of Canada.*

[2]*T. S. Hakim is a scholar of the Medical Research Council of Canada.*

The methods which are often used in the study of regional pulmonary perfusion have been discussed in detail elsewhere (2, pp. 86-158). This chapter will emphasize those studies which reported inequalities in regional pulmonary perfusion ($\dot{Q}_r$) independent of gravity and observations which cannot simply be attributed to vertical differences. We will present new data which will indicate that a gravity unrelated factor may be just as important in regional flow inequality as the gravity related vertical differences.

The injection of labelled albumin macroaggregates (MAA) or glass microspheres has been considered superior to techniques with gases because these particles become impacted in small vessels in quantities proportional to regional blood flow and remain stationary during the period of the scan for external counting (5) or even for post mortem examination in animals (6). Most earlier studies which use planar imaging of the lung or external counters have often avoided the peripheral and medial regions where difficulties arise because of the irregular shape of the lung. Regional differences in lung inflation and blood volume further complicate quantification. All these methods have assumed that differences in $\dot{Q}_r$ at the same level are minimal. Whether this indeed is true or not is the topic of this discussion.

II.   DISTRIBUTION OF FLOW UNDER THE FORCE OF GRAVITY

There is no question that in the upright man a gradient of $\dot{Q}_r$ between the apical and basal region can be demonstrated with various methods. This is generally attributed to a gradual increase in hydrostatic vascular pressure relative to alveolar pressure. This gradual increase in pressure distends the capillaries, decreasing their resistance, and hence increasing blood flow through them. This explanation was strongly supported by the histological observation that capillaries are indeed more distended in the dependent regions (7). The drawback of this argument is that an increase in $\dot{Q}_r$ from the superior to the inferior region of the lung is sometimes questionable, even in erect man (8). In the supine or prone human, Kaneko *et al.* (9) found that perfusion is relatively uniform in the ventral-dorsal direction. Amis *et al.* (10) noted a ventral-dorsal gradient in prone subjects, but not in supine subjects. Furthermore, in the upright subjects immersed to the neck in water, the vertical gradient in $\dot{Q}_r$ between the apical and basal regions disappears in spite of the continued presence of a hydrostatic pressure gradient relative to alveolar pressure (11,12). Thus there are reasons to believe that gravity or an increase in hydrostatic pressure do not always satisfactorily explain the gradient between the superior and the inferior regions in the lung.

The problem may stem from the assumption that distention of capillaries in the dependent region (7) causes the regional vascular resistance to become

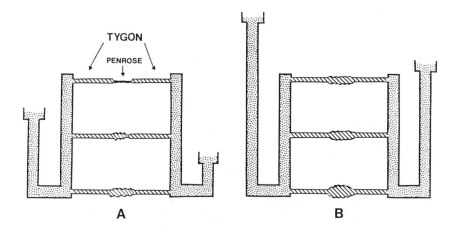

Fig. 1. A model consisting of three identical channels. In "A" the flow/channel will increase from top to bottom, while in "B", flow/channel may remain the same or may increase from top to bottom depending on the resistance of the middle segment.

smaller, and $\dot{Q}_r$ therefore higher. The validity of this precept is based on whether distention of the capillaries (after recruitment) contributes significantly to reduction in the vascular resistance. This question remains controversial. The arterial and venous occlusion technique (13) suggests that in zone 3, the capillaries contribute very little to the resistance, while the micropuncture technique suggests that they contribute at least 30% (14). The importance of this controversy can be demonstrated with a model (Fig. 1). On the left (Fig. 1A), the inflow and ouflow reservoirs are set such that the top channel is under zone 1 conditions, the middle channel under zone 2, and the bottom channel under zone 3 conditions. The penrose segments represent the alveolar vessels or the capillaries. It can easily be deduced that under these conditions, flow would increase gradually in these channels from top to bottom. A similar deduction can also be reached if all three channels were in zone 2 conditions. When the reservoirs are elevated such that all channels lie in zone 3 (Fig. 7B), it becomes more difficult to predict how the flow may be distributed unless the resistive property of the middle segment is known. If the resistance of this middle segment is negligible, then further distension would not affect the overall resistance of the channel, and therefore flow would be determined only by the resistance of the other two segments. Therefore the histologic evidence that pulmonary capillaries can distend is not necessarily an indication of lower resistance, because it depends on the contribution of the capillaries to vascular resistance.

III.   ZONE 4

A common observation which is inconsistent with the effect of gravity is zone 4, which was introduced by Hughes *et al.* (15). This zone apparently exists in most body positions (6). In this zone, there is a decrease in flow in spite of an increase in vascular pressure and potential distension of the vessels. This finding was explained by the fact that at the base of the lung, alveoli are less inflated, and thus there is less tethering effect on the extra-alveolar vessels which tends to increase their resistance. This conclusion was supported by the fact that the extent of zone 4 can be diminished (although not abolished) by lung inflation. There are, however, several pieces of evidence which do not support the argument that this zone is due to regional lung volume differences: First, and most importantly, Hughes *et al.* (16) subsequently showed that zone 4 is also present in the isolated perfused lungs which have no regional differences in inflation. Thus, while it is recognized that changes in lung volume may indeed alter the extent of zone 4 because of an effect on the extra-alveolar vessels, differences in the degree of lung inflation do not generate this zone characteristic. Besides, small differences in regional lung volume may be unimportant, because under conditions where the vascular pressure remains above the alveolar and pleural pressures (such as in the dependent regions of the lung) the effect of lung volume on the resistance and volume of the extra-alveolar vessels was found to be almost insignificant (17,18). Other factors which were thought to contribute to zone 4, *e.g.*, perivascular fluid, have also been found lacking (19).

IV.   FLOW DISTRIBUTION UNDER ZERO GRAVITY

Although flow distribution has never been directly examined under a zero gravity environment, a number of maneuvers have been used to simulate the absence of gravity. The most common approach to eliminate the gravitational gradient between the apex and the base is to study the subject in the decubitus position (supine, prone, or lateral) and to compare the flow in regions or in slices at isogravity level. This maneuver usually diminishes the gradient in $\dot{Q}_r$ between the apex and the base (9,10,20). Unfortunately, it is also associated with increases in cardiac output, pulmonary arterial and venous pressures, pleural pressure and with a decrease in lung volume (21,22). All these changes can themselves minimize the vertical gradient as demonstrated in the isolated lung (4). Unless the changes in vascular and pleural pressures are accounted for, the difference between the apical-basal gradient in $\dot{Q}_r$ in the supine and in the upright positions must be interpreted with caution.

Another attempt to circumvent gravity was the parabolic flight in a Lear jet in such a manner so as to produce zero gravity on the subject (23). During this maneuver, the radiolabelled MAA were injected intravenously and the subjects were then studied after landing. Such an approach is likely to be associated with changes in intrathoracic (vascular and pleural) pressure and cardiac output, but also provides little time (30-40s) for the redistribution of the blood to occur and for the injected material to stabilize and become fully impacted. Nevertheless, these studies reveal only a small change of the apical – basal gradient in regional blood flow during the maneuver (zero g) as opposed to normal gravity.

A third method to eliminate the effect of gravity in the lung was to fill the airway of the isolated perfused lung with saline, so that the pressures inside and outside the vessels increase equally and remain constant in the apex and in the base of the lung. In such studies, West et al. (24) demonstrated that the flow became almost but not entirely homogeneous. The validity of this observation may however be questioned after examining the pressure and flow rate ratio used in these adult dog lungs.

Therefore, in most instances, technical difficulties interfere with the interpretation of the results. A more suitable way to study the importance of gravity is to compare the vertical gradient vs. the horizontal gradient in one body position, e.g. to compare in the upright subject the apical-basal (vertical) vs. the medial-lateral (horizontal) gradient. Such studies by Newhouse et al. (25) using planar imaging following xenon injection suggested that no significant gradient exists in the horizontal direction, but that a gradient was present in the vertical direction. Amis et al. (10) on the other hand found a gradient in flow vertically as well as horizontally.

Finally, slicing of the lung post mortem, after injection of radiolabelled microspheres (glass or albumin), has been very useful in this regard. Using such a method, one can compare more reliably a vertical and a horizontal gradient. This technique has always yielded a vertical gradient favoring increased flow toward the dependent region, but almost always revealed a region with reduced blood flow (zone 4) in the most dependent region (6,19,26-30). Using the microspheres, horizontal inequalities in regional blood flow have been often identified. Some (28) found a gradient in the dorsal-ventral direction in dogs in the lateral position, whereas others (6) found no difference. The horizontal apical-basal differences at isogravity level have been documented in dogs in the supine, prone and lateral positions (6,26,28). In an attempt to analyze the distribution in more detail, Hedenstierna et al. (29) and Greenleaf et al. (28) utilized identical techniques; the former studied the animals in the supine posture, and the latter in left decubitus. The results were contrasted; the former study found neither medial-lateral, nor apical-basal inequalities at isogravity level, while the latter found the opposite: a medial-lateral, as well as apical-basal gradient. Interestingly, in Greenleaf's study the flow was highest in the slices from the center of each lung. In a more recent attempt, Beck and Rehder (27) used microspheres and found a considerable gravity nondependent inequality in blood flow, and attributed this to differences in vascular conductance. Regardless of exactly how the horizontal inequality manifests, there is usually difficulty in explaining the results. In humans, the observations of horizontal inequalities have also been inconsistent; in the upright position, the dorsal-ventral gradient was found in one study (31) but not in another (32). In the recumbent position, the differences between the basal and apical regions have been variable (10,20,32-34). Thus the horizontal inequalities are frequently present but their magnitude may depend on the body position. Most of these studies, however, agree that a gravity non-related factor was responsible. In a unique study on the snake lung (carpet python), which provides a relatively uniform tubular structure, Read and Connelly (35) reported that marked inequalities existed in the snake lung in the horizontal position, which they attributed to geometric factors in the pulmonary vasculature.

Regardless of the explanation, there is growing evidence that blood flow is not homogeneous in the horizontal direction. Thus, using an average value for $\dot{Q}_r$ at one level, such as done by an external counter, or averaging the activity within a slice, as done with post mortem examination of microspheres, may underestimate regional differences which may exist within a horizontal level.

V.   RESISTANCE OF ALVEOLAR AND EXTRA-ALVEOLAR VESSELS

The arterial and venous occlusion technique allows one to partition the pulmonary vascular resistance into upstream arterial, middle microvascular, and downstream venous segments (13). Under zone 3 condition (Pv > Palv at the top of the lung) the resistance of the middle segment contributed a small fraction ($\approx 10\%$) of the total longitudinal resistance, while the arterial and venous segments contributed a large fraction ($\approx 80\%$). Thus we hypothesized that because the conducting and collecting vessels (arteries and veins) have a considerable fraction of resistance, it is possible that in zone 3, regional resistance would be a function of the distance which blood has to travel. Thus, blood flow to the peripheral regions of the lung encounters more resistance vessels than the blood which flows to the central region of the lung. This concept would apply so long as there is only a reasonable fraction of the resistance in the conducting vessels. This is emphasized because the fractional resistance in the different segments is still a matter of controversy; the arterial and venous occlusion data in dogs suggest that there is very little resistance in the capillaries (13,17). In contrast, direct measurement of pressure in subpleural vessels using micropipettes suggests that a large fraction of the resistance resides in the capillaries (14). The disadvantage of measuring pressure on the surface of the lung is that these surface vessels have flow and pressure which may not represent that in the remainder of the lung vasculature, as will be shown in the subsequent pages.

In zone 2, a large fraction of the resistance is shifted to the alveolar vessels and flow is dominated primarily by what happens to the alveolar vessels (3,4,17). As their transmural pressure (vascular pressure – alveolar pressure) rises, they distend and the flow in them increases. Consequently, the regional blood flow in zone 2 condition increases from top to bottom because the vascular hydrostatic pressure increases gradually relative to alveolar pressure. Therefore, in zone 2, the distribution of flow will be dominated by a vertical gradient. In contrast, the distribution of flow in zone 3 may be primarily determined by the resistance of the conducting vessels. In the intact subject (especially in the supine position) the lung is primarily in zone 3, and regional blood flow may be dominated by the resistance vessels (arteries and veins). In the upright subject, the apical regions of the lung may be in zone 2 condition and the lower parts in zone 3 condition. Consequently, in the upright posture, the upper part of the lung will have a vertical gradient dominated by the vascular-alveolar pressure gradient, while the flow in the lower half will be determined by the geometric properties of the vessels.

VI.   SPATIAL DISTRIBUTION OF $\dot{Q}$ IN INTACT DOG LUNGS

A preliminary study with single photon emission computerized tomography (SPECT) in supine dogs and humans (36,37), revealed that blood flow was spatially stratified, being highest in the central region and lowest in the periphery of the lung. As a first approximation we summarized these observations with a model consisting of different size egg-shells nested within each other (Fig. 2). The smallest egg represents the region with the highest activity or blood flow. To further confirm these findings, healthy mongrel dogs ($\approx$ 30 Kg) were anesthetized (Sodium pentobarbital 25 mg/Kg) and strapped in the supine position. Cardiac output, pulmonary arterial and wedge pressures were measured via a Swan-Ganz catheter and a thermodilution cardiac output computer and found normal. When the animals were stable and breathing spontaneously, 20 mCi technetium 99m labelled albumin macroaggregates (MAA; 15-70 μ diameter) were injected into the vena cava (via the proximal port of the Swan-Ganz catheter) at end expiration over several breaths. Five minutes were allowed for the MAA to embolize the pulmonary vessels. This had no detectable hemodynamic effect. The animals were heavily sedated and exsanguinated rapidly (5 min) via a large bore catheter placed in one common carotid artery. The chest was opened, and a horizontal mark was placed on the surface of the lung. The lungs were removed,

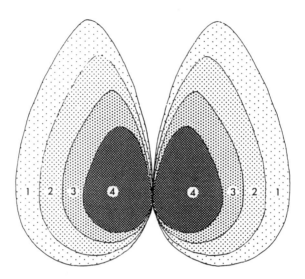

Fig. 2. A conceptual egg-shell model to describe the average distribution of blood flow in the lung. The smallest egg-shell represents the highest regional blood flow. This arrangement of egg-shells can be applied to each individual lobe.

and drained passively of their blood content. They were inflated to total capacity by blowing warm air (50° C) into them at constant pressure (35 cm H_2O) using a water overflow system. The surface of the lungs was punctured at multiple sites with a 22 gauge needle to allow the bulk of warm air to pass through the lungs. To ensure that the position of the inflated lobes remained constant relative to each other, the surface of the adjacent lobes were glued (Krazy Glue) when the lungs were inflated. This held the surfaces of the adjacent lobes in contact with each other, in a manner as it would be present in the thoracic cavity. The air drying process of the lungs continued for 18-20 hours after which time the lungs were sufficiently dry.

In three dry lungs, a mid-coronal slice (1 cm thick) was obtained and imaged directly by placing it on a large field of view gamma camera, and in three other lungs a mid-sagittal slice (1 cm thick) through the right lung was obtained and imaged directly. The activity within the direct images of the slices was expressed per unit area (3.7 x 3.7 mm).

Fig. 3a depicts a representative mid-coronal slice obtained from one lung. The distribution of activity (flow) within this slice (Fig. 3b) shows that the activity was highest near the central region of the lobes and lowest in the periphery. This was particularly obvious in the caudal lobes. The averaged activity in the apical lobes was less than in the caudal lobes. The central-

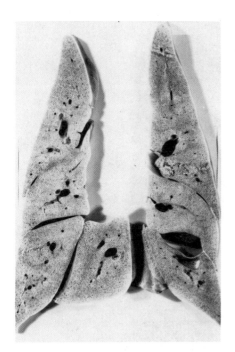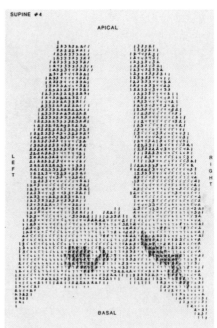

Fig. 3. A photograph of a mid-coronal slice (1 cm thick), and the activity per unit area (3.7 x 3.7 mm) in it. The distribution of flow in this slice is independent of gravity as the animal was in the supine posture. 10 is 90-100% of max activity in this slice, 9 represents 80-90%, 8 represents 70-80%, etc.

peripheral gradient in activity was present in all coronal slices, but was most striking in the middle slices.

One representative sagittal slice, and the distribution of activity within it, are shown in Fig. 4. This slice also shows a central-peripheral gradient in the individual lobes, with no indication that more flow was present in the dependent dorsal region. The pleural border of the lungs usually had the lowest activity.

VII. MICROSPHERE STUDIES

The use of radiolabelled microspheres has been widely accepted in the study of flow distribution within the lung. The activity is usually expressed per unit lung volume or per unit weight. We performed such experiments on anesthetized dogs in the supine and in the upright position, to confirm the central-

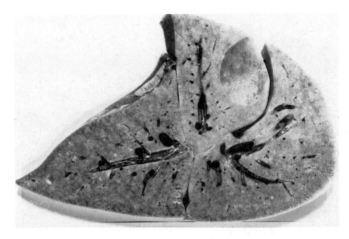

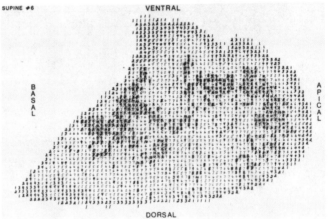

Fig. 4. A photograph of a mid-sagittal slice (1 cm thick), and the activity per unit area (3.7 x 3.7 mm) in it. The ventral-dorsal direction is in the direction of gravity. The apical-basal is isogravity. The numbers mean the same as in Fig. 3.

peripheral distribution in a coronal slice and to examine how it changed with body position. About half a million microspheres labelled with one of the following isotopes (I^{125}, Sr^{85}, Sc^{46}, Ce^{141}) were injected. The animals were strapped on a table with their hind legs folded against their abdomens with ace bandage. In one animal, the microspheres were injected while in the supine position, into the right atrium via a Swan-Ganz catheter, and, in another animal while it was suspended in the upright position. In both cases the microspheres were injected over 2 or 3 breaths during end expiration. The cardiac output, pulmonary artery pressure, and wedge pressure were measured in these animals and were normal. Five minutes after the injection, the animal was sacrificed, the lungs were rapidly removed and drained of blood and air dried at total lung capacity. When the lungs were dry a mid-coronal slice ($\approx$ 2 cm thick) was obtained from each lung for analysis. In the supine animal such a slice was horizontal, whereas in the head-up animal such a slice was vertical. The size and shape of the slice was traced on a paper for future reference. The tracing from one slice is shown in Fig. 5. Each slice was cut in wedges (A-G) as shown in the figure and each wedge was cut in 1 cm distance from the beginning of the wedge at the hilar region. Airways and vessels (> 2mm diameter) were dissected and removed from each sample. Each sample was weighed and placed in a scintillation vial and counted for 10 minutes in a multichannel well gamma counter. The activity of each sample was normalized to its dry weight. A total of about 100-120 samples free of large airways and vessels were counted in each slice. The total activity in each slice (sum of all the samples) was divided by

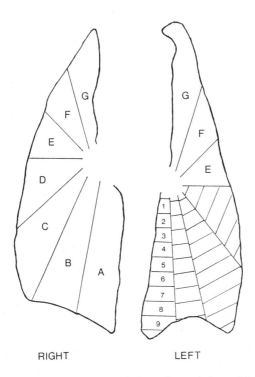

RIGHT   LEFT

Fig. 5. Outlines of the coronal slices from right and left lungs. The method of cutting the wedges and samples is shown.

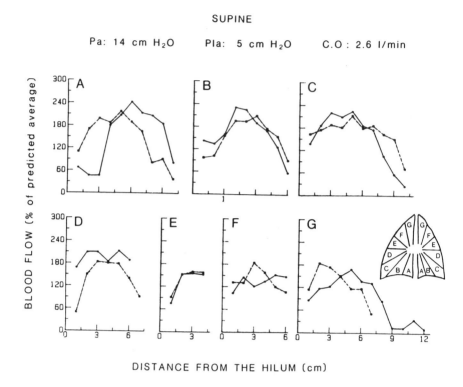

DISTANCE FROM THE HILUM (cm)

Fig. 6. The activity per unit weight in each sample in % of predicted average activity, as a function of distance from the hilar region in all wedges of a coronal slice from a supine animal.

the dry weight of each slice to obtain a predicted average activity if distribution of blood was homogeneous within each slice. The activity in each sample (normalized to the weight of each sample) was expressed as percent of the predicted average. The predicted average activity was not significantly different in the right and left sides. The dry weight of the slice which was analyzed was about 30% of the dry weight of the lung.

Figures 6 & 7 show the regional blood flow throughout each coronal slice. The plots show profiles of the activity in each wedge starting at the hilum and in 1 cm distances toward the peripheral region of each wedge (central-peripheral profiles) in the right and left lungs. Wedges A, B and C showed a peak near the middle in both lungs in the supine and in the upright animals. In wedges D, E and F this pattern was present but less consistent. In wedge G it was apparent in the supine slice (Fig. 6) but less apparent in the vertical slice (Fig. 7). In all wedges

UPRIGHT

Pa: 16.3 cm H$_2$O   Pla: 2 cm H$_2$O   C.O : 1.5 l/min

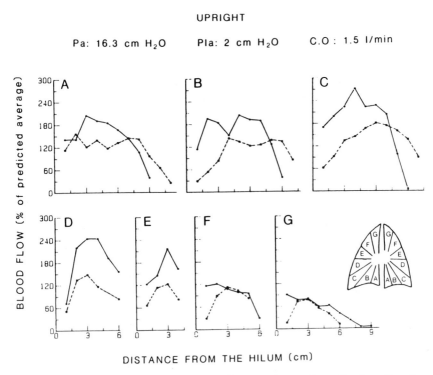

DISTANCE FROM THE HILUM (cm)

Fig. 7. The activity per unit weight in each sample in % of predicted average activity, as a function of distance from the hilar region in all wedges of a coronal slice taken from a head-up animal.

in both body positions the flow was lowest in the peripheral samples. The overall average activity was smaller in the apical regions in both supine and upright animals.

Further experiments were carried out to see if this pattern of flow distribution occurred because of regional differences in lung inflation or thoracic structures. A right lung was excised, and cannulæ were placed in the main artery and in the left atrium. The lung was suspended upright and prepared for perfusion with warmed whole autologous blood (685 ml/min) in an airtight box. Perfusion pressure was 15 cm H$_2$O and left atrial pressure was zero relative to the tip of the cannulæ. The lung was ventilated with the proper gas mixture to maintain normal blood gases. When the preparation was stable, the lung was inflated to full capacity and deflated to a transpulmonary pressure of 5 cm H$_2$O which was considered to represent end expiration in the intact lung. The alveolar pressure was

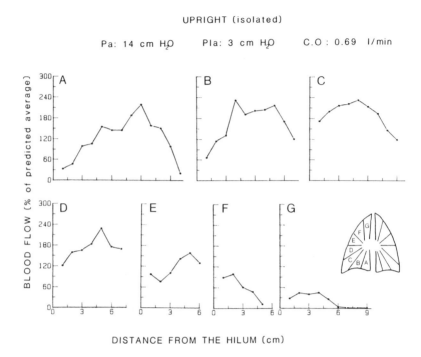

Fig. 8: The distribution of activity per unit weight (same as Fig. 6 and 7) in a right coronal slice from a head-up isolated lung.

atmospheric, while the box pressure was -5 cm H_2O. Microspheres were injected into the pulmonary artery. At the end of this experiment the lung was drained of blood and air dried while fully inflated. A mid-coronal slice was obtained and analyzed as before. The results are shown in Fig. 8, and appear to be identical with the results in the intact upright lung. The periphery had low activity in almost all wedges. These results suggest that the central-peripheral gradient in pulmonary blood flow was not related to regional differences in lung volume which exist in the intact lung, or to the effect of the diaphragm and rib cage on the lung surface.

VIII.   CONCLUSION

Both the direct images of the slices (activity expressed per unit lung volume) and the sampling technique (activity expressed per unit dry weight) consistently showed a central-peripheral (concentric) gradient independent of gravity. Conservatively, there was a gradient between the central regions and the periphery of the slice of at least 10:1 in the direct images, and about 5:1 in the samples. These results are consistent with previous studies in which we used SPECT to examine the three-dimensional distribution of pulmonary blood flow in the intact animal and human (36,37) and in the isolated lungs (unpublished observations).

   Comparison of the distribution of blood flow in coronal slices from vertical and horizontal animals revealed that a concentric gradient is also present in the upright posture but is shifted toward the dependent regions of the lung. Thus it appears that a vertical and a concentric gradient can coexist in the upright lung; in the region in which waterfall conditions exist (zone 2), vertical gradient predominates, while in the region in zone 3, the concentric gradient predominates. In the intact supine animal gravity may play a minor role because the entire lung is in zone 3 and flow distribution is determined by the resistance of the vessels, such that the periphery receives less blood flow than the central regions. In the upright posture the central-peripheral gradient is maintained but because zone 2 conditions become present in the apical regions of the lungs, the role of gravity becomes important. Figure 9 shows a model modified from Fig. 1 and demonstrates the coexistence of the vertical gradient and the central-peripheral gradient. The short channels represent the central region of the lung and the longer channels represent the peripheral regions. The reservoirs are set such that the upper half is in zone 2 condition while the lower half is in zone 3 condition. In this arrangement, (the middle segment represents the alveolar vessels), flow per channel will increase gradually from the top to the middle mainly due to a vertical gradient in hydrostatic pressure, while flow in the lower half will decrease gradually from the middle to the bottom due to the geometric properties of the channels.

   Based on the results of the present study and the previous SPECT study, we believe that the flow distribution in each lung can be described by a number of egg shells nested within each other and touching at a point which represents the entry of blood to the lungs (Fig. 2). The smallest eggshell represents the highest flow and vice versa. This conceptual model may even be applicable to the individual lobes, because microsphere studies (28) and the present study with direct images of slices show that a central-peripheral gradient exists in the individual lobes. Although a number of reasons can be proposed to explain these results, one simple explanation for the spatial stratification of pulmonary blood flow is that resistance to a region is directly proportional to its distance from the hilum because arteries and veins contribute significantly to the vascular resistance. This would be difficult to measure with accuracy because of the complex pattern of branching and change in diameter (38).

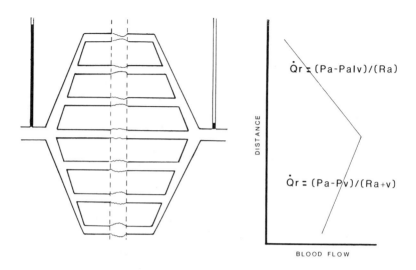

Fig. 9. A model showing the coexistence of a vertical (gravity dependent) and a concentric (gravity independent) gradient in blood flow. The distribution of flow is dominated by the effect of gravity in zone 2 (top 4 channels) and by the geometric factors in zone 3 (lower 4 channels). $\dot{Q}_r$ is regional flow per channel, R_a is resistance of the arteries, R_{a+v} is resistance of arteries and veins, P_a, $\dot{Q}_r$ and P_{alv} are inflow, outflow and alveolar pressure respectively.

Finally, it seems likely that a spatial stratification in regional pulmonary blood flow would be associated with a similar distribution in alveolar ventilation. Presently there are no data on spatial distribution of ventilation; however, it is intuitive that unless blood flow and ventilation throughout the whole lung or each lobe are stratified similarly, a large inhomogeneity in ventilation-perfusion ratio would result. If this pattern of stratification exists in both ventilation and perfusion, the lung could perform its function effectively by recruiting and de-recruiting the peripheral strata depending on the body demand. This seems mechanically more efficient in such a spatially distributed network of airways and vessels than recruiting and de-recruiting layers at varying horizontal levels. This is clearly speculative but has been demonstrated for individual lobules (39, 40).

    In conclusion we found a spatial stratification of blood flow in the lung. Blood flow was lowest in the peripheral region and tended to increase gradually toward the center of each lung. Flow stratification can be described with the egg-shells model. The length of vascular pathway may be a reasonable explanation for this pattern of blood flow. Furthermore, we suggest, that zone 4 condition is a generalized manifestation of the low perfusion in peripheral tissues in all directions, and is not necessarily limited to the most dependent region. The vertical hydrostatic pressure gradient within the lung plays an important role in flow distribution in regions under zone 2 conditions, while in zone 3, gravity plays a minor role, and flow is distributed according to the resistance of the arteries and veins. The fact that pulmonary vascular pressure is about the same in horse, man, dog, and in rat would imply that height of the lung and hence gravity is not of significant importance with regard to blood flow in intact lung. In spite of several fold difference in vertical height, the averaged vertical gradient in regional blood flow (ventral-dorsal gradient) in the horse lung (41,42) is not grossly different from the dog (6,26,30), or from man (9,10).

REFERENCES

1. Orth J. (1887) *In:* **Atiologisches und Anatomisches uber Lungen-schwindsucht.** Hirschwald, Berlin.

2. West JB. (1977) **Regional Differences in the Lung.** Academic Press: New York.

3. Permutt S, Bromberger-Barnea B and Bane HN. (1962) *Med Thorac* **19**:239.

4. West JB, Dollery CT and Naimark A. (1964) *J Appl Physiol* **19**:713.

5. Wagner HN, Sabiston DC, McAfee JG, Tow DE and Stern HS. (1964) *New Engl J Med* **271**:377.

6. Reed JH and Wood EH. (1970) *J Appl Physiol* **28**:303.

7. Glazier JB, Hughes JMB, Maloney JE and West JB. (1969) *J Appl Physiol* **26**:65.

8. Anthonisen NR and Milic-Emili J. (1966) *J Appl Physiol* **21**:760.

9. Kaneko K, Milic-Emili J, Dolovich MB, Dawson A and Bate, D. (1966) *J Appl Physiol* **21**:767.

10. Amis TC, Jones HA and Hughes JMB. (1984) *Respir Physiol* **56**:169.

11. Prefaut CH, Dubois F, Roussos CH, Amaral-Marques R, Macklem P and Ruff F. (1979) *Respir Physiol* **37**:313.

12. Arborelius M, Lopez-Majano V, Data PG, Andreoni AM and Mart R. (1982) *Physiologist* **25**, 196.

13. Hakim TS, Michel RP, Chang HK. (1982) *J Appl Physiol* **52**:710.

14. Bhattacharya J and Staub NC. (1980) *Science* **210**:327.

15. Hughes JMB, Glazier JB, Maloney JE and West J.B. (1968) *Respir Physiol* **4**:58.

16. Hughes JMB, Glazier JB, Maloney JE and West JB. (1968) *J Appl Physiol* **25**:701.

17. Hakim TS, Michel RP and Chang HK. (1982) *J Appl Physiol* **53**:1110.

18. Howell JBL, Permutt S, Proctor DF and Riley RL. (1961) *J Appl Physiol* **16**:71.

19. Ritchie BC, Schamberger G and Staub NC. (1969) *Circ Res* **24**:807.

20. Glazier JB and DeNardo GL. (1966) *Amer Rev Resp Dis* **94**:188.

21. Begin R, Epstein M, Sackner MA, Levinson R, Dougherty R and Duncan D. (1976) *J Appl Physiol* **40**:293.

22   Arborelius M and Lilger B. (1972) *Scand J Clin Invest* **29**:359.

23. Stone HL, Warren BH and Wagner H. (1965) *AGARD Conf Proc* **2**:129.

24. West JB, Dollery CT, Mathews CME and Zardini P. (1965) *J Appl Physiol* **20**:1107.

25. Newhouse MT, Wright FJ, Ingham GK, Archer NP, Hughes LB and Hopkins OL. (1968) *Respir Physiol* **4**:141.

26. Hogg JC, Holst P, Corry P, Ruff F, Housley E and Morris E. (1971) *J Appl Physiol* **31**:97.

27. Beck KC and Rehder K. *J Appl Physiol* **In press**.

28. Greenleaf JF, Ritman EL, Sass DJ and Wood EH. (1974) *Am J Physiol* **227**:230.

29. Hedenstierna G, White FC and Wagner PD. (1979) *J Appl Physiol* **47**:938.

30. Malik AB, Van Der Zee H, Neumann PH and Gertzberg NB. (1980) *J Appl Physiol* **49**:834.

31. Secker-Walker RH, Gill IS and Ho JE. (1980) *Respiration* **40**:208.

32. Bryan AC, Bentivoglio LG, Beerel F, MacLeish H, Zidulka A and Bates DV. (1964) *J Appl Physiol* **19**:395.

33. Engel LA and Prefaut C. (1981) *Respir Physiol* **45**:43.

34. Inkley SR and MacIntyre WJ. (1973) *Amer Rev Resp Dis* **107**:429.

35. Read J and Donnelly P. (1972) *J Appl Physiol* **32**:842.

36. Hakim TS, Susskind H, Zubal IG and Brill AB. (1984)*37th ACAMB Proc* **26**:114.

37. Hakim TS, Lisbona R and Dean GW. (1986) *Prog Resp Res* **21**:000.

38. Zhuang FY, Fung YC and Yen RT. (1983) *J Appl Physiol* **55**:1341.

39. Read J. (1966) *J Appl Physiol* **21**:1521.

40. Wagner P, McRae J and Read J. (1967) *J Appl Physiol* **22**:000.

41. Amis TC, Pasoe JR and Hornof W. (1984) *Am J Vet Res* **45**:1597.

42. Dobson A, Gleed RD, Meyer RE and Stewart BJ. (1985) *Q J Exp Physiol* **70**:283.

Active Regulation of the Pulmonary Circulation: A Model for Hypoxic Pulmonary Vasoconstriction

BRYAN E. MARSHALL[1]
CAROL MARSHALL
Department of Anesthesia
University of Pennsylvania School of
Medicine
Philadelphia, Pennsylvania

I.   INTRODUCTION

The active regulation of the distribution of blood flow in the pulmonary circulation has received increasing attention in the past decade. It has become apparent that hypoxic pulmonary vasoconstriction (HPV) is the most prominent of the active mechanisms and that changes in regional and general pulmonary hemodynamics are often dominated by the effects of HPV in patho-physiological conditions. A difficulty with interpretation of the published observations is that several of the variables that are known to influence HPV are often simultaneously changed and it has been difficult to identify the quantitative influences of each one. In the present work, therefore, a two compartment model has been developed incorporating all the principal variables that have been shown to influence HPV *in vivo*. The final model is useful for interpreting the separate and combined influences of multiple variables on pulmonary hemodynamics and the distribution of blood flow in the lungs.

[1]*This work supported by Grant #GM29628 from the Institute of General Medical Studies, National Institutes of Health.*

II.   DERIVATION OF THE MODEL

The basis for this model is a precise definition of the pulmonary pressure/flow relationships, during normoxia and during hypoxia. The influences of alveolar and pleural pressure, of total flow and left atrial pressure and of alveolar and mixed venous oxygen tension have been incorporated in a two compartment model which allows any combination of these variables to be examined and the results compared to those of experimental observations.

The model has been developed from several sources and these are most conveniently introduced separately as follows:

A.   Pulmonary Pressure/Flow Curves

The research of Y.C. Fung and his co-workers on the morphology and biodynamics of the pulmonary circulation of cat lungs culminated in a seminal paper (1) in which pressure/flow curves for normoxic lungs were derived. The effects of pleural, alveolar and left atrial pressure on the pressure/flow curves of lungs in conditions of normoxia were demonstrated. The mathematical basis for their derivation rests on the development of equations for flow in elastic vessels combined with detailed measurements of the number, diameter, length, compliance and apparent viscosity of blood in eleven orders of arteries, eleven orders of veins and the capillary sheet of a cat lung.

In summary, calculation of a point on the pressure/flow curve, begins at the venous outflow. The resting diameter of the vein (order #11) at the left atrium is increased by the product of the compliance and the transmural pressure, where transmural pressure is the left atrial pressure minus the pleural pressure. The pressure and diameter at the inflow end of the first venous segment is then calculated from $\dot{Q} = \text{Const } [D_{in}5 - D_{out}5]$ (equation #6 from reference 2) where $\dot{Q}$ is the flow and D the diameters at the inlet and outlet and the constant (Const.) includes the length of the vessel, apparent viscosity of blood and geometric constants. The inflow pressure to this segment becomes the outflow pressure to the next segment upstream and the process is repeated for each order of successively smaller diameter veins until the smallest venule (order #1) is reached. For the entire vascular tree, a simple symmetrical branching pattern is assumed and the flow to each vessel is calculated as the total flow divided by the number of vessels of that order. Flow in the capillaries is assumed to have the characteristics of a sheet and the pressure and diameter change across the sheet is calculated from $\dot{Q} = \text{Const } [h^4{}_{in} - h^4{}_{out}]$ (equation #2 from reference 2) where $\dot{Q}$ is the total flow and h the thickness between the capillary sheets at the inlet and the outlet. The constant (Const) includes the length and viscosity factors [corrected for hematocrit (2)] as well as corrections for posts and other geometric constants. The calculation is continued for the eleven orders of arteries, as for the veins, using the fifth power equation until the pulmonary artery pressure at the inflow to the main pulmonary artery is achieved and the calculation terminated. This calculation is repeated with increasing values of total flow and a pressure/flow curve established.

Several features of this calculation should be emphasized. The fifth power equation for calculating flow through the arteries and veins is based on Poiseuille's equation, but modified for elastic tubes that are more or less tapered according to the different transmural pressures at either end and their compliance. The transmural pressure is the difference between intravascular and extravascular pressure. The extravascular pressure is assumed to be equal to the pleural pressure for the extra-alveolar vessels (i.e., arteries of orders 5-11 and veins of orders 5-11) and equal to the alveolar pressure for the intra-alveolar vessels (i.e., arteries and veins of orders 1-4) and the capillary sheet. The fourth power equation for flow through the capillary sheet is based on a consideration of the hydrodynamics of streamlines. While others have suggested a network flow basis for capillary flow (3), it seems likely that both approaches are relevant. The sheet flow representation is more convenient for modelling because the effect of alveolar and venous pressure are clearly defined and the computation is less formidable.

An important characteristic of this model is the compliance of the vessels, for this is why the pressure/flow relationship is curved; with each increment of flow, the intravascular pressures increase, the vessels are progressively distended and the overall conductance increases. But, the second important characteristic is the limited distensibility of the vessels. For the cat, observations of compliance demonstrated that the capillary sheet and the arterioles with resting diameters less than 200 μm asymptotically approach a maximum diameter, or elastic limiting pressure at a transmural pressure of 25 cmH_2O (4), and the conductance of these vessels is not further changed by transmural pressures greater than this elastic limiting pressure. Below the elastic limiting pressure and for all other vessels, diameter increases as a function of the transmural pressure and the compliance, but at the elastic limiting pressure, the vessel or sheet diameter becomes fixed. These are the characteristics of the model described for one lung of the cat. This basic model has been modified in several respects so that it can be utilized for examining pulmonary hemodynamics in other species and other conditions.

B.   Elastic Limiting Pressure

While it is evident that the lung anatomy and detailed pulmonary hemodynamics of the cat differ from those of other species, it is reasonable to expect that the qualitative response will be the same. In fact, the pressure/flow

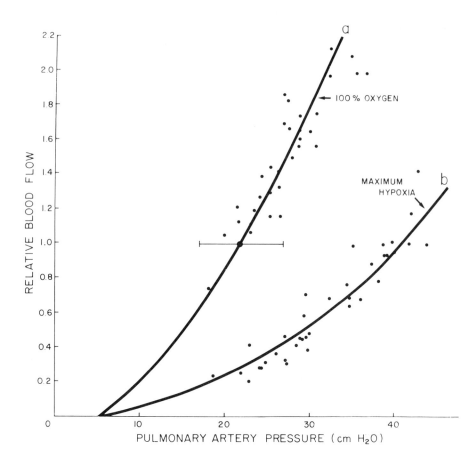

Figure 1. Pressure/flow curves derived from the model (solid lines) are compared to experimental values in dogs (solid circles and crosses) for (a) 100% oxygen ventilation and (b) maximum hypoxic conditions. The lines are calculated assuming: left atrial pressure = 5 cmH₂O; alveolar pressure = 5 cmH₂O; and pleural pressure = 0 to approximate the experimental conditions with 5 cm positive end expiratory pressure and an open thoracotomy. The elastic limiting pressure is 25 cmH₂O for both 100% oxygen and hypoxia and the constriction fraction is 0.6 during maximal hypoxia. Each data point represents the mean from series of 5-12 animals obtained during the course of experiments. The bar crossing the 100% oxygen line at a relative flow of 1.0 represents the range of mean pulmonary artery pressures obtained during 100% oxygen ventilation and normal cardiac output conditions. The experimental values with 100% oxygen are shown as solid circles. The hypoxic values (crosses) are adjusted for maximum hypoxic stimulation. It is evident that the experimental points are clustered around the appropriate curves derived from the model.

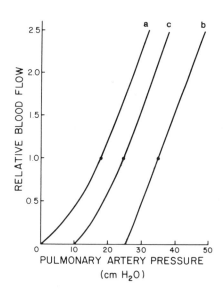

Figure 2. Pressure/flow curves for dog lung calculated from the computer model for 100% oxygen ventilation. a) Left atrial, alveolar and pleural pressures are all zero. b) Alveolar pressure = 10 cmH$_2$O while left atrial and pleural pressures are zero. c) Left atrial pressure = 20 cmH$_2$O, while alveolar and pleural pressure are zero. Because the left atrial pressure in c is equal to the elastic limiting pressure, the pressure/flow curve is truly linear. Even at the highest flow, the other curves only approach asymptotically a straight line extrapolated through their respective origins on the pressure axis.

curves for the dog can be reproduced quantitatively by two modifications of the basic model. The first is to express the flow in relative units where a flow of unity is the normal resting flow and a flow of 2 means that the flow is twice normal and so forth.

The second modification is to select the elastic limiting pressure appropriately for the species. In dogs, an elastic limit is evident at 25 cmH$_2$O for all arteries with resting diameters of less than 1600 µm and for all veins with resting diameters greater than 2000 µm (5). For the dog, the calculated and measured data, for an animal ventilated with 100% oxygen, coincide when this elastic limiting pressure is applied (Fig. la) to all vessels.

The elastic limiting pressure, in combination with the vascular compliance and the alveolar, pleural and left atrial pressures, determines the shape of the pressure/flow curve. These interactions are illustrated for the pulmonary circulation of the dog in Fig. 2. When alveolar, pleural and left atrial pressure are zero, the curvature of the line representing the pressure/flow curve when breathing 100% oxygen (Fig. 2a) is evident. Starting at the origin, each increment of pressure distends the vessels so that conductance increases towards their maximum diameter. As more orders of vessels reach this maximum diameter, the curvature becomes reduced and, at high flows, the pressure/flow curve approximates a straight line. If the left atrial pressure is less than the elastic limiting pressure, the curve will approach a straight line asymptotically, but if the left atrial pressure is equal to or greater than the elastic limiting pressure (Fig. 2b) then all the vessels are maximally distended and the system becomes a rigid one with a constant conductance and a linear pressure/flow relationship.

When alveolar pressure is greater than venous pressure, the flow across the lung becomes dependent on the arterial to alveolar pressure difference rather than the arterial to venous pressure difference. This Starling's resistance or waterfall effect is incorporated in this model at the venous end of the capillary sheet (Fig. 2c) The peculiarity of a Starling resistance is that it is self adjusting to the prevailing conditions (6). For the model, when the alveolar pressure is greater than the intravascular pressure calculated at the inlet to the smallest veins (vein order #1), then the capillary sheet narrows at its junction with these veins so that the intravascular pressure at the capillary side of the junction is equal to the alveolar pressure. As the venous pressure increases, the Starling resistance decreases until it vanishes when the inlet pressure to the smallest veins is equal to or greater than the alveolar pressure. A negative pleural pressure has the effect of increasing the distension, and hence the conductance of the extra-alveolar vessels, while a positive pleural pressure has the opposite effect.

Once the alveolar, pleural and left atrial pressures are selected, the only variable that influences the shape of the pressure/flow curve is the elastic limiting pressure. Application of the elastic limiting pressure to all vessels decreases the conductance changes at high flows and enhances the effects of left atrial pressure on the HPV response. For the large arteries and the smaller veins, this parameter does not have a precise physiological justification. However, it appears to correct for other approximations of the model and, therefore, its use as a modelling device is justified by the extent to which the model is useful.

C.   Two Compartment Model

The generalized model described so far calculates the pressure/flow curve for a single segment of a dog lung ventilated with oxygen. With relative units of flow the pressure/flow curves are the same whatever the size of the segment (Fig. 3). By utilizing two units of the basic model, the left and right lungs can be approximated. If the conditions to the two units are not identical, then a two compartment model results that can be solved by adjusting the division of flow to each side iteratively until the calculated pulmonary artery pressures to both sides are the same. With this arrangement, the effects of differential mechanical influences such as unilateral positive-end-expiratory pressure or of lateral posture can be demonstrated.

The model can be generalized further by allowing the size of the two compartments to vary. For example, if it is required to represent a segment that is one half of one lung (*i.e.*, 25% of total lungs), then the total number of vessels in two lung units are retained, but one compartment contains one and one half the

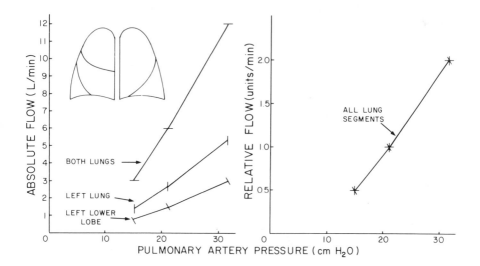

Figure 3. Lung segment size and flow units. On the left are illustrated pressure/flow curves calculated for three sizes of lung segments (both lungs, left lung and left lower lobe) with the flow expressed in absolute units. On the right, the separate pressure/flow curves become one when the flow is expressed in relative units by dividing by the normal flow to the respective unit.

number of vessels in one unit, while the other contains one half. The calculation of the pressure/flow relation proceeds iteratively exactly as before.

It is evidently possible to develop a multi-compartment model in the same manner, but this has not proven necessary in the present context.

D.   Hypoxic Pulmonary Vasoconstriction

Previous work has demonstrated that HPV results from the constriction of precapillary arterioles (7). For the computer model, the vessels sensitive to hypoxia are, therefore, arterioles of orders 1-6, the resting diameter of which are less than 500 μm. These vessels may be constricted by multiplying by a constriction fraction of less than 1.0. It is assumed that the maximum diameters to which these constricted vessels may be distended are not altered and, therefore, a greater transmural pressure than the elastic limiting pressure defined for the normoxic lung, is required before they become fully distended.

In Fig. 1b, the maximum hypoxic responses derived from experimental studies in dogs are shown to be closely approximated by a pressure/flow curve calculated with a constriction fraction of 0.6. This curve and that in Fig. 1a, therefore, define the pressure/flow curves for the dog when the ventilated gas mixture induces a maximal hypoxic response or is 100% oxygen, respectively.

The HPV response is consistent with the vascular smooth muscle being sensitive to the oxygen tension in its vicinity. These relationships can be represented as if there is a discrete sensor for HPV with an oxygen tension (P_{SO_2}) that is a function of both the mixed venous and alveolar oxygen tensions (8):

$$P_{SO_2} = [P_{AO_2}]^{0.62} \times [P\bar{v}_{O_2}]^{0.38} \tag{1}$$

A series of *in vivo* studies in dogs (8,9) have demonstrated the dose/response relationship between P_{SO_2} and HPV. Responses to HPV become detectable when the P_{SO_2} is less than 150 mmHg and are maximal at 30 mmHg. A P_{SO_2} of 55 mmHg results in a response that is 50% of maximum. The relationship between P_{SO_2} and the response, expressed as a fraction of maximum (fR_{max}) is (10):

$$fR_{max} = (P_{SO_2})^{-6.32} / [(1 \times 10^{-11}) + (P_{SO_2})^{-6.32}] \tag{2}$$

and the functional relationship between the response and the initial vascular constriction is defined by

Constriction Fraction $= 1 - 0.866[fR_{max}] + 0.801[fR_{max}]^2 - 0.33[fR_{max}]^3$ (3)

and, therefore, the pressure/flow curves are defined for all degrees of constriction from 0.6 (maximum constriction) to 1.0 (no constriction) in accordance with the P_{SO_2} resulting from any combination of alveolar and mixed venous oxygen tension (Fig. 4). Furthermore, the constriction of each compartment in the two-compartment model can be separately designated.

III.   SEQUENCE OF COMPUTATIONS

In summary, the fundamental characteristics of the pressure/flow curve derived from the original model is modified for the dog lung ventilated with oxygen only by changing the maximum vessel diameters to those achieved by an elastic limiting pressure of 20 cmH$_2$O. The pressure/flow curve for the lung in which maximum hypoxic vasoconstriction has occurred is defined by the same maximal vessel diameters together with reduction of the initial resting diameters of arterioles of order numbers 1-6 by a constriction fraction of 0.6.

The precise shape and position of the specific pressure/flow curve for each of the two compartments is specified by the alveolar, pleural and left atrial pressures together with the state of constriction as defined by the mixed venous and compartmental alveolar oxygen tensions. The distribution of blood flow and the pulmonary artery pressure in a particular set of circumstances is finally dependent on the relative size and constriction of the two compartments and the total flow.

IV.   RESULTS AND DISCUSSION

A model such as that derived herein is valuable to the extent that it reproduces experimental data, allows the identification of variables and suggests underlying mechanisms; these properties will be explored below. An attractive premise of this model is that it is both comprehensive and based fundamentally on the properties of real tissues. It is understood that modifications will be required when the anatomic and biomechanical data for the vasculature of the complete dog lung become available, but it is expected that only the details will change and not the general qualitative or quantitative performance.

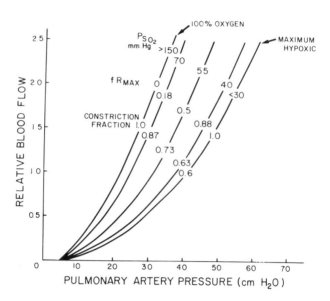

Figure 4. Response of the pressure/flow lines to graded hypoxia.
Utilizing the same conditions as in Fig. 1 (viz. left atrial pressure = 5 cmH₂O;
alveolar pressure = 5 cmH₂O; pleural pressure = 0), the pressure/flow curves have
been derived from the model simulating increasing hypoxia to illustrate the
movement of the curves from the 100% oxygen line. P_{SO_2}, the stimulus for
HPV, is derived from alveolar and mixed venous oxygen tension and, fR_{max} is the
HPV response as a fraction of the maximum response. Thus, when P_{SO_2} is >150
mmHg, HPV is not stimulated, fR_{max} is zero and the pressure/flow curve
corresponds to the 100% oxygen curve of Fig. 1. As P_{SO_2} is decreased, the HPV
response becomes apparent as a shift of the pressure/flow curve to the right. The
response is 50% of maximum (fR_{max} = 0.5) when the P_{SO_2} is 55 mmHg and
< 30 mmHg. The corresponding constriction fraction is also shown to change
from 1.0 for the 100% oxygen line to 0.6 with maximum hypoxia.

A.   Segment Size and the Dual Response to HPV

The pressure/flow relationships for different size segments of normoxic
dog lung expressed in absolute and relative units were illustrated in Fig. 3.

Consider now a dog in which different size segments of the lung are
ventilated so that they exhibit a maximal hypoxic response (P_{SO_2} ≤ 30 mmHg),
while the rest of the lung is ventilated with 100% oxygen. Assume that cardiac

output remains constant at the normal resting value throughout (Fig. 5). When the entire lung is receiving 100% oxygen, all segments are located at the point defined by the normoxic pressure/flow curve at a relative flow of 1.0 and pulmonary artery pressure of 21 cmH_2O. When the entire lung becomes maximally hypoxic, constriction occurs, but because the cardiac output is constant and the relative flow remains at 1.0, the pulmonary artery pressure increases along the horizontal line and the new pressure/flow point is defined on the maximal hypoxic pressure/flow curve at the relative flow of 1.0 and pressure of 40 cmH_2O. In contrast, if a small lung segment, say 25% of the total lung, becomes maximally hypoxic while the rest is ventilated with 100% oxygen, the constriction of this segment results in a marked reduction of blood flow and a small increase in pulmonary artery pressure so that the line on the pressure/flow plot defining these changes will be more vertical. For hypoxic segments of intermediate size such as 45%, the figure shows that pressure and flow changes occur that are intermediate between these two extremes.

It is evident that two responses to hypoxia (the relative magnitude of which is dependent on the segment size) can be distinguished. These responses are reduction of blood flow to the hypoxic segment with diversion of the flow to the rest of the lung, and an increase in pulmonary artery pressure. This dual response, defined by the model, is compared in Fig. 6 to the results published previously (9) for different size dog lung segments. It is apparent that the model closely approximates the empirical polynomial that was defined as the best fit to the data.

Further examination of the two compartment model reveals the basis for these responses. When constriction occurs in the hypoxic segment, the blood flow that is diverted away from that segment must flow through the normoxic segment if cardiac output is to remain constant. The larger the hypoxic segment, the greater the absolute flow of blood that needs to be accommodated by the smaller remaining lung segment and, therefore, the greater the increase of pulmonary artery pressure. However, as pulmonary artery pressure increases, the driving pressure increases and, therefore, the blood flow across the hypoxic segment becomes greater and the effective diversion of blood flow is reduced. These effects for both the 100% oxygen and hypoxic lung are illustrated in Fig. 7 for a situation where the cardiac output is increased to 1.3 times the resting value and 75% of the lung becomes maximally hypoxic. The hypoxic constriction of this segment causes relative blood flow to decrease from 1.3 on the 100% oxygen pressure/flow line to 0.87 on the hypoxic pressure/flow line. The blood that is directed away from this hypoxic lung results in an increase of flow to the 25% of the lung that remains ventilated with oxygen, the relative flow of which increases from 1.3 to 2.58 on the 100% oxygen pressure/flow line. The final pulmonary artery pressure (37 cmH_2O is the same for both lung compartments and it is evident that the

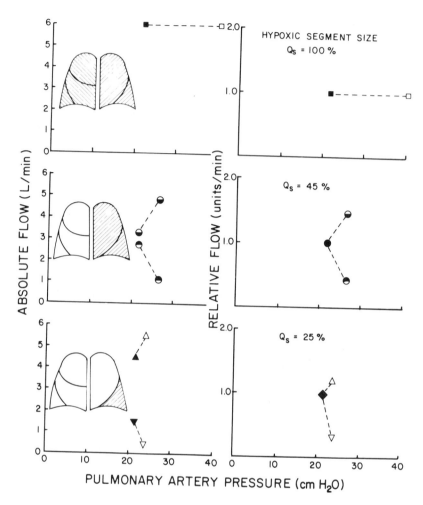

Figure 5. The dual response to HPV. The diagram illustrates the effects
when different size segments (Qs) of lung become maximally hypoxic (shaded
areas of lung) while the rest of the lung remains ventilated with oxygen. For the
panels on the left, the flow is expressed in absolute units. In the middle panel,
flows to the individual lungs are initially 2.7 l/min to the left (Qs = 45%) and 3.3
l/min to the right lung with the common pulmonary artery pressure at 21
cmH$_2$O. When the left lung becomes hypoxic, flow to this segment decreases to
1.0 l/min and flow to the right lung correspondingly increases to 5.0 l/min, while
the pulmonary artery pressure increases to 27 cmH$_2$O. These simultaneous
changes of pulmonary artery pressure and blood flow distribution constitute the

distribution of blood flow between the 100% oxygen and hypoxic segments follows from the shape and position of their respective pressure/flow lines.

The actual blood flows can be readily computed for each segment from the relative blood flow to the test segment during hypoxia multiplied by the product of absolute cardiac output and the relative blood flow to the test segment during 100% oxygen under the same conditions of pleural, alveolar and left atrial pressures. The effects on arterial oxygen tension can also be approximated utilizing the alveolar oxygen tension for each segment.

B.   Variation of P_{SO_2} in the Two Compartments

In the preceding discussion, the hypoxic or test segment was stimulated with a maximal hypoxic stimulus by a P_{SO_2} of 30 mmHg, while the rest of the lung was ventilated with 100% oxygen so that its P_{SO_2} was >600 mmHg and HPV was not stimulated. In practice, all other combinations can be simulated.

A study from Benumof *et al.* (11) generated observations on dog lung in two compartments when many variables were changed simultaneously. When these variables were entered in the computer model, the observed changes of blood flow distribution were reproduced and, furthermore, the underlying mechanism, which had previously been uncertain, could be identified.

In that study, the left lower lobe (LLL) was ventilated throughout with air while the rest of the lung (REST) was ventilated at first with 100% oxygen and then subsequently the oxygen concentration was reduced in steps to 6%. With

dual response to HPV. The magnitude of the response varies with segment size. Thus, as shown in the lower panel, when a smaller lung segment, i.e. left lower lobe (Qs = 25%), is hypoxic, the flow is diverted to the rest of the lung with a smaller increase in pressure. Conversely, the upper panel illustrates the limiting exception when the entire lung becomes hypoxic so no diversion of flow can occur and a maximal increase of pulmonary artery pressure is the only response. The panels on the right column show the same data, but, in relative units, the different segments all start from the same point (i.e. relative flow = 1.0 and pulmonary artery pressure = 21 cmH$_2$O). However, during maximal hypoxia all the points for the hypoxic segments will move from the 100% oxygen pressure/flow curve to the hypoxic one defined in Fig. 1 while the points for the oxygen containing remainder of the lung will move along the 100% oxygen pressure/flow curve. The value of the relative unit format is that all of these relationships can be expressed graphically on the same plot.

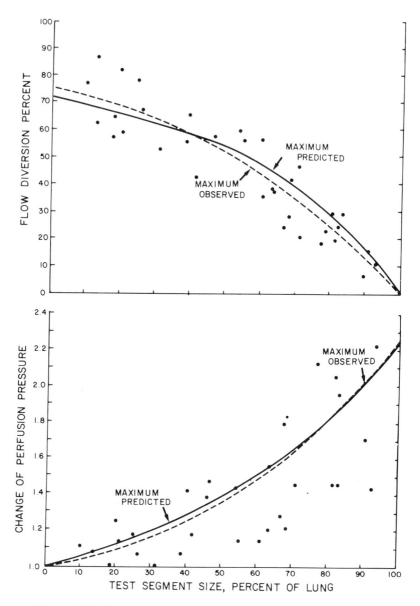

Figure 6. Influence of segment size on HPV in canine lung. The dual response of a) flow diversion and b) perfusion pressure change is shown when different size lung segments are stimulated with maximum hypoxia while the rest of the lung receives 100% oxygen. In both figures, the solid circles are the values previously reported for individual dogs (4) and the dashed lines represent the best fit curves for these observations. The solid lines were calculated from the model with

each reduction of inspired oxygen, the PA_{O_2} to the REST obviously decreased, but in addition, the $P\overline{v}_{O_2}$ decreased and, hence, the PA_{O_2} of the LLL also decreased. To complicate matters further, the cardiac output progressively increased from its initial value of 1.64 l/min to 3.03 l/min when ventilated with 6% oxygen. The experimental data are shown in the table inset of Fig. 8 for three of the conditions (viz. REST ventilated with 100, 12 and 6% oxygen, respectively). The flow to the LLL, measured with an electromagnetic flow probe, was 20% of the cardiac output when the REST received 100% oxygen, increased to 29% of the cardiac output when the REST was ventilated with 12% oxygen, but decreased again to 20% when the REST was ventilated with 6% oxygen. This same sequence of LLL flow changes was reproduced by the model simulation as shown in the final column of the table.

The basis for these changes can be appreciated from the simulated data shown on the pressure/flow plot in Fig. 8. At the start, both segments are close to their resting 100% oxygen values and only a small HPV response is evident because the LLL at point "a" is ventilated with air. The flow to each segment is proportional to its size. When the REST is ventilated with 12% oxygen (point "b"), the Ps_{O_2} in that segment becomes 38 mmHg and a strong HPV response (91% of maximum) is stimulated. The Ps_{O_2} of the LLL also decreases to 54 mmHg and an HPV response (52% of maximum) is stimulated also in the LLL, but since the HPV is greater in the REST segment, blood flow is diverted to the

alveolar pressure = 5 cmH_2O; pleural pressure = 10 cmH_2O; left atrial pressure = 10 cmH_2O; constriction fraction = 0.6 for the hypoxic segment.

The ordinates of flow diversion and change of perfusion pressure are used for ease of comparison with the previous reports (9,17). Flow diversion is calculated as the difference between the flows to the test segment with oxygen and hypoxic expressed as a percent of the flow with oxygen. The greater the flow diversion, the more effective the HPV response in diverting blood away from the hypoxic segment. The perfusion pressure is calculated as the pulmonary artery pressure minus the left atrial pressure and the change of perfusion pressure is the ratio of the perfusion pressure during hypoxia with that during 100% oxygen. The greater this value, the more of the hypoxic response is manifest as pulmonary artery pressure increase.

The figure demonstrates a close agreement between the curves generated by the model and those observed. They show that as more of the lung becomes hypoxic, the effectiveness of HPV to divert blood flow away from the hypoxic segment is reduced while the pulmonary artery pressure is increased.

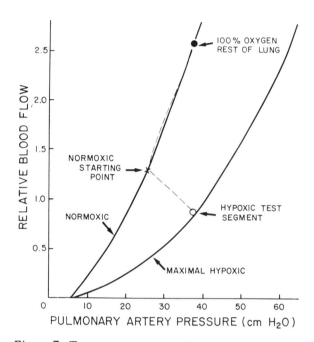

Figure 7. Two compartment model HPV responses. A test segment
consisting of 75% of the lung and the 25% segment representing the rest of the
lung are both ventilated with 100% oxygen. With the cardiac output increased 1.3
fold, the starting point for the relative flow (1.3) and the pulmonary artery pressure
(25 cmH_2O) for both segments coincide on the 100% oxygen pressure/flow curve
at the (x). If maximal HPV is stimulated in the 75% test segment with a PsO_2
≤30mm Hg the relative blood flow will decrease in this segment to 0.87 (open
circle on the hypoxic pressure/flow curve) and the diverted blood will increase the
relative blood flow to the 100% oxygen rest of the lung from 1.3 to 2.58 (closed
circle on the normoxic pressure/flow curve). The pulmonary artery pressure is the
same for both. For this simulation, the alveolar and left atrial pressures are 5
cmH_2O and the pleural pressure is zero.

LLL and its proportional flow increases. The lines on the pressure/flow curve are
shifted up because the cardiac output has increased by 1.3 fold and the cross on the
100% oxygen pressure/flow curve at "b" indicates the new hypothetical origin for
the LLL and the REST if they were both ventilated with 100% O_2.

When the REST is ventilated with 6% oxygen and the cardiac output
increases further to a relative total flow of 1.85, the lines for "c" originate at this
new hypothetical point on the 100% oxygen pressure/flow curve. The PsO_2 of the

REST is now 14 mmHg, a value inducing a maximal HPV response. However, the $P\overline{v}O_2$ is now so reduced that the PsO_2 of the LLL is 37 and an HPV response of 92% of maximum is stimulated there also. The change from point "b" to point "c" is, therefore, associated with a much greater increase in HPV for the LLL than for the REST. Both segments are, therefore, constricted, but to a more similar extent and the blood flow of the LLL decreases accordingly while pulmonary artery pressure increases.

A further simulation is included in Fig. 8 as "d" assumes that all the conditions of point "c" remain constant except that the PAO_2 of the REST is increased to 657 as it was in "a". In these circumstances, a 91% maximal HPV response occurs unopposed in the LLL and its flow decreases to 9% of cardiac output. The effect is further contrasted in the figure; the changes for the LLL and REST are shown for "d" on the dashed lines radiating from the same point on the 100% oxygen curve as "c". The separation between the points for 100% oxygen to the REST and the hypoxic LLL is apparent and, further, it can be intuitively seen that comparing "c" and "d" as the REST is rendered hypoxic, at a constant cardiac output, the lines connecting the LLL and the REST will move towards the hypoxic pressure/flow line and, therefore, will converge until at the same PsO_2 they will superimpose. It is evident that the complex interactions that underlie experimental observations such as these can be conveniently analyzed with this approach and allow more confident conclusions to be advanced.

C.   Cardiac Output Effects

It has been reported on numerous occasions (12), that pulmonary shunt increases when cardiac output increases and several explanations have been advanced for this effect. Several variables inevitably change simultaneously when cardiac output is altered and, therefore, no one hypothesis has been preferred (13).

If the cardiac output is increased twofold, pulmonary artery pressure will increase along the appropriate pressure/flow curve and, assuming oxygen consumption remains constant, the mixed venous oxygen tension will also increase. It was shown above that the mixed venous oxygen tension influences the PsO_2, particularly when the alveolar oxygen tension is reduced and, in fact, in regions of atelectasis the PsO_2 corresponds to the mixed venous oxygen tension. Therefore, it follows that in areas of the lung with zero ventilation/perfusion ratios corresponding to pulmonary shunt, increasing the mixed venous oxygen tension will result in increased shunt flow.

In Fig. 9a, the effects of cardiac output on pulmonary shunt are shown for published data (14) and for the model simulation at the same conditions. The analyses simulated in Fig. 9b demonstrate that essentially all of the changes in

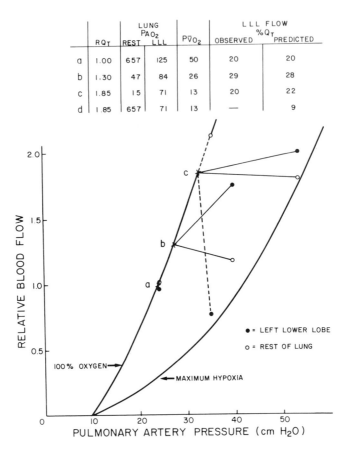

	R_{Q_T}	LUNG P_{AO_2} REST	LUNG P_{AO_2} LLL	$P_{\bar{V}O_2}$	LLL FLOW %Q_T OBSERVED	LLL FLOW %Q_T PREDICTED
a	1.00	657	125	50	20	20
b	1.30	47	84	26	29	28
c	1.85	15	71	13	20	22
d	1.85	657	71	13	—	9

• = LEFT LOWER LOBE

o = REST OF LUNG

100% OXYGEN

MAXIMUM HYPOXIA

RELATIVE BLOOD FLOW

PULMONARY ARTERY PRESSURE (cm H_2O)

Figure 8. Comparison of experimental data and model simulation for hypoxic vasoconstriction for two compartments simultaneously. The experimental data are from dogs (18) in which the left lower lobe (LLL) was ventilated with air throughout while the rest of the lung (REST) was ventilated with a) 100% oxygen, b) 12% oxygen or c) 6% oxygen. The data for the relative cardiac output (R · Qt), alveolar oxygen tension (P_{AO_2}, mmHg) in the REST and LLL, the mixed venous oxygen tension ($P\bar{v}O_2$ mmHg) and the observed LLL flow as a percent of cardiac output are shown in the table insert together with the LLL flow predicted from the computer model with the same conditions. It was assumed that the alveolar pressure was 5 cmH_2O in both segments, the left atrial pressure was 9.7 cmH_2O and the pleural pressure was zero throughout. The predicted relative flows and pressure for the REST and the LLL are also shown for each condition on the pressure/flow plot. The interpretation of this material is discussed in the text, but, in summary, as the inspired oxygen to the REST is

pulmonary shunt can be accounted for by changes in mixed venous oxygen tension and not by changes in pressure or flow themselves.

D.   Left Atrial Pressure

In Fig. 10, normoxic and hypoxic pressure/flow curves are calculated for conditions in which the left atrial pressure was changed from 9.7 to 34 cmH_2O. The separation between the respective normoxic and hypoxic curves is a direct measure of the HPV response and it is clear that the response is reduced at the greater left atrial pressure. For both curves, the simulated hypoxic constriction was the same (constriction fraction = 0.69), but the increased venous and capillary distension associated with the increased left atrial pressure reduced the vascular resistance change that could result for this initial constriction and, therefore, the pressure and flow responses were reduced. The conditions used to generate these pressure/flow lines were the same as those reported in dogs (15). For the experimental series, the blood flow to the LLL was measured during normoxia and hypoxia while the rest of the lung was ventilated with oxygen. The left atrial pressure was then increased to 34 cmH_2O either by infusing fluids during which cardiac output increased 2.9 fold or by inflating a left atrial balloon during which cardiac output decreased to 0.7 of the normal value. With both procedures, the hypoxic response of LLL blood flow was reduced. With the normal left atrial pressure, the hypoxic response of LLL reduced its blood flow by 52%, but with either procedure associated with increasing the left atrial pressure, the change of blood flow during hypoxia was reduced to about 14%. It is evident that the results are reproduced quite precisely by the simulation shown in Fig. 10. The basis of this effect of the left atrial pressure is revealed by analysis of the simulation and is due to the predominant influence of the left atrial pressure on the distension of the

decreased, the LLL flow at first increases and then decreases as a result of the different extent to which HPV is stimulated in the two segments. At "a", the two segments are close because HPV is minimal in both while in "c" they also become close because HPV approaches the maximum in both.

The condition "d", shown on the last row in the table and by the dashed lines in the figure, illustrated the hypothetical situation where the conditions are as in "c" except for the PAO_2 of the REST which is normoxic as in "a". The result is a near maximal HPV in the LLL unopposed by HPV in the REST, and this is demonstrated by the much reduced LLL flow and the wide separation in the dashed lines.

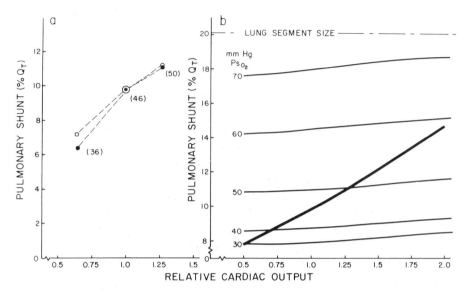

Figure 9. Relationship between pulmonary shunt and cardiac output. Panel a: The data (filled circles) from Smith, et al. (10) for pulmonary shunt shows that it increases as cardiac output increases. The figures in parentheses are the observed $P\bar{v}O_2$ values. Under the same conditions (alveolar pressure = 5 cmH_2O, pleural pressure = -3 cmH_2O) of oxygen tensions, releative cardiac output and left atrial pressure, the model predicts (open circles) essentially the same changes assuming that a 21.7% segment of the lung is hypoxic (atelectatic). Panel b: The effects of PsO_2 and cardiac output changes are separated in this simulation, while all other variables are maintained constant to a 21.7% atelectatic test segment. The fine lines predict that blood flow to this segment, or pulmonary shunt, changes little if PsO_2 is maintained constant while cardiac output changes. Thus, the line for PsO_2 40 is almost horizontal. The thick line in contrast shows the effect expected if oxygen consumption remains constant so that $P\bar{v}O_2$ and hence PsO_2 increased with increasing cardiac output. In these circumstances, as the relative cardiac output increases from 0.5 to 2.0, the PsO_2 increases from 30 to 58 mmHg and pulmonary shunt increases from 8 to 14% as the stimulation of HPV declines. In practice, panel a, the flow to the hypoxic or atelectatic segment, is determined primarily by the PsO_2, but modified also by changes in left atrial pressure that may accompany changes in flow.

venous end of the bed (Fig. 11). As the left atrial pressure increases, the vascular bed distends so that the conductance increases and the slope of the pressure/flow

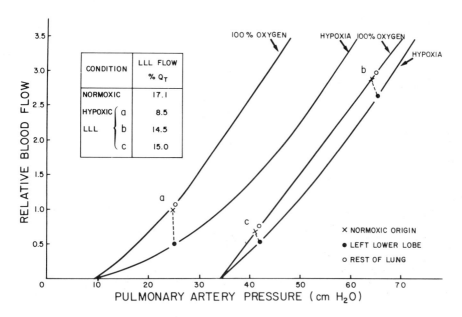

Figure 10. Influence of left atrial pressure on HPV responses. The solid lines are the normoxic and hypoxic pressure/flow curves calculated for left atrial pressures of both 9.4 and 34 cmH₂O. The remaining conditions are: alveolar pressure = 5.4 cmH₂O; pleural pressure = 0; and constriction fraction = 0.69. The HPV response of a lung segment corresponding to the left lower lobe (17.1% of total lung) is simulated. When the left atrial pressure is 9.4 cmH₂O, hypoxia causes a 50.2% decrease in LLL blood flow, but when the left atrial pressure is 34 and hypoxia is induced, the blood flow only decreases by 15.2% and by 13.3% when the cardiac output is increased (2.9 times normal) and decreased (0.2 times normal), respectively. The insert tabulates the calculated LLL flow for each of the conditions and these effects are essentially identical to those reported experimentally (10). See text for further discussion.

curve becomes steeper; but, as the vessel diameter increases, the successive increments have less effect on pressure and flow and so the normoxic and hypoxic curves will approach each other even in the absence of an elastic limit. This process is enhanced by the presence of the elastic limit because each order of vessel eventually reaches its maximum diameter, so that the pressure/flow curves eventually approach the same straight line. The result of these relationships is the prediction that all responses to HPV will be progressively reduced as the left atrial pressure is increased.

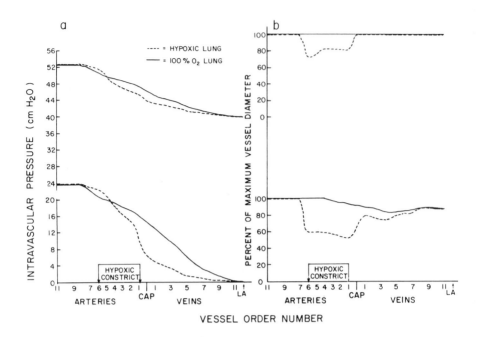

Figure 11. Basis for reduction of HPV response with increased left atrial pressure. In this simulation (alveolar pressure = 5 cmH₂O; pleural pressure = 0 cmH₂O), the left lung was stimulated with maximum hypoxia and the right lung remained normoxic while the left atrial pressure was maintained at zero or at 40 cmH₂O and the relative cardiac output was 1.0. Panel a shows the detailed changes in the intravascular pressures across each of the 23 orders of vessels from the left atrium (LA) to the final pulmonary artery pressure at the order #11 artery. Hypoxic constriction at the orders 1-6 arteries results in a pulmonary artery pressure that is higher than in the normoxic segment in those vessels upstream from the middle of the constricted vessels. Conversely, the intravascular pressure is reduced in all vessels downstream from the constricted vessels. When the left atrial pressure is zero, these effects are large, but at a left atrial pressure of 40 cmH₂O, the differences between the hypoxic and normoxic segment are reduced. The reason for this becomes clearer in panel b, where the diameter at the flow end of each vessel segment is expressed as a percent of its maximum diameter when fully distended. In the lower figure, with the left atrial pressure at zero, the diameters of both the normoxic and the hypoxic lung segments (except for the largest arteries) are not fully distended and there is a large difference between the constricted and non-constricted small arterioles which extends well into the small and medium sized veins. When the left atrial pressure is increased to 40 cmH₂O (upper figure), all the vessels, are maximally distended whether hypoxic or

V.   SUMMARY AND CONCLUSIONS

The theory of the physiological basis for the responses of hypoxic pulmonary vasoconstriction that is advanced here possesses the advantage that it is based on anatomic, biodynamic and physiologic data and that it consistently accounts for experimental results from a wide variety of conditions. The effects of gravity have been ignored for this presentation because all of the experimental data were from animals in the prone or supine position. However, the influence of gravity is easily incorporated and the well known changes of blood flow in the vertical lung correspond to regional shifts of the pressure/flow curves.

The model provides a conceptual framework for understanding complex interactions and it appears to be particularly useful for the interpretation of data when several variables are simultaneously altered. On this basis, active pharmacologic effects are convincingly suggested where previously conclusions were uncertain (16), and it is evident, for example (Fig. 11), that hypoxic pulmonary vasoconstriction is unlikely to provide protection from hydrostatic pulmonary edema.

It should be emphasized that, while predictions of the model are remarkably consistent with the mean results of experimental series, this version of the model should not be expected to project the results for an individual subject. The nature and range of individual variability suggests that additional, presently unknown factors will have to be incorporated before the performance of an individual animal can be reliably predicted.

ACKNOWLEDGMENTS

The authors are grateful to the following colleagues who contributed both to the collection of data and to the development of the ideas on which this analysis is based: Karen Domino, Steven Glasser, Linda Chen, Christian Alexander, Frank Miller, Leena Lindgren and Seong Dok Kim. The authors also thank Jonathan Reed for technical expertise and Cathi Mercer Gan for the preparation of the manuscript.

normoxic, except for the arterioles of orders #1-6 during hypoxia. Even the constricted arterioles are re-expanded by the increased transmural pressure so that their diameter is nearer the maximum. It is, therefore, evident that blood flow in the hypoxic and normoxic segments will be more similar when the left atrial pressure is 40 cmH₂O and, therefore, the responses to HPV are reduced.

REFERENCES

1.   Zhuang FY, Fung YC and Yen RT. (1983) *J Appl Physiol* **55**:1341.
2.   Yen MRT and Fung YC. (1973) *J Appl Physiol* **35**:510.
3.   Warrel DA, Evans JW, Clark RO, Kingaby GP and West JB. (1972) *J Appl Physiol* **32**:346.
4.   Fung YC. (1984) *In* **Biodynamics: Circulation.** Springer Verlag:New York.
5.   Maloney JE, Rooholamini SA and Wexler L. (1970) *Microvasc Res* **2**:1.
6.   Dawson CA. (1984) *Physiol Rev* **64**:544.
7.   Fishman AP. (1976) *Circ Res* **38**:221.
8.   Domino KB, Wetstein L, Glasser SA, Lindgren L, Marshall C, Harken A and Marshall BE. (1983) *Anesthesiology* **59**:428.
9.   Marshall BE, Marshall C, Benumof J and Saidman LJ. (1981) *J Appl Physiol* **51**:1543.
10.   Marshall BE and Marshall C. (1985) *In* **Effects of Anesthesia.** Amer Physiol Soc:Bethesda, MD.
11.   Benumof JL. (1981) *J Appl Physiol* **51**:871.
12.   Cheney FW and Colley PS. (1980) *Anesthesiology* **52**:496.
13.   Breen PH, Schumacker PT, Sandouan J, Mayers I, Oppenheimer L and Wood LDM. (1985) *J Appl Physiol* **59**:1313.
14.   Smith G, Cheney FW and Winter PM. (1974)*Br J Anaesth* **46**:337.
15.   Benumof JL and Wahrenbrock EA. (1975) *J Appl Physiol* **38**:846.
16.   Angle M, Ducas J, Schick U, Girling L and Prewitt RM. (1984) *J Appl Physiol* **57**:1498.
17.   Marshall BE and Marshall C. (1980) *J Appl Physiol* **49**:189
18.   Marshall BE and Marshall C. (1983) *J Appl Physiol* **55**:711.
19.   Marshall C and Marshall BE. Submitted to J Appl Physiol, 1986.

Pulmonary Hemodynamics: Summary

The discussion of pulmonary hemodynamics emphasized a new appreciation of the relationship between structure and the detailed hemodynamic properties of the pulmonary circulation. Furthermore, it has become clear that changes in the distribution of blood flow and volume in acute pathophysiologic conditions are attributable to active regulatory processes, particularly hypoxic pulmonary vasoconstriction.

Chris Dawson (Medical College of Wisconsin, Milwaukee) presented an overview of the work by himself and his coworkers concerning the changes in pulmonary pressure and volumes that follow independent or simultaneous occlusion of the pulmonary arteries and veins. Utilizing a series of black box mathematical models of increasing complexity they have identified, both quantitatively and qualitatively, variables that allow observations from in vivo preparations to be reproduced. In particular, this work has suggested that pulmonary microvasculature, including the capillaries and possibly adjacent small arteries and veins, is the principal site of intrapulmonary vascular compliance, while changes in vascular resistance occur upstream or downstream from this region. This conclusion accounts for most of the experimental observations, but, with the addition of model elements representing viscoelasticity and volume dependent compliance and resistance, it was possible to model more precisely the time sequence for the changes in pressures and volume observed after vascular occlusion.

For the black box modelling approach, all of the parameters representing the internal properties of the lungs are assigned by the investigator. In contrast, the model developed by Y.C. Fung (University of California, San Francisco) and his associates is a deterministic one in which they have systematically attempted to define and measure all of the relevant properties of the pulmonary vasculature, and to combine these with equations derived rigorously from hydrodynamic theory. In his discussion, Dr. Fung utilized this model to examine the basis for pulmonary flow changes in Zone 2 conditions. The critical factor was the identification that pulmonary veins are so tethered by surrounding structures that they do not collapse even when the transmural pressure is compressive. The site of flow restriction in Zone 2 condition was shown to be the venous end of the capillary sheet, therefore, the transmural pressure determining waterfall or sluicegate like behavior is at this site. A further conclusion from this formulation was that additional energy is required to reopen the collapsed vessels and, therefore, that experimental observations should be interpreted in the light of the immediately preceeding history. Perhaps, in analogy with studies of the mechanics of the air spaces wherein the lung is often hyperinflated in order to reduce variability prior to the observations, the pulmonary vasculature might need to be perfused in Zone 3 conditions prior to performing an experiment.

Two subsequent presentations utilized modification of the deterministic model of Y.C. Fung and his coworkers with in vivo and in vitro animal model preparations. Wayne Mitzner (Johns Hopkins University, Baltimore) reexamined previously published data on pulmonary vascular pressure/flow curves from pig lungs exposed to normoxic and hypoxic conditions. They compared the observed data to two models. The curves could be approximated by a rigid tube model incorporating multiple Starling resistances or by the distensible morphometric model, described by Fung for the cat lung, scaled to reproduce the pressure and flow characteristics observed in pigs. The key observation was that in order for the shift in the pressure flow curves seen with hypoxia to be accounted for by the distensible vessel model the distensibility of the resistance vessels had to be increased as their resistances increased. Such behavior is not unlike that of a Starling resistance, suggesting that the two models are part of the same continuum rather than diametrically opposed.

The presentation by Bryan Marshall (University of Pennsylvania, Philadelphia) also utilized the Fung model, but the data from the cat were generalized by normalizing the flow and a two compartment model was shown capable of reproducing a variety of experimental observations concerning hypoxic pulmonary vasoconstriction from dogs in vivo. Marshall's group has argued that this approach may allow quantitative identification of which variables influence pulmonary hemodynamics when several variables are changes simultaneously.

These studies using the deterministic modeling reemphasized the need for detailed biodynamic measurements of the pulmonary vasculature in different species to allow discrimination of which specific variables change with animal size and in different conditions.

The role of gravity in the distribution of pulmonary perfusion has been a major contributor to understanding in this area since it was popularized by the work of J.B. West and S. Permutt and others in the past 20 years. However, detailed observations have suggested that gravity alone is not a sufficient explanation for the inhomogeneity of flow distribution that is observed even in normal lungs. This was the theme of the presentation by Tawfic Hakim (McGill

University, Montreal) who utilized single photon emission computerized tomography and radioactive microspheres to generate three dimensional maps of the distribution of pulmonary perfusion. These maps revealed a consistent pattern of increased central and diminished peripheral flow in all lung lobes. The possible explanations for these observations remain to be confirmed.

Overall, the emerging view of the pulmonary circulation is, therefore, one that superimposes more complex and actively regulated flow and volume characteristics onto the passive mechanical properties that have long dominated thinking in this area. Such a deeper appreciation has already stimulated contributions to the basic understanding and management of pathophysiologic processes.

BRYAN E. MARSHALL

Pulmonary Blood Flow and Gas Exchange

Pulmonary Blood Flow and Gas Exchange: Introduction

I.   THE SPEAKERS

In his opening remarks one of the chairmen quoted Dr. Bill Briscoe, an eminent physiologist and colleague of Dr. André Cournand who, while taking issue with Dr. P. P. Wagner, said in a letter:

"At least we agree that the lung is an organ whose main function is gas exchange rather than the production of macrophages or the manufacture of angiotensin converting enzyme to regulate blood pressure" (Bull. Europ. Physiopath. Resp. 16:152P, 1980)

While we did not mean these remarks to be taken seriously, gas exchange is the raison d'étre of the pulmonary circulation!

In his overview, Dr. J.M.B. Hughes discussed the role of molecular diffusion, firstly in the gas phase within the acinus, and then in the tissue phase. He pointed out (as had Dr. Briscoe in his letter, *vide supra*) situations where heterogeneity of diffusion-perfusion ($D/\dot{Q}$) ratios may play the major role in the development of arterial hypoxaemia and an abnormal alveolar-arterial gradient. The hematocrit and transit time through the microcirculation were also considered. Dr. David Dantzker dealt with the pertinent question of gas exchange in conditions affecting primarily the pulmonary vessels. He discussed the use of the multiple inert gas infusion technique for measuring the heterogeneity of $\dot{V}_A/\dot{Q}$ distribution. $\dot{V}_A/\dot{Q}$ mismatching was not particularly bad in primary pulmonary hypertension (though made worse by vasodilator drugs) and the development of hypoxæmia on exercise was attributed mainly to a low cardiac output and gross desaturation of the mixed venous blood. Dr. Brian Whipp gave a very clear exposition of the coupled response of pulmonary blood flow and ventilation at the onset of exercise. The increase in blood flow in the first 15 seconds contributes, by itself, significantly to the increase in oxygen uptake (even if ventilation is not allowed to change). Will pulmonary vasodilator drugs improve the performance of transient exercise in patients with respiratory disease? Dr. Sylvester considered the old but intriguing question of the site of hypoxic vasoconstriction as illustrated by the effects of lung inflation on pressure-flow relations in normoxia and hypoxia in two species, the ferret and the pig, with different patterns of pulmonary vascular smooth muscle (see article by Dr. J. M. Kay, this volume). In the ferret, hypoxic vaso-constriction occurs in upstream extra-alveolar vessels, but in the pig some of the responsive vessels are influenced by alveolar pressure; the mechanism remains speculative! Since the classic article of von Eular and Liljestrand (Acta. Phys. Scand. 12:301-320, 1946), hypoxic vasoconstriction has been considered a potentially important mechanism for reducing the heterogeneity of $\dot{V}_A/\dot{Q}$ ratios. In an elegant analysis, using control theory, Dr. Brydon Grant showed that because of the shape of the oxygen dissociation curve, this mechanism can only compensate at best for 60% of any imposed local fall of alveolar PO_2. Worse than that, the efficiency is optimal at alveolar PO_2's c. 70 mmHg ($\dot{V}_A/\dot{Q}$ 0.4) dropping away at very low $\dot{V}_A/\dot{Q}$ ratios where it is most needed.

II.   POSTER COMMENTARY

Dr. Hervé and colleagues from Hôpital Antoine Béclere in Paris had measured the compliance of large pulmonary arteries using a coneangiographic technique during cardiac catheterisation in man. They showed that almitrine bismesylate, a carotid body agonist which also increases PVR, decreased arterial distensibility. In response to questions, they were not clear how this related to the improvement in $\dot{V}_A/\dot{Q}$ distribution which has been observed with this drug. Dr. Marrone and colleagues from Palermo presented interesting data on pulmonary artery pressure (PAP) and SaO_2 (oximetry) in humans with the obstructive sleep apnoea syndrome. The rise in PAP and fall in SaO_2 in sleep (more severe in REM sleep) was completely reversed by the application of continuous positive airway pressure by face-mask. The presentation of Dr. Melst and colleagues from Brussels extended Dr. Brydon Grant's analysis of the efficiency of hypoxic vasoconstriction (HPV) to normal human volunteers. They reached similar conclusions to those drived by Dr. Grant from his work in the coati mundi (South American raccoon)! HPV was not very effective in limiting the arterial hypoxaemia induced by lowering inspired oxygen to 12.5%. Dr. Prefaut and his colleagues from Montpellier in southern France have reported previously on the effect of water immersion (to the neck) on pulmonary gas exchange. They have shown that airway closure occurs in the dependent half of the lung. Thus immersion is a good human model for HPV. Intriguingly, they showed that the hypoxæmia and inversion of the normal gradient of regional blood flow (studied with radioisotopic techniques) induced by immersion could be reversed by deep breathing. There was also a tendency for the immersion-induced hypoxæmia to diminish with time; this may reflect an effect of HPV but other explanations are possible. The only non-European poster presentation was from Dr. Schuster and the team in St. Louis, Missouri, who have been using positron emission tomography (PET) to measure regional blood flow water volumes and protein (transferrin) permeability in dogs with oleic acid acute lung injury. PET is a major step forward in defining structure-function relationships within and between lung regions The measurements are non-invasive and relatively exact since the geometric conditions are defined precisely. Dr. Schuster also had measurements in two patients after recovery from ARDS which indicated that microvascular permeability to transferrin remained abnormal.

JMB HUGHES

Pulmonary Blood Flow and Gas Exchange: An Overview

J.M.B. HUGHES
Department of Medicine,
Royal Postgraduate Medical School
Hammersmith Hospital
London, W12 OHS, United Kingdom.

I.   INTRODUCTION

In this overview I shall focus on the microvasculature as the site of gas exchange. Within the acinus, diffusion-perfusion imbalance may be more important as a cause of impaired gas exchange than ventilation-perfusion inhomogeneity.

II.   BLOOD FLOW AND GAS EXCHANGE WITHIN THE ACINUS.

The human lung consists of approximately 23,000 acini each with a diameter of 6.7 mm (1) and containing c. 1-2000 alveolar sacs. At the present time the spatial resolution of external imaging techniques is insufficient to distinguish functional differences between acini. With rapid freezing techniques static measurements, such as the volume of blood and number of patent capillary vessels, within and between acini can be determined. In perfused dog lungs, Warrell *et al.* (2) concluded that inhomogeneity of vascular volume and recruitment occurred within rather than between arteriolar domains. Does this imply inhomogeneity of blood flow and gas exchange within the acinus? Presumably for blood flow, but probably not for gas exchange, for the following reasons. The acinus begins at Weibel's generation 15; respiratory bronchioles terminate at

The Pulmonary Circulation
in Health and Disease

281

generation 18 and alveolar ducts and sacs continue until generation 26. The branching is asymmetric and the majority of sacs appear from generations 20-26 (3 mm difference in axial distance). In the normal lung at rest, inspired gas is transported by convection to generations 16-18 with further penetration into alveolar sacs predominantly by molecular diffusion (3). Although the expanding surface area favours rapid diffusion, the furthest sacs because of the longer distance have a lower concentration (as much as 6% for a foreign gas) at end-inspiration which persists even after 10 sec breath-holding (3). In terms of an alveolar-arterial gradient for oxygen for the acinus (assuming uniform intra-acinar blood flow) the diffusion-based gradient of alveolar PO_2 contributes little (<0.2 mmHg; 4). Is the distribution of blood flow uniform? It is not, but available evidence suggests the proximal part of the acinus is better perfused than the distal *i.e.*, a) from washout of inhaled versus i.v. ^{13}N (5), b) from the intra-acinar distribution of radiolabelled albumin particles (6), and c) from the improvement in A-a DO_2 when SF_6 replaces N_2 as the carrier gas for inspiration (7). The explanation for the latter is that in the presence of the heavy gas (SF_6) the convective front penetrates deeper but diffusive mixing with the distal (by implication more poorly perfused) sacs is reduced. Finally, analysis of single expirations suggest that units which empty late are the least well perfused (8,9). Thus the inhomogeneity of acinar blood flow which occurs normally would tend to match the serial distribution of ventilation and favor gas exchange.

There are grounds for believing that in the normal lung the acinus is the functional unit for pulmonary gas exchange. Young *et al.* (10) found that arterioles of at least 150 μm diameter had to be blocked (with beads) to produce high $\dot{V}_A/\dot{Q}$ regions detectable by the MIGET technique. Beads of similar size (but not smaller ones) produced inhomogeneity of clearance of inhaled $C^{15}O_2$ uptake and impaired diffuse equilibrium of injected $H_2^{15}O$ in perfused lobes (11). Swinburne *et al.* (11) calculated that the domain of such vessels would have a diameter of 4 mm *i.e.*, close to acinar size.

III.   DIFFUSION-PERFUSION RATIO

The previous section has related diffusion in the gas phase to the distribution of pulmonary blood flow; tissue diffusion is another step which intervenes between the alveolus and the red cell. Assuming no impairment of tissue diffusion, alveolar and end-capillary partial pressures are in equilibrium, the actual value (at fixed inspired and mixed venous values) being determined by the local $\dot{V}_A/\dot{Q}$ ratio. Nevertheless, capillary PO_2 starts at the mixed venous level. What factors determine its rate of rise towards alveolar PO_2 (and the inverse for

PCO_2)? The major factor is the Bohr integral or $D/\dot{Q}$ ratio. This is a dimensionless number (like $\dot{V}_A/\dot{Q}$) which relates diffusing capacity (or diffusive conductance) to perfusive conductance ($\dot{Q} \times \beta$) where β is the instantaneous slope of the dissociation curve ($\Delta C/\Delta P$) of blood for gas. Since $\dot{Q} = Q_c/t_c$ where Q_c is capillary blood volume and t_c is capillary transit time the Bohr integral can be rewritten: $DL \cdot t_c/Q \cdot \beta$ (12). Alveolar-end-capillary disequilibrium, expressed as Pc'/P_A, is >0.95 for Bohr integral values >3 (all inert gases and oxygen in normoxia), 0.6 for a value of 1.0 (oxygen in hypoxia) and 0.04 for a value of 0.03 (carbon monoxide). Thus equilibration is nearly instantaneous for inert gases such as nitrous oxide and acetylene which are used to measure cardiac output (perfusion dependent alveolar removal) but never occurs for carbon monoxide (diffusion dependent uptake). The differences between gases are actually determined by the β_{tiss}/β_b ratio where the subscripts tiss and b refer to the solubility of gas in lung tissue and blood respectively; this ratio is 1.0 for inert gases but <0.01 for carbon monoxide (13). From the Bohr integral the factors favouring alveolar-capillary disequilibrium or "block" for oxygen are a low diffusing capacity, short capillary transit time, large capillary volume and a position on the steepest portion of the oxygen dissociation curve ($PO_2 < 45$ mmHg). There are several physiological and clinical situations where alveolar-capillary block occurs.

A.   Gas Exchange at Altitude

The observation that when man exercises at a low inspired PO_2 his cyanosis deepens is quite old (14). Lilienthal et al. (15) found that the alveolar-arterial (A-a) PO_2 gradient in normal subjects averaged 9 mmHg at rest and 16 mmHg on exercise both breathing air and during hypoxia (alveolar PO_2 33 mmHg); if $\dot{V}_A/\dot{Q}$ inhomogeneity had continued to play the major role during hypoxia the gradient should have diminished considerably. West et al. (16) have reported some unique observations from the 1981 American Medical Research Expedition to Mt Everest on climbers acclimatized at an altitude of 6,300 m (inspired PO_2 64 mmHg) exercising when inspired oxygen was only 14% (inspired PO_2 43 mmHg, equivalent to that on the summit). In two subjects arterial oxygen saturation fell from 60% (rest) to 48% (exercise at VO_2 1.0 l/min). Using data from an Italian expedition (17) Piiper (12) has calculated that maximal exercise in acclimatized subjects at 5,350 m (P_IO_2 72 mmHg) is associated with a Bohr integral value of 0.44 compared with 2.1 at rest; this value of 0.44 suggests a large degree of diffusion limitation and a substantial alveolar- end-capillary PO_2 gradient. Although D_LO_2 increases on exercise (from 54 to 65 ml/min/mmHg) (18), and may be even higher in climbers, the Bohr integral falls because $\dot{Q}$ (25 l/min) and β (in deep hypoxia) are so high.

B.   Clinical Alveolar-Capillary Block

The occurrence of cyanosis on exercise in patients with fibrotic and granulomatous lung disease was described and analysed in classic articles from the Bellevue Hospital Cardiopulmonary Laboratory (19,20). All patients had a low oxygen diffusing capacity and an alveolar-arterial oxygen tension gradient which did not fall when they breathed hypoxic gas mixtures (*vide supra*). Although these patients do have some $\dot{V}_A/\dot{Q}$ inhomogeneity at rest (21), the low $D_L O_2$ in relation to $\dot{Q}$ on exercise is the main reason for the development of cyanosis.

Severe hypoxæmia can occur in chronic liver disease, generally attributed to intrapulmonary arterio-venous shunts but actually caused by severe $D/\dot{Q}$ imbalance (22) in a pulmonary microvasculature where the gas-exchanging vessels have become grossly (tenfold) dilated (23). The carbon monoxide diffusing capacity in such patients is low, presumably because of an unfavourable surface area/thickness ratio and large diffusion distance into the middle of the vessel lumen. Singh *et al.* (24) have presented an interesting mathematical analysis of pulmonary oxygen transport which predicts that the distance along the capillary for complete oxygen equilibrium to occur increases more than threefold as capillary diameter increases from 10 to 20 µm; since capillary length is finite, alveolar-capillary disequilibrium must occur as capillaries enlarge pathologically.

IV.   PULMONARY MICROHEMATOCRIT

The diameter of stationary red cells is often larger than that of the pulmonary capillaries and they may assume a "parachute" configuration (25) in traversing them. Plasma is thus squeezed to the edge of small vessels where it forms a relatively stationary cuff, the Fåhraeus-Lindqvist phenomenon (26). The corollary is that pulmonary microvascular hematocrit (Hct) must be less than large vessel Hct since red cells accelerate relative to plasma in the capillary bed (but decelerate when they reach the pulmonary veins). In normal dogs, analysis of the quantity of red cells versus plasma in lung homogenates (27) and of their different transit times (28) suggests that lung hematocrit is 15% less than large vessel Hct. Recently, in man, the Hct in the lung periphery has been measured with positron emission tomography using ^{11}C-labelled red cells and ^{11}C-methyl albumin (29), and a ratio of 0.9 between lung and heart chamber or peripheral venous Hct found. To the extent that 70% of pulmonary blood in the field of view is in larger vessels with a normal hematocrit, the capillary Hct will be 0.67 of the large vessel value or about 0.3 absolutely. Using similar methods the hematocrit in human brain is at 0.69 of the arterial value (30). The Roughton-Forster technique (31) for calculating pulmonary capillary volume using carbon monoxide yields volumes of about 100 ml. If a microhematocrit of 0.3 is assumed, the resulting values (150 ml) are somewhat closer to morphometric estimates (150-250 ml) reported by Weibel (32).

V.   PULMONARY VASCULAR TRANSIT TIMES

Capillary transit time is one of the components of the Bohr integral. Using inhaled carbon monoxide to measure pulmonary capillary volume (31) Johnson et al. (33) calculated an average capillary transit time of 0.8 s decreasing to 0.5 s on exercise. Regional measurements using inhaled $C^{15}O$ and $C^{15}O_2$ suggest a 50% decrease in transit times during moderate exercise (50 W) in both upper and lower zones in seated subjects (34). These measurements refer to red cell transit only, though this is the most relevant for oxygen exchange. Plasma transit has been measured more directly by recording photometrically the passage of fluorescein isothio-cyanate in arterioles and venules (<20 μm diam.) on the pleural surface of anæsthetized dogs (35). Mean transit times were 12.7 ± 3.2 s at low pulmonary artery pressures falling to 4.0 s at elevated pressures. The fastest transit was 0.3 s. The slow transit for a plasma marker is not surprising in view of the Fåhraeus-Lindqvist effect.

Using a positron camera and inhaled ^{11}CO to measure vascular volume (36) L.H. Brudin (personal communication) in the MRC Cyclotron Unit at this hospital has calculated vascular transit times in the periphery of the supine human lung. The spatial resolution was 17 mm^3 and the vascular volume contained blood in small arteries and veins (c.70%) as well as capillaries (c.30%). Vascular volumes were corrected for microhematocrit differences. In the supine lung at rest the vertical gradients (ventral to dorsal) of blood flow (12.2 to 19.9 ml/min/g lung tissue) and blood volume (1.2 to 1.7 ml/g) are well matched so that peripheral transit times vary little (4.3 to 6.4 s) and not in any systematic way. In chronic airflow obstruction, peripheral regions with very low extravascular density (by implication emphysematous) had prolonged peripheral vascular transit times (7-18 s) but in patients with a more bronchitic pattern (normal or high extravascular density), peripheral transit times were sometimes reduced (1.3 - 4.2 s). In stable asthmatics, transit times in abnormal, *i.e.* poorly ventilated, regions also tended to be prolonged. The significance of the prolonged transit times in emphysema and asthma is not clear but hyperinflation may play a part.

REFERENCES

1. Hansen JE and Ampaya EP. (1975) *J Appl Physiol* **38**:990.
2. Warrell DA, Evans JW, Clarke RO, Kingaby GP and West JB. (1972) *J Appl Physiol* **32**:346.
3. Paiva M and Engel LA. (1983) *J Appl Physiol* **56**:418.
4. Paiva M and Engel LA. (1985) *Respir Physiol* **62**:257.
5. Ewan PW, Jones HA, Nosil J, Obdrzalek J and Hughes JMB. (1978) *Resp Physiol* **34**:45.
6. Wagner P, McRae J and Read J. (1967) *J Appl Physiol* **22**:1115.
7. Gledhill N, Froese AB, Buick FJ and Bryan AC. (1978) *J Appl Physiol* **45**:512.
8. Read J. (1966) *J Appl Physiol* **21**:1521.
9. West JB, Maloney JE and Castle BL. (1972) *J Appl Physiol* **32**:357.
10. Young IRW, Mazzone RW and Wagner PD. (1980) *J Appl Physiol* **49**:132.
11. Swinburne AJ, MacArthur CGC, Rhodes CG, Heather JD and Hughes JMB. (1982) *J Appl Physiol* **52**:1535.
12. Piiper J. (1982) *Bull Europ Physiopath Resp* **18**(suppl 4):29.
13. Piiper J and Scheid P. (1981) *Respir Physiol* **46**:193.
14. Barcroft J, Binger CA, Bock AV, Doggart JH, Forbes HS, Harrop G, Meakins JC and Redfield AC. (1923) *Phil Trans Roy Soc (London)* **B:211**:351.
15. Lilienthal JL, Riley RL, Proemmel DD and Franke RE. (1946)*Am J Physiol* **147**:199.
16. West JB, Boyer SJ, Graber DJ, Hackett PH, Maret KH, Milledge JS, Peters RM, Pizzo CJ, Samaja M, Sarnquist FH, Schoene RB and Winslow RM. (1983) *J Appl Physiol* **55**:688.
17. Cerretelli P. (1976) *J Appl Physiol* **40**:658.
18. Meyer M, Scheid P, Riedl G, Wagner H-J and Piiper J. (1981) *J Appl Physiol* **51**:1643.
19. Baldwin E de F, Cournand A and Richards DW. (1949) *Medicine* **28**:1.
20. Austrian R, McClement JH, Renzetti AD, Donald KW, Riley RL and Cournand A. (1951) *Am J Med* **11**:667.
21. Finley TN, Swenson EW and Comroe JH. (1962) *J Clin Invest* **41**:618.
22. Arndt H, Buchta I and Schomerus H. (1975) *Respiration* **32**:21.
23. Davis HH, Schwartz DJ, Lefrak SS, Susman N and Schainker BA. (1978) *Chest* **73**:507.
24. Singh MP, Khetarpal K and Sharan M. (1980) *J Math Biol* **9**:305.
25. Miyamoto Y and Moll WA. (1971) *Respir Physiol* **12**:141.

26.   Fåhraeus R and Lindqvist T. (1931) *Am J Physiol* **96**:562.
27.   Gibson JG, Seligman AM, Peacock WC, Aub JC, Fine J and Evans RD. (1946)*J Clin Invest* **25**:848.
28.   Rapaport E, Kuida H, Haynes FW and Dexter L.(1956) *Am J Physiol* **185**:127.
29.   Brudin LH, Valind SO, Rhodes CG, Turton DR and Hughes JMB. (1986) *J Appl Physiol* **60**:1155.
30.   Lammertsma AA, Brooks DJ, Beaney RP, Turton DR, Kensett MJ, Heather JD, Marshall J and Jones T. (1984) *J Cereb Blood Flow Metab* **4**:317.
31.   Roughton FJW and Forster RE. (1957) *J Appl Physiol* **11**:290.
32.   Weibel ER. (1980) *In* **Assessment of Pulmonary Function**. (AP Fishman ed) McGraw-Hill:New York.
33.   Johnson RL Jr, Spicer WS, Bishop JM and Forster RE. (1960) *J Appl Physiol* **15**:893.
34.   Pande JN and Hughes JMB. (1983) *Clin Physiol* **3**:491.
35.   Wagner WW, Latham LP, Gillespie MN, Guenther JP and Capen RL. (1982) *Science* **218**:379.
36.   Rhodes CG, Wollmer P, Fazio F and Jones T. (1981) *J Comput Assist Tomogr* **5**:783.

Gas Exchange in Pulmonary Vascular Disease

D. R. DANTZKER
*University of Texas Health
Science Center
Houston, Texas 77030*

I. INTRODUCTION

The pulmonary vascular bed is involved in a large number of pathological processes either as protagonist or innocent bystander. In all of these situations, abnormal pulmonary gas exchange is an invariant finding. In order to focus more clearly on the role that the pulmonary vascular involvement plays in the abnormalities which are seen, this discussion will confine itself to three entities in which the pulmonary vascular disease is the predominant pathological process.

II. ACUTE PULMONARY VASCULAR OCCLUSION: PULMONARY EMBOLISM

Acute pulmonary embolism almost always results in abnormal pulmonary gas exchange. Only 11.5% of patients with significant pulmonary embolism entered into the Urokinase Pulmonary Embolism Trial had an arterial oxygen tension (PaO_2) greater than 80 torr (1). Combined data from three well documented series of patients with acute pulmonary embolism, revealed that only 13% of patients had a PaO_2 greater than 80 torr and in only 6% was it greater than 90 torr (2-4). Even those patients with a relatively normal PaO_2 had a widened alveolar to arterial gradient for oxygen (A-a DO_2). A significant percentage (32%)

Copyright © 1987 by Academic Press, Inc.
All rights of reproduction in any form reserved.

had severe hypoxemia with a PaO_2 less than 60 torr and in patients without a prior history of cardiopulmonary disease there was a good correlation between the degree of hypoxemia and the extent of the pulmonary vascular bed which was occluded (2). This relationship between the degree of vascular occlusion and the severity of the hypoxemia was not apparent in patients with preexisting disease (5). Hypocarbia, while common, was not as universally found although even in patients with severe underlying lung disease, a reduction in the arterial carbon dioxide tension ($PaCO_2$) is often seen following an acute embolic event (6).

Studies designed to define the physiological mechanisms responsible for these abnormalities in pulmonary gas exchange have produced conflicting results. This is not surprising; animal models of embolic events probably do not adequately mirror the situation in humans. Differences in the coagulation and thrombolytic systems as well as in the putative mediators which are released following embolization are the most likely reasons. In addition, anesthetized animals have a blunted respiratory drive and are often studied while mechanically ventilated making any potential respiratory difficult or even impossible to evaluate. Finally, variations in the size and composition of the embolic material guarantee a diversity of findings. Human studies have posed an equally formidable challenge, both to accomplish and to compare one to another. It is difficult to obtain accurate and reproducible data from acutely ill patients and they often have concomitant medical problems such as pneumonia, congestive heart failure and chronic underlying lung disease which by themselves cause significant alterations in pulmonary gas exchange. In addition, the variables measured in these studies have often been inadequate to differentiate between various physiological mechanisms with sufficient sensitivity. Finally, poor documentation as to the time the patient was studied relative to the embolic event as well as poor definition as to the extent of the pulmonary vascular bed involved have further clouded the picture. Despite these roadblocks, the probable mechanisms of the abnormal gas exchange have now been worked out and include right-to-left shunt, ventilation-perfusion ($\dot{V}_A/\dot{Q}$) inequality, impaired diffusion and mixed venous desaturation. One or more of these abnormalities appears to be operative, to variable degrees, in different clinical settings. We will look in detail at the evidence for each.

A.   Shunt

Animals studies have demonstrated the development of right-to-left shunting subsequent to embolization with both homologous blood clots and foreign material (Fig. 1; 7-9). In a group of patients without prior heart or pulmonary disease and in whom pulmonary emboli had been proven angiographically, shunting, as measured by the breathing of 100% O_2 accounted

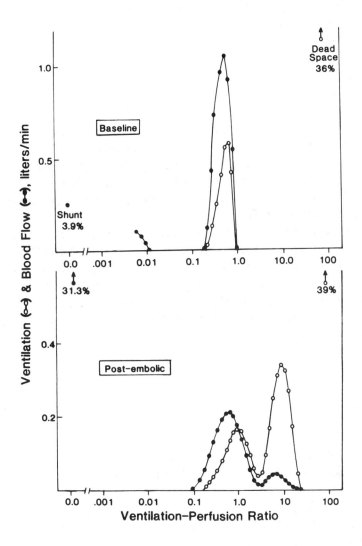

Fig. 1. The distribution of ventilation—perfusion ratios in a dog at baseline and following glass bead embolization. The post-embolic distribution shows a dramatic increase in shunt and the appearance of lung units with high ventilation—perfusion ratios but no significant change in dead space. [From Dantzker DR and Bower JS. (1982) Alterations in gas exchange following pulmonary thromboembolism. Chest **81**:495; with permission]

for most of the hypoxemia which was observed (4). An intracardiac location for the shunt was ruled out in all but one subject by dye dilution curves. In a subsequent study (10), two patients with massive embolic disease had their $\dot{V}_A/\dot{Q}$ distributions measured using the multiple inert gas elimination technique (11) and were found to have large shunts as the etiology of their hypoxemia. The similarity between the $\dot{V}_A/\dot{Q}$ distributions in these patients (Fig. 2) and the experimental findings in animals is obvious.

The etiology of the shunt has not been clearly defined although many possibilities have been proposed. One suggestion has been that the rise in pulmonary artery pressure leads to the opening of preexisting pulmonary arterial—venous anastomoses (12). However, specific studies designed to reveal such channels found no arterial—venous connections despite four-fold elevations of pulmonary artery pressure (13).

Post-embolic atelectasis distal to the embolized vessels has also been postulated (4,7). Later dissolution or distal migration of the emboli with reperfusion of the atelectic and thus unventilated lung units would result in shunting. In both laboratory animals and patients, post-embolic hypoxemia has been ameliorated by short periods of positive pressure ventilation or hyperventilation lending credence to this hypothesis (4,7,13). The atelectasis, itself, may be due to a number of events which are known to occur subsequent to pulmonary embolization. The release of humoral mediators, demonstrated in animal studies, has been implicated as an early cause of bronchoconstriction (14,15). Bronchiolar and pneumoconstriction has also been shown to occur subsequent to regional hypocapnia in the non- or under-perfused embolized lung regions (16). Finally, the occlusion of pulmonary blood flow leads to the loss of surfactant activity and may result in hemorrhagic atelectasis (17).

The development of pulmonary edema may also play a role in the production of the shunt. Two mechanisms for the production of the edema have been suggested. The first involves the effect of the increased pulmonary artery pressure on the unobstructed vessels causing either physical damage to the endothelium (18) or an alteration in the Starling forces (19). This would cause leakage from the unobstructed micro-vessels or from larger vessels upstream from the occlusion (20). In one study, using glass beads, the degree of shunt produced was closely correlated with the increase in pulmonary artery pressure produced (8). A second possible mechanism involves the release of vasoactive mediators leading to increased vascular permeability. This was suggested by experiments in which aqnimals pretreated with heparin failed to develop edema in the embolized lung regions while those not previously treated, did (21). Which mechanism is dominant may depend on the size of the vessel occluded. When glass beads were used to embolize sheep, the mechanism of pulmonary edema differed depending on

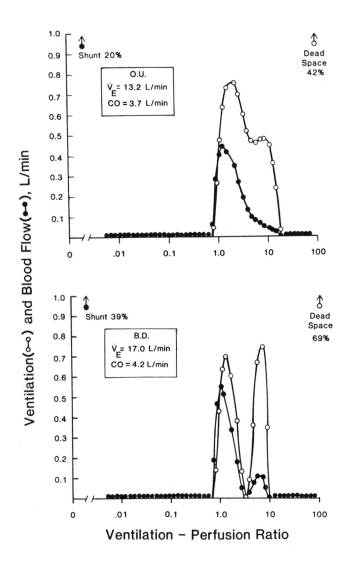

Fig. 2. The distribution of ventilation—perfusion ratios in two patients with acute, massive pulmonary embolism. Similar to the findings in Figure 1, the major abnormalities are the large shunt and the presence of lung units with high ventilation—perfusion ratios. VE is the minute ventilation and CO the cardiac output. [From D'Alonzo GE, Bower JS, DeHart P and Dantzker DR. (1983) The mechanisms of abnormal gas exchange in acute massive pulmonary embolism. Am Rev Resp Dis 128:170; with permission]

the size of the beads which were used. Smaller beads (200 µm) altered downstream permeability while the larger ones (500 µm) appeared to increase vascular pressure in the unobstructed vessels leading to hydrostatic pulmonary edema (19).

A final possibility is the development of an intracardiac shunt through a patent foramen ovale subsequent to the development of pulmonary hypertension, right ventricular failure and elevated right atrial pressures. Since 15% of people are thought to have a potentially patent foramen ovale this is a distinct possibility in patients with acute cor pulmonale and has been demonstrated recently in two patients (22).

B.   Ventilation—Perfusion Inequality

Alterations in the distribution of ventilation and blood flow have now been shown to occur following pulmonary emboli in a total of 17 patients who have had their $\dot{V}_A/\dot{Q}$ distributions measured utilizing the multiple inert gas

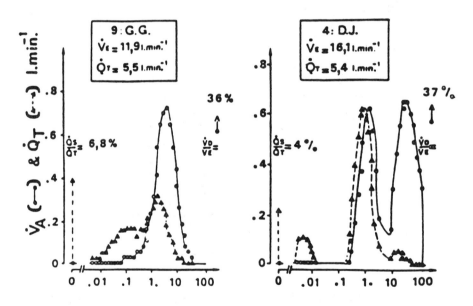

Fig. 3. The distribution of ventilation—perfusion ratios in two patients with acute pulmonary embolism. Two different patterns can be seen. Patient GG has a large amount of blood of lung units with very low ventilation—perfusion ratios while the major abnormality in patient DJ is the presence of high ventilation—perfusion units. Both patients have a small amount of shunt but no increase in dead space. $\dot{V}_A$ is alveolar ventilation, $\dot{V}_E$ is minute ventilation and $\dot{Q}_t$ is cardiac output. (From 23; with permission).

BEFORE EMBOLIZATION

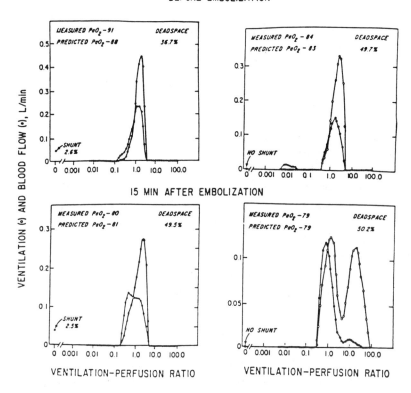

Fig. 4. *The distribution of ventilation—perfusion ratios in two dogs before and after pulmonary embolization with autologous clood clot. Despite equal increases in pulmonary artery blood pressure, suggesting equal degrees of embolization, two different patterns of ventilation—perfusion inequality developed similar to that shown in Fig. 3. The animal shown on the left side of the figure developed predominantly long units with low ventilation—perfusion ratios while the dog on the right developed predominantly high ventilation—perfusion units. (From 25; with permission).*

elimination technique (23,24). The patterns of $\dot{V}_A/\dot{Q}$ inequality varied from patient to patient and included unimodal distributions only slightly wider than normal, a predominance of low or high $\dot{V}_A/\dot{Q}$ units or distributions demonstrating modes of both high and low $\dot{V}_A/\dot{Q}$ units (Fig. 3). In general, shunt played a relatively minor role in the abnormal gas exchange which was found, although in some patients shunts as high as 15% were found. The dead space (ventilated but unperfused lung units) varied from a low of 26.5% to a high of 63.4%.

This heterogeneity of patterns of $\dot{V}_A/\dot{Q}$ inequality was predicted by studies done in dogs in whom emboli were created with autologous blood clot (25). Following embolization, a variety of $\dot{V}_A/\dot{Q}$ distribution patterns were noted despite equal degrees of embolization. Most animals developed broad bimodal patterns consisting of both high and low $\dot{V}_A/\dot{Q}$ units. However, similar to the patient studies, some dogs developed only low $\dot{V}_A/\dot{Q}$ units and others only high (Fig. 4). Neither shunt nor an increase in the ventilation of totally unperfused lung units (*i.e.*, dead space) were found. The absence of an increase in dead space suggested that either complete vascular occlusion was uncommon or that compensatory mechanisms were at work, decreasing ventilation to poorly perfused alveoli. Using a simple two compartment model, it was demonstrated that the diversity of patterns which were found could be simply explained by the manner in which emboli lead to a redistribution of blood flow from embolized to nonembolized units (Fig. 5). Almost total occlusion of blood flow from a relatively small number of lung units would results in lung units with high $\dot{V}_A/\dot{Q}$ ratios but no significant increase in low $\dot{V}_A/\dot{Q}$ units and thus, no hypoxemia. By contrast, if flow to a larger compartment was reduced by a lesser percentage and diverted to the small compartment, then an increase in low $\dot{V}_A/\dot{Q}$ units along with hypoxemia would be seen without a significant increase in high $\dot{V}_A/\dot{Q}$ units. In order to reverse the hypoxemia created by this mechanism, a dramatic increase in minute ventilation (more than 21 L/min in the example shown in Fig. 5) would be required. This degree of hyperventilation would lead to marked hypocapnia which would almost certainly blunt full compensation.

In addition to this simple explanation for the observed $\dot{V}_A/\dot{Q}$ inequality, it is likely that mechanisms other than simple mechanical obstruction are at work further adding to the heterogeneity of the resultant $\dot{V}_A/\dot{Q}$ distributions. In work already described, marked changes in pulmonary mechanics have been seen following pulmonary embolization with an increase in airways resistance and fall in pulmonary compliance (14,16). In addition, conservative physiological reflexes [hypoxic vasoconstriction (26) and hypocapnic bronchoconstriction (27)] are probably operating and may explain the rapid normalization of the $\dot{V}_A/\dot{Q}$ distributions seen in some of the animal studies and the relatively normal distributions found in some patients.

In general, the $\dot{V}_A/\dot{Q}$ inequality which is found following pulmonary embolism fully explains the hypoxemia which is present, suggesting that impaired diffusion is not contributing to the abnormal gas exchange. However, in a recent study, it was suggested that diffusion impairment could explain up to 13% of the measured A-a DO_2 (23). Thus, incomplete alveolar end-capillary equilibration,

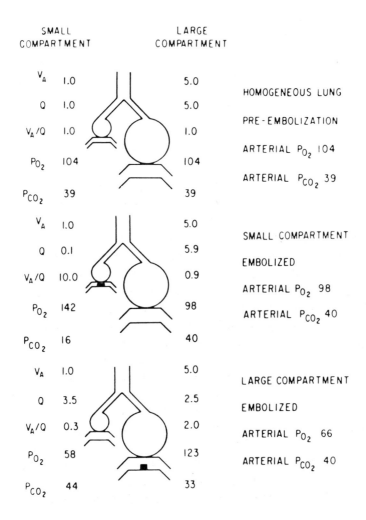

Fig. 5. Ventilation and perfusion are matched in the two-compartment lung model demonstrated in the top panel. In the middle panel small compartment blood flow has been reduced by 90 per cent and diverted to the large compartment, resulting in the development of a high $\dot{V}_A/\dot{Q}$ unit but a minimal decrease in the $\dot{V}_A/\dot{Q}$ of the larger compartment (1.0 to 0.9). Thus, no significant hypoxemia would develop (104 to 98 mmHg). In the bottom panel, larger compartment blood flow has been reduced by 50 percent and diverted to the small compartment. This leads to 58 percent of the blood flow distributed to a lung unit with a $\dot{V}_A/\dot{Q}$ of 0.3, and significant hypoxemia develops (104 to 66 mmHg). Mixed venous gas tensions remained constant and physiologic. (From 25; with permission).

probably as a result of the rapid transit time of blood through the reduced pulmonary vascular bed, could be playing an additional small role.

C.   Non-Pulmonary Factors

For any lung unit, the resultant end-capillary PO_2 will be influenced by the mixed venous PO_2 ($P\bar{v}O_2$) although the magnitude of the effect will depend on the $\dot{V}_A/\dot{Q}$ of the unit (28). In the case of shunt, any change in the $P\bar{v}O_2$ will be directly translated into an altered end capillary PO_2. For lung units that are ventilated, the effect will be greatest for lung units with a $\dot{V}_A/\dot{Q}$ of 1.0 or less and decrease as the $\dot{V}_A/\dot{Q}$ increases above 1.0. The ultimate effect on the arterial PO_2 will depend on the overall $\dot{V}_A/\dot{Q}$ distribution. In the presence of significant $\dot{V}_A/\dot{Q}$ inequality or shunt, a low $P\bar{v}O_2$ can lead to considerable hypoxemia. With normal lungs an increase in minute ventilation markedly attenuates the influence of a low $P\bar{v}O_2$ on the arterial PO_2 by increasing the overall $\dot{V}_A/\dot{Q}$ of the distribution, as is seen during exercise (29). However, in the presence of $\dot{V}_A/\dot{Q}$ inequality, this is much less effective, and thus despite the hyperventilation which usually accompanies pulmonary embolic disease, a low $P\bar{v}O_2$ could make a major contribution to the observed hypoxemia. In patients with pulmonary thromboembolism, the $P\bar{v}O_2$ may be low because of a decrease in cardiac output, or the inability of the cardiac output to keep up with increased metabolic demands.

A low $P\bar{v}O_2$ has now been shown to be a common finding in acute pulmonary embolic disease and, in fact, to contribute in large part to the observed hypoxemia (23,24). In a recent reported series only one patient out of ten would still have been hypoxemic if their $P\bar{v}O_2$ had been normal. Thus the widened A-a DO_2 seen with acute pulmonary embolism may well overestimate the amount of shunt or degree of $\dot{V}_A/\dot{Q}$ inequality which is present and variations in the arterial PO_2 are as likely to represent alterations in cardiac output as a change in lung function.

D.   Hypocapnia

The mechanism responsible for the ubiquitous finding of hypocapnia is much less clearly worked out. The increase in minute ventilation is beneficial to gas exchange by returning the $\dot{V}_A/\dot{Q}$ ratio of the overperfused, uninvolved lung units towards normal and thus correcting the hypoxemia. In addition, it would blunt, to some degree, the depressing effect of the low $P\bar{v}O_2$ on the PaO_2. However, it is unlikely that abnormal gas exchange is the stimulus for the increased ventilation since hyperventilation is seen even when the resultant hypoxemia would appear to be well below the level usually though to elicit a response from the carotid chemoreceptors.

Non-chemical stimuli are more likely to be playing the dominant role (30). Following glass bead embolization, an increase in medullary respiratory neuronal discharge with a subsequent increase in minute ventilation has been demonstrated (31). Presumably this is due to lung receptor stimulation and increased vagal afferent activity. In addition, increases in right ventricular pressure, independent of flow, lead to significant increases in minute ventilation (32). The combination of stretch receptor and baroreceptor drive is the most likely explanation for the respiratory alkalosis.

III. CHRONIC PULMONARY VASCULAR OCCLUSION: PRIMARY PULMONARY HYPERTENSION AND RECURRENT PULMONARY EMBOLI

Patients with chronic pulmonary vascular occlusion characteristically have mild to moderate hypoxemia which worsens during exercise as well as a chronic respiratory alkalosis. The hypoxemia was initially ascribed to the reduced transit time of blood through a restricted pulmonary capillary bed with resultant failure of end-capillary equilibration for O_2. Recent studies, however, have now shown that the abnormal gas exchange is due to mechanisms similar to those seen in acute pulmonary vascular occlusion.

Measurements of $\dot{V}_A/\dot{Q}$ distributions in these patients demonstrates that despite the marked vascular occlusion, there is only mild to moderate $\dot{V}_A/\dot{Q}$ inequality and small amounts of intrapulmonary shunt (Fig 6; 33). Unlike the patients with acute vascular occlusion, there is usually no clear cut mode of high $\dot{V}_A/\dot{Q}$ units or significant increase in dead space. The pattern of $\dot{V}_A/\dot{Q}$ inequality is similar for patients with primary pulmonary hypertension and recurrent pulmonary emboli and there is no evidence that impaired diffusion plays a significant role in the resultant hypoxemia in either group of patients. In each patient, the degree of hypoxemia is significantly greater than one might expect form the degree of $\dot{V}_A/\dot{Q}$ inequality alone. The amplifying factor is a low $P\overline{v}O_2$ which is present uniformly due to a low cardiac output. As in the patients with acute pulmonary embolism, if the patients had maintained a normal $P\overline{v}O_2$, it would have significantly decreased and in some patients even abolished the hypoxemia.

The etiology of the shunt and low $\dot{V}_A/\dot{Q}$ units in these patients is unclear, but is probably due to the overperfusion of lung units as a result of the decreased number of open pulmonary vessels as well as to alterations in the

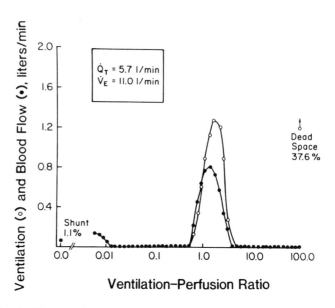

Fig. 6. The distribution of ventilation and blood flow in a 35-year old patient with chronic, recurrent pulmonary emboli and severe pulmonary hypertension. Despite the presence of extensive angiographically documented pulmonary embolism, the $\dot{V}_A/\dot{Q}$ distribution is essentially normal. (From 33; with permission).

distribution of ventilation. The latter may be ascribed to the presence of interstitial pulmonary edema due to the high pulmonary vascular pressure (34) or results from airway occlusion secondary to bronchial compression by adjacent dilated pulmonary arteries (35). When severe hypoxemia is seen it is often due, in part, to intracardiac shunting through a patent foramen ovale.

The absence of an increased dead space in patients with chronic pulmonary vascular occlusions suggests that either total vascular occlusion is unusual or that the vessels which are occluded do not supply a functionally distinct gas exchanging unit (8). Alternatively, there may be compensatory mechanisms at work to minimize $\dot{V}_A/\dot{Q}$ inequality. This latter possibility may also explain the absence of a significant amount of blood flow to low $\dot{V}_A/\dot{Q}$ units and shunt. A pharmacologically induced reduction in pulmonary vascular tone is often accompanied by an increase in the degree of $\dot{V}_A/\dot{Q}$ inequality (36,37) suggesting that at least some of the pulmonary vascular tone which is present contributes to minimizing the abnormal blood flow distribution in these patients. Whether or not similar mechanisms exist with regards to ventilation is not yet known with certainty. It should be pointed out that this increase in $\dot{V}_A/\dot{Q}$ inequality subsequent to pharmacological therapy does not usually lead to worsening hypoxemia since it is invariable accompanied by an increase in cardiac output and thus a rise in $P\bar{v}O_2$. This is usually able to offset the detrimental effects of the increased $\dot{V}_A/\dot{Q}$ inequality and result in no change in the PaO_2 or in some cases even an increase.

As in patients with acute pulmonary vascular occlusion, the mechanism(s) responsible for the chronic hyperventilation and respiratory alkalosis is unclear. Presumably, as in the acute situation, it is due to increased afferent activity from intrapulmonary stretch receptors or intravascular baroreceptors (38) since the blood gases are not abnormal enough to postulate a significant contribution from the chemoreceptors.

A further widening of the A-a DO_2 during even low level exercise is characteristically seen in patients with chronic pulmonary vascular occlusive disease. This is due almost entirely to a further decrease in the $P\bar{v}O_2$ as increased metabolic requirements require a greater O_2 extraction by the tissues (39). The fall in $P\bar{v}O_2$ during exercise in these patients is an exaggeration of the normal response since their abilities to increase O_2 delivery are limited by the high right ventricular afterload. There is no increase in the degree of $\dot{V}_A/\dot{Q}$ inequality during exercise and, in fact, it usually improves (39). Impaired diffusion is also not an important contributor to the increased hypoxemia.

These patients also have an abnormal ventilatory response to exercise with an increase in the slope of the relationship between minute ventilation and increased CO_2 production. By increasing the overall $\dot{V}_A/\dot{Q}$ ratio this exaggerated response tends to mitigate some of the $P\bar{v}O_2$ induced fall in PaO_2 which would otherwise be seen. It is unlikely, however, that abnormal gas exchange is the cause of the excessive minute ventilation. Normal subjects maintain their baseline $PaCO_2$'s during exercise even if they begin with baseline values significantly lower than normal (40,41). The lower the starting $PaCO_2$, the greater is the increase in ventilation required for any increased CO_2 production (40). Since patients with obliterative pulmonary vascular disease have a chronic respiratory alkalosis at rest, it is not surprising that they also attempt to maintain their baseline hypocapnia and therefore require a similar increased ventilatory response. Recently it has been shown that patients with primary pulmonary hypertension have a decrease in their ventilatory responses to exercise following heart-lung transplantation and that this decrease is not correlated with changes in the resting $PaCO_2$ (42). This suggests that, the exaggerated ventilatory response during exercise is not fully explained by a lowering of the baseline set point and may also be due to direct exercise-induced respiratory stimulation originating from within the diseased cardiopulmonary system; perhaps an exaggeration of mechanisms postulated as the etiology of the resting hyperventilation.

   To summarize, the abnormal pulmonary gas exchange in both acute and chronic pulmonary vascular disease is predominantly due to the redistribution of blood flow in the lungs creating units with low $\dot{V}_A/\dot{Q}$ ratios and shunt which is often modified by conservative reflexes. The hypoxemia which is seen is as much doe to the presence of mixed venous desaturation (as a result of inadequate cardiac output) as it is to the abnormal distribution of blod flow and ventilation. The characteristic respiratory alkalosis is predominantly due to increased baroreceptor and stretch receptor activity. Alterations in arterial blood gases secondary to drug therapy or exercise are determined by the manner in which they influence these factors.

REFERENCES

1.   Urokinase pulmonary embolism trial. A national cooperative study. (1973) *Circulation* (Suppl II).
2.   McIntyre KM and Sasahara AA. (1971) *Am J Cardiol* **28**:288.
3.   Stanek V, Reidel M and Widimsky J. (1978)*Bull Eur Physiopathol Respir* **14**:561.
4.   Wilson JE, Pierce AK, Johnson RL, Winga ER, Harrell WR, Curry GC and Mullins CG. (1971) *J Clin Invest* **50**:481.
5.   McIntyre KM and Sasahara AA. (1973)*In* **Pulmonary Thromboembolism**. (K Moser and M Stein, eds). Year Book Medical Publishers:Chicago.
6.   Lippmann M and Fein A. (1981) *Chest* **79**:39.
7.   Caldini P. (1965) *J Appl Physiol* **20**:184.
8.   Young I, Mazzone RW and Wagner PD. (1980) *J Appl Physiol* **49**:132.
9.   Johnson A and Malik AB. (1981)*J Appl Physiol* **51**:461.
10. D'Alonzo GE, Bower JS, DeHart P and Dantzker DR. (1983) *Am Rev Resp Dis* **128**:170.
11. Wagner PD, Saltzman HA and West JB. (1974) *J Appl Physiol* **36**:588.
12. Niden AH and Aviado DM. (1956) *Circ Res* **4**:67.
13. Cheney FW, Pavlin J, Ferens BS and Allen D. (1978) *J Thoracic Cardiovasc Surg* **76**(Part 2):473.
14. Nadel JA, Colebatch HJ and Olsen CR. (1964). *J Appl Physiol* **19**:387.
15. Levy SE and Simmons DH. (1975) *J Appl Physiol* **39**:41.
16. Levy SE and Simmons DH. (1974)*J Appl Physiol* **36**:60.
17. Cherniak V, Hudson WH and Greenfield LJ. (1966)*J Appl Physiol* **21**:1315.

18. Ohkuda K, Nakahara K, Weidner WJ, Binder A and Staub NC. (1978) *Circ Res* **43**:152.
19. Johnson A and Malik AB. (1981) *J Appl Physiol* **51**:461.
20. Albert RK, Lakshminarayan S, Huang TW and Butler J. (1978) *J Appl Physiol* **44**:759.
21. Malik AB and Van der Zee H. (1978)*Circ Res* **42**:72.
22. Herve L and Rokseth R. (1983) Letter to the Editor. *Am Rev Resp Dis* **128**:1101.
23. Manier G, Castaing Y and Guenard H. (1985) *Am Rev Resp Dis* **132**:332.
24. Huet Y, Lemaire F, Brun-Buisson C, *et al.* (1985) *Chest* **88**:829.
25. Dantzker DR, Wagner PD, Tornabene VW, Alazraki NP and West JB. (1978) *Circ Res* **42**:92.
26. Grant BJB, Davies EE, Jones HA and Hughes JMB. (1976) *J Appl Physiol* **40**:216.
27. Swenson EW, Finley TN and Guzman SV. (1961) *J Clin Invest* **40**:828.
28. West JB. (1977) *Am Rev Resp Dis* **116**:919.
29. Gledhill N, Froese AB and Dempsey JA. (1977) *In* **Muscular Exercise and the Lung.** (JA Dempsey and CE Reeds, eds) University of Wisconsin Press:Madison.
30. Whitteridge D. (1950) *Physiol Rev* **30**:475.
31. Katz S and Horres AD. (1972) *J Appl Physiol* **33**:390.
32. Jones PW, Huszczuk A and Wasserman K. (1982) *J Appl Physiol* **53**:218.
33. Dantzker DR and Bower JS. (1979) *J Clin Invest* **64**:1050.
34. West JB, Dollery CT and Heard BE. (1964) *Lancet* **II**:181.
35. Stranger P, Lucas RV and Edwards JE. (1969) *Pediatrics* **43**:760.
36. Dantzker DR and Bower JS. (1981) *J Appl Physiol* **51**:607.
37. Melot C, Naeije R, Mols P, Vandenbossche J and Denolin H. (1983) *Chest* **83**:203.
38. Guz A, Noble MIM, Eisele JH and Trenchard D. (1970) *In* **Breathing, Hering-Breuer Centenary Symposium.** J&A Churchill Ltd:London.
39. Dantzker DR, D'Alonzo GE, Bower JS, Popet K and Crevey BJ. (1984) *Am Rev Resp Dis* **130**:412.
40. Oren A, Wasserman K, Davis JA and Whipp BJ. (1981) *J Appl Physiol* **51**:185.
41. Mitchell GS, Smith CA and Dempsey JA. (1984) *J Appl Physiol* **57**:1894.
42. Theodore J, Robin ED, Morris AJR, Burke CM, Jamieson SW, Van Kessel A, Stinson EB and Shumway NE. (1986) *Chest* **89**:39.

Pulmonary Circulation in Exercise

BRIAN J. WHIPP
KATHY E. SIETSEMA
*Division of Respiratory Physiology and
Medicine
Harbor-UCLA Medical Center
Torrance, California 90509, USA*

I. INTRODUCTION

Almost three quarters of a century ago, Krogh and Lindhard recognized that the increase of oxygen uptake, ($\dot{V}O_2$) within the first few seconds of the onset of dynamic muscular exercise must have resulted from an increase in pulmonary blood flow ($\dot{Q}c$), as the mixed venous blood entering the pulmonary capillaries would not yet have had time to have been influenced by the widened arterio-venous (a-$\bar{v}$) O_2 difference across the contracting muscle bed. Thus, after the onset of exercise, there exists a small temporal window through which the dynamics of the changes in pulmonary blood flow may be inferred from the concomitant response profile of $\dot{V}O_2$. This is represented by the Fick equation as shown in equations 1 - 4:

$$\dot{V}O_{2r} = \dot{Q} \cdot (C_aO_2 - C_{\bar{v}}O_2) \ldots\ldots \quad \emptyset 3_r \tag{1}$$

$$k_r \qquad k'_r$$

$$\dot{V}O_2 = \dot{Q} \cdot (C_aO_2 - C_{\bar{v}}O_2) \ldots\ldots \quad \emptyset 1 \tag{2}$$

$$v \qquad k'_r$$

$$\dot{V}O_2 = \dot{Q} \cdot (C_aO_2 - C_{\bar{v}}O_2) \quad \ldots\ldots \quad \text{\o}2 \tag{3}$$

$$\underset{k_x}{\overset{v}{\dot{V}O_{2x}}} = \dot{Q} \cdot (\underset{k'_x}{\overset{v'}{C_aO_2 - C_{\bar{v}}O_2}}) \quad \ldots\ldots \quad \text{\o}3_x \tag{4}$$

For example, equation 1 indicates that for a subject sitting quietly at rest, $\dot{V}O_2$ is constant when both cardiac output ($\dot{Q}$) and the arterial–to–venous O_2 difference ($C_aO_2 - C_{\bar{v}}O_2$) are constant ($\underline{k}_r$ and $\underline{k}'_r$, respectively). But as shown in equation 2, immediately following the onset of exercise, as the a–$\bar{v}$ difference remains constant for some period of time, the changes in $\dot{V}O_2$ are consequently determined by the changes in cardiac output ($\underline{v}$). Subsequently (equation 3), as the mixed venous O_2 content ($C_{\bar{v}}O_2$) begins to fall, the developing $\dot{V}O_2$ response becomes determined both by any residual change in cardiac output and the widening a–$\bar{v}$ O_2 difference ($\underline{v}$ and $\underline{v}'$, respectively). And finally, in equation 4, a new steady state is established during exercise within which $\dot{V}O_2$ is again constant reflecting the new constant levels of cardiac output ($\underline{k}_x$) and of the a–$\bar{v}$ O_2 difference ($\underline{k}'_x$).

II.   PHASES OF $\dot{V}O_2$ KINETICS

The period during which the a–$\bar{v}$ O_2 difference remains relatively constant after the onset of exercise has been termed "phase 1" of the $\dot{V}O_2$ kinetics. This response profile is shown in Figure 1, for a subject beginning cycle-ergometer exercise at 75 Watts from a prior background of rest. $\dot{V}O_2$ is seen to increase abruptly at exercise onset, as do CO_2 output ($\dot{V}CO_2$) and ventilation ($\dot{V}_E$). The respiratory exchange ratio (R) remains relatively constant; this indicates that despite both $\dot{V}CO_2$ and $\dot{V}O_2$ increasing, they do so in proportion. This constance of R supports the contention that pulmonary gas exchange in this phase of exercise is caused primarily by the increase in pulmonary blood flow; *i.e.*, propelling blood with an unchanged composition more rapidly through the pulmonary capillaries will not alter R when arterial blood gas tensions are regulated. Similarly, the rapid increase in ventilation in this phase results in a relative constancy of end-tidal PCO_2 ($P_{ET}CO_2$).

Phase 1 ends when the composition of the blood entering the pulmonary capillaries begins to change as a result of the exercise. This is shown in Figure 1 as the point at which R begins to fall transiently — reflecting the tissue

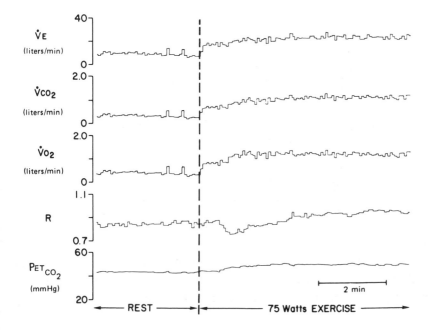

Figure 1. Breath-by-breath time course of $\dot{V}_E$, $\dot{V}CO_2$, $\dot{V}O_2$, R and $P_{ET}CO_2$ in response to 75 Watts exercise undertaken from rest by a normal male. The vertical dashed line indicates exercise onset. Taken from ref. 20.

capacitance for CO_2 being appreciably greater than for O_2 — and also by the beginning of an increase in $P_{ET}CO_2$ which reflects the increased mixed venous CO_2 content causing an increase in the slope of the alveolar phase of the expiratory PCO_2 profile. "Phase 2", or the period in which the a–$\bar{v}$ O_2 difference is changing, continues until both R and $P_{ET}CO_2$ become constant. At this time $\dot{V}O_2$, $\dot{V}CO_2$ and $\dot{V}_E$ have all established their steady-state or "phase 3" levels.

Several investigators using impedence plethysmographic or pulse-Doppler techniques (2-4) have attempted to determine the temporal characteristics of the cardiac output response to moderate-intensity exercise. For example, Cummin *et al.* (2) found that the time course of cardiac output and ventilation were well correlated in phase 1 of rest-to-exercise transitions (Figure 2). This observation, coupled with the stability of end-tidal gas tensions in this phase, provides support for pulmonary gas exchange during phase 1 being "cardiodynamic" in origin.

It is important to point out here, however, that — with the proviso that the algorithm which computes $\dot{V}O_2$ corrects for changes in pulmonary gas stores

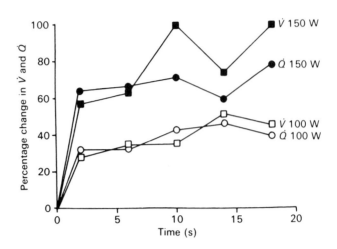

Figure 2. Percentage changes in $\dot{V}_E$ and $\dot{Q}$ (aortic blood flow or systemic blood flow) following the onset of exercise at both 100 Watts and 150 Watts in a normal subject. "0" represents exercise onset. Taken from ref. 2.

(*i.e.*, computing the <u>alveolar</u> exchange of O_2) — ventilatory changes will not themselves influence $\dot{V}O_2$ during phase 1 (except to the extent that changes of ventilation might alter pulmonary blood flow). Thus, Weissman *et al.* (5) have demonstrated that $\dot{V}O_2$ can increase abruptly at the onset of moderate exercise, despite ventilation being volitionally constrained to its resting level for a period of some 40 seconds (Figure 3). And because cardiac output increases in this phase, note that end-tidal PO_2 ($P_{ET}O_2$) falls rapidly and $P_{ET}CO_2$ rises rapidly in this condition. It is further shown in Figure 3 that the magnitude of the change in $\dot{V}O_2$ during phase 1 is relatively independent of the work rate.

In summary, therefore, as the change in $\dot{V}O_2$ during phase 1 is caused by a change in cardiac output and pulmonary blood flow, the change in $\dot{V}O_2$ during phase 1 may therefore be used to represent both the pattern and magnitude of the immediate change in pulmonary blood flow which occurs at the onset of exercise.

III.   REST-TO-EXERCISE TRANSITIONS

Whipp *et al.* (6) therefore investigated the time course of $\dot{V}O_2$ for rest-to-exercise transitions in normal subjects in the upright position, and compared these changes with the corresponding response of $\dot{V}O_2$ to an exercise transition performed to the same work rate but undertaken from prior light exercise (*i.e.*,

unloaded pedaling or "0" Watts; Figure 4). This design allowed use to be made of
the fact that for moderate exercise undertaken from rest, the stroke volume
increases by approximately 50% within the first few breaths of exercise. In
contrast, for a background of light exercise in which the stroke volume is already
at or near its subsequent exercise level, the immediate change in cardiac output

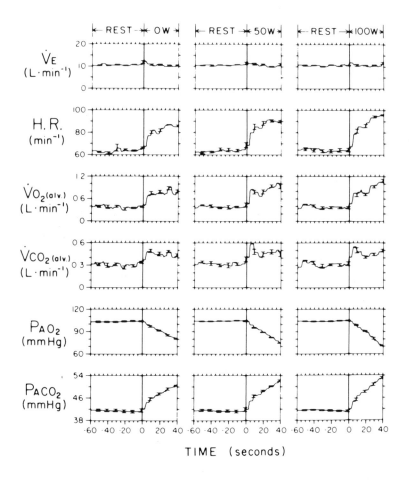

Figure 3. Mean time course of $\dot{V}_E$, heart rate, alveolar $\dot{V}O_2$ ($\dot{V}O_2[alv]$),
alveolar $\dot{V}CO_2$ ($\dot{V}CO_2[alv]$), alveolar (end-tidal) PO_2 and PCO_2 in response to
exercise (0, 50 & 100 Watts) undertaken from rest by a normal male during
volitionally-controlled breathing. Solid vertical line indicates exercise onset.
Taken from ref. 5.

during phase 1 was expected to be slower. This was clearly borne out in these experiments. Similar results have also been reported by Linnarsson (7).

Karlsson *et al.* (8) and Weiler-Ravell *et al.* (9) utilized a different strategy for modifying the stroke volume response at exercise onset. These investigators compared the responses of normal subjects performing rest-to-exercise transitions

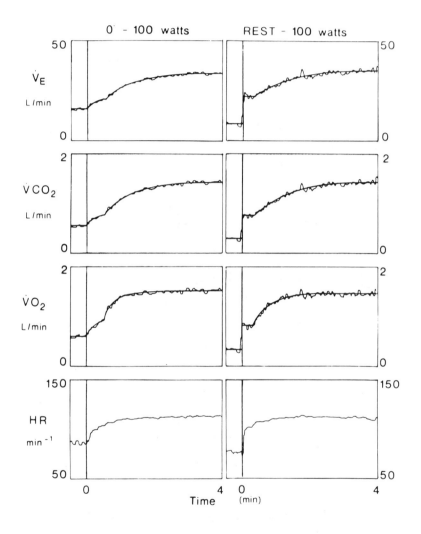

Figure 4. Mean time course of $\dot{V}_E$, $\dot{V}CO_2$, $\dot{V}O_2$ *and heart rate in response to 100 Watts exercise undertaken from rest (right panels) and from "0" Watts (left panels) by a normal male. Solid vertical line indicates exercise onset. Taken from ref. 6.*

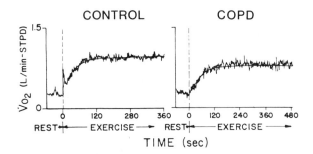

Figure 5. Breath-by-breath time course of $\dot{V}O_2$ *in response to 40 Watts exercise undertaken from rest by a normal subject (left) and a patient with COPD (right). Dashed vertical line indicates exercise. Taken from ref. 10.*

in the upright and also in the supine posture. They argues that stroke volume would be elevated to or near its exercise level in the supine condition at rest; consistent with this notion, these authors demonstrated that there was a rapid increase in $\dot{V}O_2$ at exercise onset in the upright posture, but a relatively slow response in the supine posture.

If indeed the pattern and magnitude of the phase 1 change in $\dot{V}O_2$ represents the time course of the change in pulmonary blood flow, then one might expect that in certain diseases involving the lungs and/or the heart, rapid changes in pulmonary blood flow would be unlikely to result at exercise onset. For example, Nery *et al.* (10) studied patients with chronic obstructive pulmonary disease and demonstrated that the rapid component of the phase 1 $\dot{V}O_2$ response was appreciably slowed in these patients compared to control subjects (Figure 5). These authors attributed these small and relatively slow phase 1 responses of $\dot{V}O_2$ to a high pulmonary-vascular resistance, a compromised ability of the pulmonary vascular bed to dilate and thus to accomodate the sudden increase in venous return, and also possibly some primary myocardial dysfunction (11-13).

Sietsema *et al.* (14) have recently reported findings on the phase 1 $\dot{V}O_2$ kinetics for a group of patients in which the responses of the systemic and pulmonary circulation were congenitally dissociated. Thirteen patients with abnormal pulmonary perfusion owing to cyanotic congenital heart disease were studied: eleven had obliterative pulmonary vascular disease and pulmonary hypertension; one patient had elevated (though sub-systemic) pulmonary artery pressures; and another patient had normal pulmonary artery pressures but moderate pulmonic stenosis. The results from this group were compared with nine normal volunteers of similar ages with no known history of cardiac or pulmonary disease.

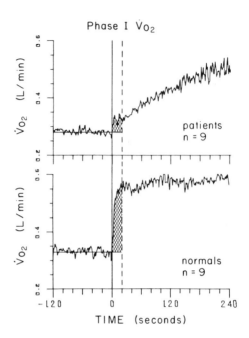

Figure 6. Mean time course of $\dot{V}O_2$ in response to "0" Watts exercise undertaken from rest by nine patients with cyanotic congenital heart disease and pulmonary hypertension (upper panel) and by nine normal subjects (lower panel). The solid vertical line indicates exercise onset. The dashed vertical line at 20 sec into the work represents the end of "phase 1". The shaded area is the total volume of O_2 (above resting levels) taken up across the lung during this phase. Taken from ref. 14.

As nine of the patients were only able to exercise to the lightest degree (*i.e.,* "0" Watts cycling), we show in Figure 6 the results of these nine patients compared with the group of nine normal controls. It is clear that the mean $\dot{V}O_2$ response during phase 1 is appreciably smaller than normal for the patients, despite the fact that — when corrected for body size — there was no difference in either the resting or the steady-state exercise levels of $\dot{V}O_2$.

The total additional amount of oxygen taken up across the alveolar capillary bed (above resting levels) in these patients averaged only 15 ml for the entire initial 20 seconds ascribed to phase 1 (14); and in three of the patients there was no increase at all. This figure should be compared with the significantly higher average uptake of about 50 ml in the normal subjects. A further point worth noting is that in the normal subjects — because the immediate increase in pulmonary blood flow and cardiac output achieved during phase 1 effectively equalled the $\dot{V}O_2$ required for the task — the subsequent phase 2 O_2 uptake response was virtually indistinguishable (14); this is predictable from the Fick equation presented earlier (equations 1 - 4). On the other hand, the attenuated phase 1 $\dot{V}O_2$ in the patients that resulted from the presumed smaller pulmonary blood flow response required a significant further increase in $\dot{V}O_2$ during phase 2, as the a-$\bar{v}$ O_2 difference continues to widen; this was clearly apparent in Figure 6.

It is important to recognize, however, that in patient populations of the kind which Sietsema et al. (14) studied there is a dissociation between the systemic cardiac output and the pulmonary blood flow: a significant right-to-left shunt was present in these patients. The onset of exercise resulted in a virtually instantaneous decrease in arterial oxygen saturation, indicating an abrupt, further increase in the right-to-left shunt fraction (14). Thus, the reduced $\dot{V}O_2$ response in phase 1 observed in this group of patients must have reflected a reduced pulmonary blood flow response. We believe that the small phase 1 $\dot{V}O_2$ increase in these patients is not due to the narrowing of the a-$\bar{v}$ O_2 difference (with systemic arterial O_2 content being decreased and mixed venous O_2 content being unchanged), but rather a compromised pulmonary blood flow response with a relatively unchanged pulmonary arterial to pulmonary venous O_2 content difference. Supporting this argument is the observation that $P_{ET}O_2$ actually consistently increased during phase 1 in these patients as a result of alveolar hyperventilation.

It is perhaps surprising, therefore, that the use of the phase 1 $\dot{V}O_2$ response as a gas exchange probe of the pulmonary circulatory kinetics has received such little attention since Krogh and Lindhard's (1) cogent perception in 1913. Part of this undoubtedly reflects the technological requirements for tracking these rapid $\dot{V}O_2$ changes accurately (7,15) and also for correcting the measurements for changes in lung O_2 stores (7,16-19). But the ability to make breath-to-breath pulmonary gas exchange measurements across exercise transients and to time-align and average the results of several responses allows these patterns of change to be made with great precision. This, coupled with our knowledge of the influence of the tissue gas stores on O_2 and CO_2 exchange dynamics at the lung (20, 21), allows one now to discern the time at which phase 1 is complete; i.e., from the onset of the transient decrease in R and the beginning of the increase in $P_{ET}CO_2$ (e.g., Figure 1) and the associated decrease in $P_{ET}O_2$.

Consequently, the duration of the temporal window within which the $\dot{V}O_2$ response reflects the kinetics of the pulmonary circulation may now be determined. And although (as shown in Figures 5 and 6) the $\dot{V}O_2$ responses in phase 1 observed in patients with impaired pulmonary circulatory function are clearly aberrant (14), there still remains the task of establishing both the values and the

TABLE I. Factors modifying direct proportionality between $\dot{V}O_2$ and $\dot{Q}$ during Phase 1 (ø1).

$\dot{V}O_2$	Changes in lung O_2 stores, *i.e.*, Δ FRC, hyperventilation or hypoventilation. The $\dot{V}O_2$ algorithm must therefore compute "alveolar" O_2 exchange.
‖	Transient disparity between right-sided cardiac output and pulmonary capillary blood flow, *i.e.*, resulting from a change in pulmonary arterial blood volume.
$\dot{Q}$	Conditions which dissociate cardiac output and pulmonary capillary blood flow, *e.g.*, right-to-left intracardiac shunt.
X	Decrease in CaO_2 during ø1 owing to right-to-left shunt. (Pulmonary venous O_2 content is the appropriate variable for this analysis.)
CaO_2	Increase in CaO_2 in ø1 resulting from acutely improved $\dot{V}_A/\dot{Q}$ distribution, or from hyperventilation, in a hypoxemic subject.
$\mid$	
$C\bar{v}O_2$	$C\bar{v}O_2$ changing within "phase 1" because of mixing of superior and inferior vena caval blood with appreciably different CvO_2's.

determinants of the normal distribution of the phase 1 $\dot{V}O_2$ response in order to establish the appropriate frame of reference for what may be statistically justifiable as an abnormal response.

As with most non-invasive techniques, certain caveats apply to the use of the phase 1 $\dot{V}O_2$ kinetics as being representative of pulmonary circulatory or cardiac output responses; these are given in Table I. With these in mind, it seems that the phase 1 $\dot{V}O_2$ response kinetics provide a potentially useful non-invasive probe of pulmonary circulatory function associated with the stress of the onset of muscular exercise. The utility of the $\dot{V}O_2$ response as an index of pulmonary circulatory function effectively ends when the a-$\bar{v}$ O_2 difference begins to widen. And consequently, the phase 2 $\dot{V}O_2$ response reflects in large part the influence of tissue O_2 exchange (*i.e.*, as a result of changes in the $\dot{V}O_2$-to-$\dot{Q}$ ratio of the muscle).

IV.   STEADY STATE (PHASE 3)

There has been a recent surge in interest in pulmonary circulatory function during phase 3 of exercise; previously widely-held views regarding both how well ventilation and perfusion were matched in the lung and also how effectively the lung subserved its function its function of "alveolarizing" the pulmonary-capillary blood have been challenged. It had been generally assumed that normal subjects maintained arterial O_2 saturation and PO_2 at or close to the resting values throughout the entire range of work rates. Also, as the topographic distribution of $\dot{V}_A$ and $\dot{Q}$ appeared to improve with exercise, it was therefore assumed that the distribution of alveolar ventilation-to-perfusion ($\dot{V}_A/\dot{Q}$) within the lung was improved and that the lung was a more efficient organ at gas exchange during exercise than at rest. This hypothesis appeared to be confirmed for light exercise, in that the alveolar-to-arterial PO_2 difference either remained unchanged or decreased (22,23).

More recently, however, Gledhill et al. (24) have utilized the multiple-inert-gas technique of Wagner and West and their associates (25) during exercise to determine the dispersion profile of $\dot{V}_A/\dot{Q}$ throughout the lung. They demonstrated that although the mean $\dot{V}_A/\dot{Q}$ for the lung increased during steady-state exercise (as necessary for a system that maintains arterial oxygenation associated with a reduced mixed venous O_2 saturation), their index for the dispersion of the $\dot{V}_A/\dot{Q}$ ratios throughout the lung actually widened (Figure 7). This was considered to be a major contributing factor to the normal widening of the alveolar-to-arterial PO_2 difference with moderate and heavy exercise. These authors recognized the — at

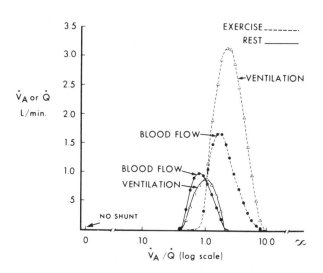

Figure 7. Distributions of ventilation and blood flow at rest (solid lines) and during moderate exercise (dashed lines). Taken from ref. 24.

first — apparently contradictory conclusion that the distributions of $\dot{V}_A$ and $\dot{Q}$ have been shown to become more uniform topographically during exercise (26-28), but at the same time the distribution of $\dot{V}_A/\dot{Q}$ ratios becomes more dispersed. They argue, therefore, that the radioactive-tracer techniques were relatively insensitive for accurate assessment of the $\dot{V}_A/\dot{Q}$ distribution, in that they reflect relatively large, two-dimensional planar representations of the lung with the average $\dot{V}_A/\dot{Q}$ assigned to all regions within that region. However, the multiple-inert-gas technique would reflect the intra-regional inhomogeneities of $\dot{V}_A/\dot{Q}$ ratios.

Using these same techniques, however, Gale *et al.* (29) and Hammond *et al.* (30) did not find statistically significant changes in their indices of either $\dot{V}_A$ or of $\dot{Q}$ dispersion in the steady-state of moderate exercise ($\dot{V}O_2$ < approx. 2 l/min) in normal subjects at sea level. This was consistent with earlier results of Derks (31) who found that the perfusion distribution was either unchanged or even narrowed somewhat at these work rates. At higher work rates, however ($\dot{V}O_2$ > 3 l/min), Hammond *et al.* (30) did find evidence of increased $\dot{V}_A/\dot{Q}$ inequality. These authors furthermore found that at these higher work rates the $\dot{V}_A/\dot{Q}$ inequality alone was not sufficient to account for the widened alveolar-to-arterial PO_2 difference (30).

V.   PULMONARY GAS EXCHANGE EFFICIENCY DURING EXERCISE

This conclusion leads to the second recent point of concern regarding the efficiency of pulmonary gas exchange in normal subjects exercising at sea level. Dempsey *et al.* (32) demonstrated that some highly-fit subjects (*i.e.*, subjects who could attain high levels of $\dot{V}O_2$, and therefore high levels of cardiac output and pulmonary blood flow) became hypoxemic at high work rates; they postulated that the subjects were developing a pulmonary diffusion limitation consequent to the high pulmonary blood flow not allowing adequate time for diffusion equilibrium to be attained, at least in some parts of the lung. Hammond *et al.* (30) therefore utilized highly-fit subjects exercising in "the steady state" at 300 Watts and demon-strated (using the multiple-inert-gas technique) that the increased dispersion of $\dot{V}_A/\dot{Q}$ which they demonstrated at high work rates (Figure 8) was no longer sufficient to explain the widening of the alveolar-to-arterial PO_2 difference. These authors argued persuasively against an increased post-pulmonary shunt component, and therefore support the contention of Dempsey and his associates (32) that with a high-enough cardiac output some subjects may develop functional diffusion impairments. It should be noted here that the degree of arterial hypoxemia observed in the study of Hammond *et al.* (30) was modest compared with that

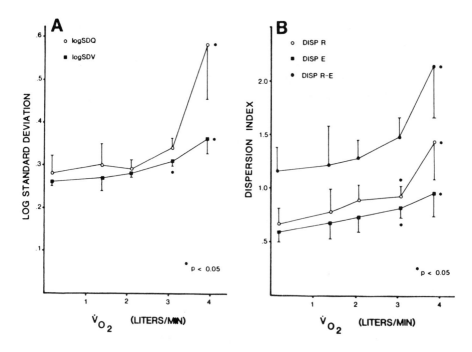

Figure 8. Indices of ventilation-perfusion inequality as a function of
$\dot{V}O_2$. *These indices are expressed as the log standard deviation of $\dot{Q}$ and $\dot{V}$ (panel
A) and as dispersion indices derived form retention (R) and excretion (E) data (panel
B). Taken from ref. 30.*

reported by Dempsey *et al.* (32), although the exercise levels were not maximal in
the former case. This diffusion-impairment component of the widened alveolar-to-
arterial PO_2 difference clearly should therefore be exacerbated by high altitude in
normal subjects.

Consequently, for arterial oxygenation to be maintained during exercise,
the pulmonary capillary volume must expand such that the required cardiac output
for the $\dot{V}O_2$ does not traverse appreciable portions of the pulmonary vascular bed
so rapidly that alveolar-to-pulmonary endcapillary equilibrium has not had time to
occur. This may be simply demonstrated by the fact that the mean transit time of
pulmonary capillary blood flow at a cardiac output of 20 l/min (equivalent to a
$\dot{V}O_2$ of "only" 3 l/min or so) will be about 0.5 seconds for a pulmonary capillary
blood volume of 150 ml, but only 0.3 seconds for a volume of 100 ml which will
encroach upon the minimum time normally required for diffusion equilibrium.
Consequently, the more rapid components of the distribution of pulmonary
capillary transit times will predispose to arterial hypoxemia. And therefore the

pulmonary circulatory dimensions, and hence the "diffusing capacity" (and $D/\dot{Q}$ distribution) for O_2, have important implications for the ability for the highly-trained athlete to perform very heavy exercise without developing arterial hypoxemia (30,32-34) which further stresses the already-taxed tissue energy exchange and ventilatory control mechanisms. The mechanisms of the further gas-exchange 'impairment' implicit in the wider dispersion of $\dot{V}_A/\dot{Q}$ at high work rates remain to be elucidated.

REFERENCES

1. Krogh A and Linghard J. (1913) *J Physiol* **47**:112.
2. Cummin ARC, Iyawe VI, Mehta N and Saunders KB. (1986) *J Physiol* **370**:567.
3. Miyamoto Y, Nakazono Y, Hiura R and Abe Y. (1983) *Jap J Physiol* **33**:971.
4. Loeppky JA, Greene ER, Hoekenga DE, Caprihan A and Luft UC. (1981) *J Appl Physiol* **50**:1173.
5. Weissman ML, Jones PW, Oren A, Lamarra N, Whipp BJ and Wasserman K. (1982) *J Appl Physiol* **52**:236.
6. Whipp BJ, Ward SA, Lamarra N, Davis JA and Wasserman K. (1982) *J Appl Physiol* **52**:1506.
7. Linnarsson D. (1974) *Acta Physiol Scand* **415** (suppl):1.
8. Weiler-Ravell D, Cooper DM, Whipp BJ and Wasserman K. (1983) *J Appl Physiol* **55**:1460.
9. Karlsson H, Lindborg B and Linnarsson D. (1975) *Acta Physiol Scand* **95**:329.
10. Nery LE, Wasserman K, Andrews JD, Huntsman DJ, Hansen JE and Whipp BJ. (1982) *J Appl Physiol* **53**:1594.
11. Khaja F and Parker JO. (1971) *Am Heart J* **83**:319.
12. Matthay RA and Berger HJ. (1981) *Med Clin N America* **65**:489.
13. Slutsky RA, Ackerman W, Karlinger IS, Ashburn WL and Moser KM. (1980) *Am J Med* **68**:197.
14. Sietsema KE, Cooper DM, Perloff JK, Rosove MH, Child JS, Canobbio MM, Whipp BJ and Wasserman K. (1986) *Circulation* **73**:1137.
15. Beaver WL, Wasserman K and Whipp BJ. (1973) *J Appl Physiol* **34**:128.
16. Auchincloss JH Jr, Gilbert R and Baule GH. (1966) *J Appl Physiol* **21**:810.
17. Wessel HU, Stout RL, Bastanier CK and Paul MH. (1979) *J Appl Physiol* **46**:1122.

18. Beaver WL, Lamarra N and Wasserman K. (1981) *J Appl Physiol* **51**:1662.

19. Swanson GD, Sodal IE and Reeves JT. (1981) *IEEE Trans on Biomed Engineering* **BME-28**:749.

20. Whipp BJ. (1981) *In* **The Regulation of Breathing**. (T Hornbein ed.) Dekker:New York.

21. Hughson RL and Morrisey M. (1982) *J Appl Physiol* **52**:921.

22. Hesser CM and Matell G. (1965) *Acta Physiol Scand* **63**:247.

23. Whipp BJ and Wasserman K. (1969). *J Appl Physiol* **27**:361.

24. Gledhill N, Froese AB and Dempsey JA. (1977) *In* **Muscular Exercise and the Lung**. (JA Dempsey and CE Reed, eds). Univ of Wisconsin Press:Madison.

25. Wagner PD, Laravuso RB, Uhl RR and West JB. (1977) *J Clin Invest* **54**:54.

26. Bake B, Bjure J and Widimsky J. (1968) *Scand J Clin Lab Invest* **22**:99.

27. Bryan AC, Bantivagio BL, Beerel F, MacLeish H, Zidulka A and Bates DV. (1964) *J Appl Physiol* **19**:395.

28. West JB and Dollery CT. (1960) *J Appl Physiol* **15**:405.

29. Gale GE, Torre-Bueno J, Moon R, Saltzman H and Wagner PD. (1985) *J Appl Physiol* **58**:978.

30. Hammond MD, Gale GE, Kapitan KS, Ries A and Wagner PD. (1986) *J Appl Physiol* **60**:1590.

31. Derks CM. (1980) *Bull Eur Physiopathol Resp* **16**:145.

32. Dempsey JA, Hanson PG and Henderson KS. (1984) *J Physiol* **355**:161.

33. Johnson RL Jr, Spicer WS, Bishop JN and Forster RE. (1960) *J Appl Physiol* **15**:893.

34. Shepherd RH. (1958) *J Appl Physiol* **12-13**:487.

Effects of Hypoxic Vasoconstriction on the Mechanical Interaction between Pulmonary Vessels and Airways

J.T. SYLVESTER
R.G. BROWER
S. PERMUTT
Johns Hopkins Medical Institutions
Francis Scott Key Medical Center
Baltimore, Maryland

I.   INTRODUCTION

The mechanical interaction between the airways and blood vessels has fascinated physiologists for over a hundred years (1, 2). Particular experimental attention has been paid to the effects of lung volume (V_L) on the resistance of the pulmonary vasculature to blood flow. After some initial confusion caused by differences in experimental technique, such as the use of positive versus negative-pressure ventilation and the location of reservoirs in extracorporeal perfusion systems (3), a consensus has emerged (1-5). In the normal lung under physiologic conditions, inflation from residual volume to approximately functional residual capacity will either decrease or not change vascular resistance. Continued inflation, however, will cause resistance to rise.

The generally accepted explanation for these effects depends upon the categorization of pulmonary vessels into two functional types (1-5). Alveolar vessels are surrounded by alveolar pressure and are therefore externally compressed as the lung inflates. Extra-alveolar vessels are surrounded by the difference between alveolar pressure and the pressure generated by the outward-acting pull exerted on them by tissue attachments to the lung parenchyma. The decompressive effects of this outward-acting pull exceed the compressive effects of alveolar pressure (6-7) and thus extra-alveolar vessels are externally decompressed as the lung inflates. It should be emphasized that the definitions of alveolar and extra-alveolar vessels are functional, not anatomic. Alveolar vessels may include small arteries and veins, as well as septal capillaries. Extra-alveolar vessels may include capillaries at the junction between alveolar septæ (the so-called "corner vessels"), as well as large arteries and veins.

With these definitions in mind, the effects of inflation on vascular resistance can be explained as follows. At low lung volumes, the major component of vascular resistance is provided by extra-alveolar vessels. With inflation, these vessels become externally decompressed and enlarge, causing resistance to fall. Simultaneously, however, alveolar vessels become externally compressed and smaller. Thus, at some lung volume the increase in alveolar vessel resistance will begin to exceed the decrease in extra-alveolar resistance and further increases in lung volume will cause resistance to rise. These concepts are supported by studies of the effects of inflation on vascular volume (8-10) and morphology (11-13), as well as resistance (14-19).

Recently, our work has focused on the effects of hypoxic pulmonary vasoconstriction on the interaction between lung volume and vascular resistance. In particular, we have found that these effects differ markedly between the pig and the ferret, two species which respond equally vigorously to hypoxia (20). In addition, we have described and made some initial attempts to elucidate the mechanism by which hypoxic vasoconstriction alters the inflation-deflation hysteresis in the relationship between lung volume and vascular resistance.

II.   EFFECTS OF HYPOXIC VASOCONSTRICTION
         IN THE PIG AND FERRET

From the definitions of alveolar and extra-alveolar vessels, it is reasonable to expect that the site of hypoxic vasoconstriction should have important effects on the interaction between lung volume and vascular resistance. For example, if hypoxia increased resistance by constricting alveolar vessels, inflation could cause a further increase in resistance, since the compressive effects of inflation on these vessels would be expected to add to the effects of vasoconstriction. If, on the other hand, constriction occurred in extra-alveolar vessels, increasing lung volume could subtract from the effects of vasoconstriction because of the external decompression of these vessels caused by inflation.

To determine the relationship between transpulmonary pressure and vascular resistance, we used isolated lungs perfused with a constant flow of autologous blood under zone II conditions (alveolar pressure > left atrial pressure). Under these conditions, pulmonary artery pressure (P_{pa}) was a direct measurement of the flow-resistive properties of the vasculature and alveolar pressure (P_{alv}) was

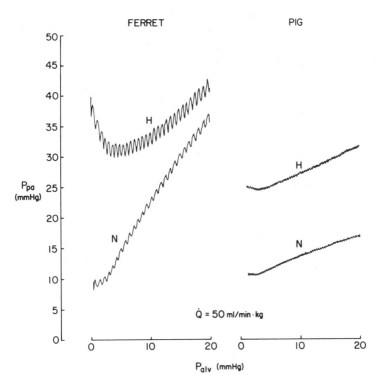

Figure 1. Recording of pulmonary artery pressure (Ppa) versus alveolar pressure (Palv) obtained from isolated, blood-perfused ferret and pig lungs during normoxia (N) and hypoxia (H) as Palv was slowly reduced from 20 to 0 mmHg. Blood flow ($\dot{Q}$) was constant at 50 ml/min·kg. Outflow perfusion pressure was subatmospheric.

equal to transpulmonary pressure. Figure 1 shows results typical of those obtained during slow deflation of ferret and pig lungs from total lung capacity to residual volume. In the ferret, Ppa was not influenced by Palv < 2.5 mmHg during normoxia; however, Ppa and Palv were directly proportional at Palv > 2.5 mmHg. As described above, these results suggest that at higher Palv there was an increasing contribution to total resistance by alveolar vessels which were compressed as Palv increased. Hypoxia markedly altered the Palv-Ppa relationship. Ppa increased at all Palv, consistent with vasoconstriction, and varied inversely with Palv at Palv 0-5 mmHg. Although Ppa and Palv were directly proportional at Palv > 5 mmHg, the slope of this relationship was less than that observed during normoxia. In other words, the higher the alveolar pressure, the closer the hypoxic curve was to the normoxic curve. These results are similar to those reported by

Suggett *et al.* (21) and suggest that hypoxic constriction occurring in extra-alveolar vessels was progressively cancelled by the decompressive effects of inflation. At the highest levels of Palv, the hypoxic curve became parallel to the normoxic curve, but remained slightly higher. These findings suggest that some hypoxic constriction occurred in alveolar vessels; however, the predominant site of constriction appears to have been the extra-alveolar vessels.

Results in the pig were quite different (Figure 1). Even at the highest lung volumes, Palv had less effect on Ppa than in the ferret, suggesting that the alveolar vessels were somehow protected from alveolar pressure. Moreover, hypoxia caused a virtually parallel shift in the Palv-Ppa curve to higher Ppa; *i.e.*, inflation did not progressively cancel the effects of hypoxic constriction as was observed in the ferret. This suggests that hypoxic constriction occurred predominantly in alveolar vessels (22, 23).

To gain further insight, we repeated the above measurements at different flow rates. This allowed us to construct the relationship between Ppa and flow ($\dot{Q}$) at different alveolar pressures. Because these relationships were well described by straight lines, we analyzed the data in terms of slope ($\Delta Ppa/\Delta \dot{Q}$) and pressure-axis

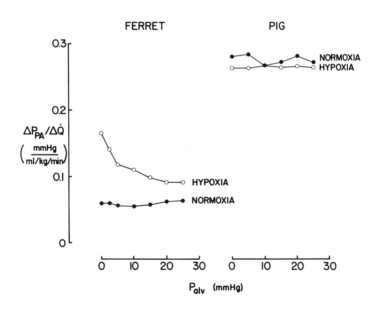

Figure 2. Effects of alveolar pressure (Palv) during slow deflation of isolated ferret and pig lungs on the slope of the pulmonary artery pressure-flow relationship ($\Delta Ppa/\Delta \dot{Q}$) during normoxia and hypoxia.

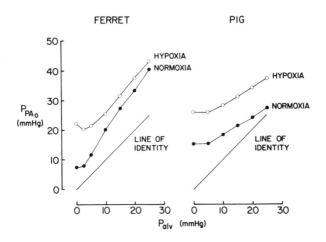

Figure 3. Effects of alveolar pressure (Palv) during slow deflation of isolated ferret and pig lungs on the pressure-axis intercepf the pulmonary artery pressure-flow relationship (Ppaₒ) during normoxia and hypoxia.

intercept (P_{pa_0}), as shown in Figures 2 and 3. In the ferret during normoxia, Palv did not affect the slope of the Ppa-$\dot{Q}$ line (Figure 2), indicating that inflation had either no effect or equal but opposite effects on the alveolar and extra-alveolar vessels which determined the slope. Hypoxia increased $\Delta Ppa/\Delta\dot{Q}$ indicating vasoconstriction of the vessels which determined the slope. Moreover, $\Delta Ppa/\Delta\dot{Q}$ now varied inversely with Palv, suggesting that these vessels were extra-alveolar. In the pig, $\Delta Ppa/\Delta\dot{Q}$ was higher than in the ferret, unchanged by hypoxia and independent of Palv. Thus, in the pig the vessels contributing to the slope were relatively smaller and/or fewer than in the ferret and unresponsive to hypoxia.

Figure 3 illustrates the effects of hypoxia and Palv on the intercept (P_{pa_0}) of the Ppa-$\dot{Q}$ line in these two species. Qualitatively, the effects were similar to those on Ppa (Figure 1) and indicate that in both species the vessels which determined P_{pa_0} were responsive to hypoxia; however, these vessels were predominantly extra-alveolar in the ferret and alveolar in the pig.

Under the Zone II conditions of these experiments, P_{pa_0} can be interpreted to represent the mean back-pressure to flow through the pulmonary circuit provided by the critical pressures of a vascular waterfall (22-25). When vasomotor tone is low and alveolar pressure high, these critical pressures will be located predominantly in alveolar vessels. Thus, during normoxia at high Palv, P_{pa_0} should vary directly and equally with Palv. Yet, as shown in Figure 3, P_{pa_0} increased more than Palv in the ferret lung, but less than Palv in the pig lung.

How can these results be explained? One possibility is illustrated in Figure 4. Perhaps in the ferret the connective tissue fibers surrounding the alveolar septal vessels were arranged like a tubular net which exerted a compressive force as it was stretched during inflation, thereby adding to the compressive effect of P_{alv}. Perhaps in the pig these fibers were arranged as longitudinal cables. Under increased tension at high lung volumes, these cables would resist deformation and therefore cancel to some extent the compressive effects of P_{alv}. Alternatively, the results might be explained by the effects of surface tension on the transmission of alveolar pressure to the septal interstitium. In the ferret, septal vessels might bulge into the alveolar lumen. In this case, interfacial surface tension would add to the compressive effect of alveolar pressure. In the pig, alveolar vessels might

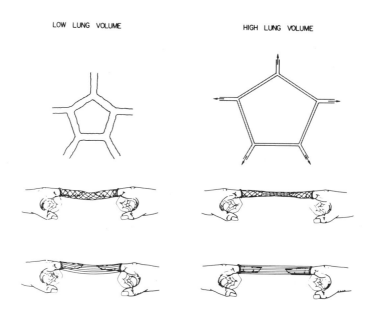

Figure 4. Possible explanation for the observation that the change in P_{pa_o} per unit change in P_{alv} exceeded 1.0 in the Zone II ferret lung but was less than 1.0 in the Zone II pig lung. As the alveolus enlarges with increasing P_{alv} (top row), the septus stretched. In the ferret lung (second row), a net-like arrangement of connective tissue fibers surrounds the septal capillary (finger) and subjects it to a compressive force which adds to that of P_{alv} as lung volume increases. In the pig lung (third row), the fibers are arranged around the septal capillary like longitudinal cables and thus resist the compressive effects of P_{alv} when stretched by increases in lung volume.

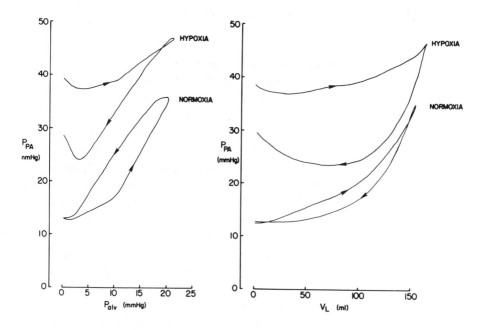

Figure 5. Simultaneous recordings of pulmonary artery pressure (Ppa) versus alveolar pressure (Ppa) and lung volume above residul volume (V_L) obtained during normoxia and hypoxia by slow inflation and deflation of an isolated ferret lung perfused with autologous blood at 100 ml/min·kg. Outflow perfusion pressure was subatmospheric. The direction of the hysteresis is indicated by the arrows.

be contained within a septum whose interface curves toward the alveolar lumen, causing interfacial tension to subtract from the effect of alveolar pressure. Whether these or other less fanciful explanations account for the Ppa_0 data in Figure 3 remains to be determined.

Our results indicate that hypoxic pulmonary vasoconstriction occurred predominantly in extra-alveolar vessels in the ferret and in alveolar vessels in the pig; therefore, the effects of lung volume on vascular resistance differed markedly between the two species. Inflation of a hypoxic lung region could increase regional perfusion in the ferret, but decrease it in the pig. The mechanism and physiologic significance of this species difference remain unclear.

III.   HYSTERESIS BETWEEN LUNG VOLUME
         AND VASCULAR RESISTANCE

The studies described above employed slow deflation of the lung from a state of maximum inflation. During these studies, it became apparent that the effects of inflation differed considerably from those of deflation and, further, that this difference was altered by hypoxic vasoconstriction. Typical hysteresis loops measured in isolated ferret lungs are shown in Figure 5. During normoxia P_{pa} was less at the same P_{alv}, during inflation than deflation; *i.e.,* there was a closed, counterclockwise hysteresis loop in the P_{alv}-P_{pa} relationship. When P_{pa} was plotted against the simultaneously measured change in lung volume above residual volume (V_L), the hysteresis loop was clockwise; *i.e.,* P_{pa} was greater at the same V_L during inflation. Similar changes in vascular resistance and volume have been previously reported (9,16,26,27). These loops were generated during a total cycle time of about 200 seconds. Previous experiments in this preparation indicated that this rate of change produced relationships no different from those generated by static changes in P_{alv} and V_L. Thus, time-dependent processes seem unlikely to account for the hysteresis observed during normoxia.

During hypoxia, the results were quite different. The loops occurred at higher levels of P_{pa} because of vasoconstriction. More interestingly, the loops were now clockwise for both the P_{alv}-P_{pa} and V_L-P_{pa} relationships and did not close at P_{alv} and $V_L = 0$. Preliminary experiments indicate that loop closure does occur under static conditions but the clockwise hysteresis persists. This suggests that the hysteresis seen during hypoxia was caused by both time-dependent and time-independent processes.

In general, there are two possible explanations for inflation-deflation hysteresis in the interaction between pulmonary vessels and airways. First, it could result from hysteresis of the forces exerted on the vessels via the airways and nonvascular parenchyma. This seems highly likely. The well-recognized hysteresis in the static relationship between transpulmonary pressure and lung volume is thought to result from the viscoelastic properties of lung tissue and the presence of surfactant in the liquid lining the airspaces, which causes surface tension at the gas-liquid interface to be higher on inflation than on deflation at the same transpulmonary pressure (28). Because of these factors, fewer airways will be open at a given transpulmonary pressure during inflation and the volume of those which are will be less. As a result, the compressive effect of P_{alv} on alveolar vessels and the decompressive effects of the outward-acting tissue pressure on extra-alveolar vessels will also be less during inflation.

Second, the hysteresis in vascular resistance could be caused by hysteresis in the response of the vessels to the forces exerted on them by the lung. This also seems likely. Hysteresis of vascular pressure- diameter or pressure-volume relationships has been described for both isolated vessels (29) and vessels within the pulmonary parenchyma (7). Undoubtedly, this hysteresis is partly the result of the passive viscoelastic properties of vascular smooth muscle. It is also possible that external stresses could trigger active changes in the state of vasomotor tone by mechanisms intrinsic to the vessel or by release of vasoactive mediators from the surrounding lung parenchyma. For example, Sasaki and Hoppin (30) found that distention of contracted, isolated airways caused marked relaxation of bronchial smooth muscle and counterclockwise hysteresis in the relationship between transmural pressure (abscissa) and bronchial diameter (ordinate). Although the mechanism of this effect is unknown, it was obviously intrinsic to the airway. Perhaps similar events occur in vascular smooth muscle. With respect to possible nonintrinsic mechanisms, it has been found that inflation of the lung can release vasodilator prostaglandins (31).

As an initial approach to the problem of the mechanism by which hypoxic vasoconstriction altered the Palv-Ppa hysteresis, we performed a model analysis to assess whether our results in the ferret lung could be explained simply by hysteresis of the passive mechanical forces acting on the vasculature. In our model, we assumed that (a) the relationship between Palv and V_L during inflation and deflation could be described by power functions, as shown in Figure 6; (b) $Ppa = \dot{Q} (\Delta Ppa/\Delta \dot{Q}) + Ppa_o$, where $\dot{Q}$, the blood flow through the lung, was constant at 100 ml/kg/min; (c) $Ppa_o = V_L P_A + (1-V_L)P_E$, where V_L was lung volume

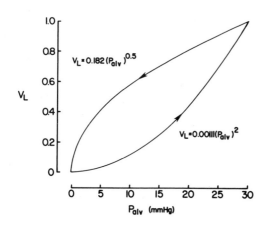

Figure 6. Relationships between alveolar pressure (Palv) and lung volume (V_L) used in the model analysis of the Palv-Ppa and V_L-Ppa hysteresis shown in Figure 5.

expressed as a decimal fraction of total lung volume, V_L and $(1-V_L)$ expressed the fractional conductances of the pathways leading to the alveolar and extra-alveolar vessels, respectively, providing back-pressures to flow, and P_A and P_E were the respective back-pressures of the alveolar and extra-alveolar vessels; and (d) left atrial pressure was zero.

During normoxia, we assumed further that the vessels were without tone; thus, under the Zone II conditions of our experiments the back-pressure to flow provided by alveolar vessels was Palv while that provided by extra-alveolar vessels was left atrial pressure, or zero. In addition, $\Delta Ppa/\Delta\dot{Q}$ was constant, as we observed (Figure 2) at an arbitrary value of 0.1 mmHg ml^{-1}·min·kg. Thus, during normoxia $Ppa = 10 + V_L Palv$. The graphical solution of this equation is shown in Figure 7. Consistent with our experimental results (Figure 5), the model predicted a counterclockwise hysteresis in the Palv-Ppa relationship and a clockwise hysteresis in the V_L-Ppa relationship. These results indicate that the hysteresis

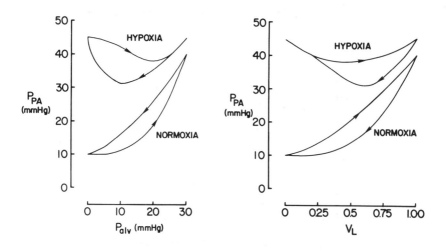

Figure 7. Predictions of the model analysis for the normoxic and hypoxic Palv-Ppa and V_L-Ppa relationships obtained during inflation and deflation of the lung. For explanation, see text. Note similarity to experimental observations in Figure 5.

during normoxia can be explained by poor transmission of Palv to the alveolar vessels during inflation because of a smaller number of open airways and/or a greater surface tension of the air-liquid interface in those alveoli which are open.

During hypoxia, we assumed that vasoconstriction increased $\Delta Ppa/\Delta \dot{Q}$ and that $\Delta Ppa/\Delta \dot{Q}$ decreased with increasing V_L, as we observed experimentally in the ferret lung (Figure 2). This decrease was described by the equation, $\Delta Ppa/\Delta \dot{Q} = 0.3 - 0.15 V_L$. We also assumed that hypoxic vasoconstriction caused the formation of critical pressures (Pc) which varied indirectly with V_L, such that $Pc = 15 - 10V_L$. This is also consistent with our observations (Figure 3). These critical pressures acted as outflow pressures in all vascular pathways when Palv < Pc. When Palv $\geq$ Pc, however, Palv became the back-pressure provided by alveolar vessels. Thus, $Ppa = 45 + 25V_L$ when Palv < Pc and $45 - V_L(40-Palv) + 10V_L^2$ when Palv $\geq$ Pc. The graphical solution to these equations is shown in Figure 7. Again, the predictions of the model are consistent with the experimental results (Figure 5): clockwise rotation in both the Palv-Ppa and V_L-Ppa loops at higher values of Ppa. This indicates that hypoxic reversal of the normoxic Palv-Ppa hysteresis can be explained by V_L- dependent reductions in the degree of hypoxic constriction of extra-alveolar vessels due to the outward pull exerted on these vessels by the lung parenchyma.

Obviously, the accuracy of the model's predictions indicates only that it is possible to explain the hysteresis of the Palv-Ppa relationship by hysteresis of the forces acting on the vasculature. It does not rule out other possible explanations. Indeed, the model did not predict that during hypoxia the Palv-Ppa loop would not close at Palv = 0 (Figures 5 and 7). Possibly, this result was due to stretch-induced relaxation of constricted extra-alveolar vessels. As mentioned above such an effect has been previously observed in airways (30).

We have also begun experiments to assess the possibility that the hysteresis may reside in the vessels themselves rather than in the forces imposed on the vessels by the lung. For example, we treated isolated ferret lungs with papaverine to obliterate smooth muscle tone. As shown in Figure 8, papaverine did not significantly alter the hysteresis observed during normoxia, suggesting that changes in smooth muscle tone did not play a role under these conditions. During hypoxia, however, papaverine caused the Palv-Ppa loop to revert to a normoxic configuration, indicating that smooth muscle tone did play an important role under these conditions. In other experiments, indomethacin, given in concentrations sufficient to block cyclooxygenase, had no effect on the Palv-Ppa loops during normoxia or hypoxia, suggesting that prostaglandins were not involved in the generation of the hysteresis.

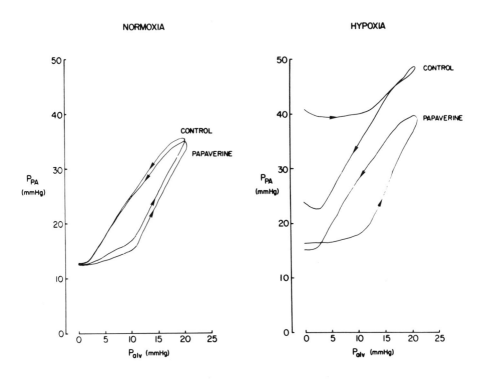

Figure 8. Effects of the smooth muscle relaxant, papaverine, on the P_{alv}-
P_{pa} relationship obtained during normoxia and hypoxia by slowly inflating and
deflating isolated ferret lungs perfusd with autologous blood at
100 ml/min·kg. Outflow perfusion pressure was subatmospheric. The direction
of the hysteress is indicated by the arrows.

IV.   CONCLUSIONS

Our results indicate that the resistive properties of the pulmonary vasculature depend markedly on the volume history of the lung and that these volume-dependent effects in turn depend on the direction, degree and locus of changes in vasomotor tone. The mechanisms of these effects and their physiological significance await elucidation. It seems likely that the mechanical interaction between the blood vessels and airways of the lung will fascinate scientists for another hundred years.

REFERENCES

1. Mead J and Whittenberger JL. (1964) *In* **Handbook of Physiology.** **Respiration Vol. 1** (WO Fenn and H Rahn, eds) American Physiological Society:Washington, D.C.
2. Culver BH and Butler J. (1980)*Ann Rev Physiol* **42**:187.
3. Permutt S. (1979)*In* **Pulmonary Edema.** (AP Fishman and EM Renkin, eds). American Physiological Society:Bethesda.
4. Dawson CA. (1984) *Physiol Rev* **64**:544.
5. Permutt S and Wise RA. (1986) *In* **Handbook of Physiology: Section 3: The Respiratory System. Vol. III, Mechanics of Breathing, Part 2.** (AP Fishman ed). American Physiological Society:Bethesda.
6. Lai-Fook SJ. (1979) *J Appl Physiol* **46**:419.
7. Smith JC and Mitzner W. (1980) *J Appl Physiol* **48**:450.
8. Howell JBL, Permutt S, Proctor DF, Riley RL. (1961) *J Appl Physiol* **16**:71.
9. Rosenzweig DY, Hughes JMB and Glazier JB. (1970) *J Appl Physiol* **28**:553.
10. Quebbeman EJ and Dawson CA. (1979) *J Appl Physiol* **43**:8.
11. Glazier JB, Hughes JMB, Maloney JE and West JB. (1969) *J Appl Physiol* **26**:65.
12. Mazzone RW. (1980) *Microvascular Res* **20**:295.
13. Gil J. (1980) *Ann Rev Physiol* **42**:177.
14. Burton AC and Patel DJ. (1958) *J Appl Physiol* **12**:239.
15. Lloyd TC Jr and Wright GW. (1960)*J Appl Physiol* **15**:241.
16. Whittenberger JL, McGregor M, Berglund E and Borst HG. (1960) *J Appl Physiol* **15**:878.
17. Roos A, Thomas LJ Jr, Nagel EL and Prommas DC. (1961) *J Appl Physiol* **16**:77.
18. Baile EM, Paré PD, Brook LA and Hogg JC. (1982) *J Appl Physiol* **52**:914.
19. Beck KC and Lai-Fook SJ. (1985) *J Appl Physiol* **58**:2004.
20. Peake MD, Harabin AL, Brennan NJ and Sylvester JT. (1981) *J Appl Physiol* **51**:1214.
21. Suggett A, Mohammed F, Barer G, Twelves C and Bee D. (1981) *Resp Physiol* **46**:89.
22. Mitzner W and Sylvester J. (1981) *J Appl Physiol* **51**:1065.
23. Sylvester JT, Mitzner WA, Ngeow Y and Permutt S. (1983) *J Appl Physiol* **54**:1660.
24. Permutt S and Riley RL. (1963) *J Appl Physiol* **18**:924.

25. Rock P, Patterson GA, Permutt S and Sylvester JT. (1985) *J Appl Physiol* **59**:1891.

26. Thomas LJ Jr, Griffo ZJ and Roos A. (1961) *J Appl Physiol* **16**:451.

27. Bruderman I, Somers K, Hamilton WK, Tooley WH and Butler J. (1964) *J Appl Physiol* **19**:707.

28. Radford EP Jr. (1964) *In* **Handbook of Physiology. Respiration. Vol. 1.** (WO Fenn and H Rahn, eds). American Physiological Society:Washington DC.

29. Murphy RA. (1980) *In* **Handbook of Physiology. The Cardiovascular System. Vol II. Vascular Smooth Muscle.** (DF Bohr, AP Somlyo and HV Sparks Jr, eds). American Physiological Society:Washington DC.

30. Sasaki T and Hoppin FG Jr. (1979) *J Appl Physiol* **47**:1251.

31. Leffler CW, Hessler JR and Terragno NA. (1980) *Am J Physiol* **238**:H282.

Vasomotor Tone and Optimization of Gas Exchange

BRYDON J. B. GRANT[1]
Department of Medicine,
State University of New York at
Buffalo,
Buffalo, NY 14215

I. INTRODUCTION

The idea that pulmonary vascular tone can optimize gas exchange was first introduced by Von Euler and Liljestrand in their landmark paper of 1946 (1). They argued that a reduction in ventilation to a lung region will decrease local alveolar oxygen tension which will cause an increase pulmonary vascular tone. As a result of the localized increase in vascular tone, pulmonary blood flow decreases to the poorly ventilated lung region and is diverted to better ventilated areas of the lung. In the succeeding years, the importance of this mechanism for pulmonary gas exchange became a matter of some dispute. Because of this controversy, we became interested in the quantification of the effects of alveolar oxygen tension on local pulmonary blood flow on pulmonary gas exchange.

II. APPLICATION OF CONTROL THEORY

One approach to this problem is to consider the effect of alveolar oxygen tension on local pulmonary blood flow as a controlling mechanism in a feedback

---

[1]*Some of the work described herein was supported by a grant-in-aid from the American Heart Association and the West Palm Beach Chapter. BJB Grant is a recipient of a research career development award HL-01418.*

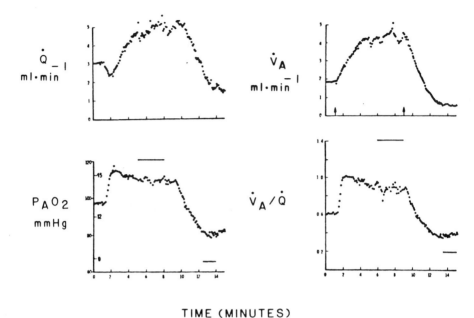

TIME (MINUTES)

Figure 1. Experimental results of alveolar ventilation ($\dot{V}_A$), alveolar oxygen tension ($P_A O_2$), pulmonary blood flow ($\dot{Q}$) and local ventilation–perfusion ratio ($\dot{V}_A / \dot{Q}$) of a small group of lung lobules that comprised less than one percent of the lungs of the coati mundi obtained over a period of just under fifteen minutes. $\dot{V}_A$ is increased then subsequently decreased. The bars in the panels displaying $P_A O_2$ and $\dot{Q}$ indicate the extremes which these variables would have reached had it not been for the effect of $P_A O_2$ on local $\dot{Q}$. Thus hypoxic pulmonary vasoconstriction has the effect of minimizing changes of $P_A O_2$ and $\dot{V}_A / \dot{Q}$ under these experimental conditions.

loop. There are two lines of evidence to support this idea: the first is experimental, the second is theoretical.

The experimental evidence was obtained in the coati mundi or South American raccoon (2). We used this animal to study the strength of the hypoxic response in small lung units because of its lack of collateral ventilation. This feature enabled us to wedge a catheter into a small group of lobules, and alter the local alveolar ventilation by modulating the amount of fresh inspired gas delivered to the group of lobules. From continuous measurements of their expired gas composition and knowing the inspired and mixed venous blood gas tensions, we were able to calculate local alveolar ventilation, local alveolar oxygen tension, local pulmonary blood flow and local alveolar ventilation-perfusion ratio. Figure 1 shows the time course of the response when we altered local alveolar ventilation. As ventilation is increased, alveolar oxygen tension increases. There is also an increase in the local ventilation-perfusion ratio but it is not as great as would have been expected from the increase in ventilation. The expected increase in local ventilation-perfusion ratio did not occur because the increased local alveolar oxygen tension reduces local vascular tone and results in a concomitant increase of local pulmonary blood flow. A similar sequence of events occurs when local alveolar ventilation is reduced. The ability of the system to minimize changes of variables such as the local alveolar oxygen tension and ventilation-perfusion ratio that is the hallmark of a negative feedback system.

The theoretical evidence is based on the analysis of relations between gas exchange variables in a single lung unit in which hypoxic pulmonary

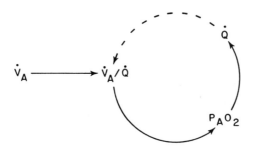

Figure 2. Symbol–arrow diagram of the working relations for pulmonary gas exchange in a single homogeneous lung unit in which hypoxic pulmonary vasoconstriction is operating. The arrows represent the sequence of events in a relation between two variables. For example, hypoxic pulmonary vasoconstriction is represented by $P_A O_2$ - - -> $\dot{Q}$. This arrow indicates that it is the change in alveolar oxygen tension ($P_A O_2$) that results in a change of pulmonary blood flow ($\dot{Q}$). Solid arrows represent a direct relation between two variables which means that the sign of the first derivative will be positive; interrupted arrows represent an inverse relation between two variables which means that the sign of the first derivative will be negative. $\dot{V}_A$ and $\dot{V}_A/\dot{Q}$ represent alveolar ventilation and ventilation–perfusion ratio, respectively. A negative feedback loop is indicated by the fact that the sign of the product of the first derivatives around the feedback loop is negative.

vasoconstriction is operating. A symbol–arrow diagram of these working relations is shown in Figure 2. A decrease of alveolar ventilation ($\dot{V}_A$) reduces the ventilation–perfusion ratio ($\dot{V}_A/\dot{Q}$) which, in turn, results in a decrease of alveolar oxygen tension (P_AO_2). The decrease in local P_AO_2 causes a decrease in local blood flow ($\dot{Q}$) due to hypoxic pulmonary vasoconstriction which, in turn, results in the $\dot{V}_A/\dot{Q}$ ratio increasing back toward its initial value. Therefore, hypoxic pulmonary vasoconstriction has had the effect of minimizing changes of local ventilation-perfusion ratio through a sequence of unidirectional relations, thus fulfilling Rigg's definition of a feedback system (3).

The techniques to assess the efficiency of a feedback system are readily available in control theory and have been adapted for their application in physiological systems (4). Gain due to feedback (G_{fb}) provides a suitable measure of the effectiveness of the local pulmonary $\dot{Q}$ control by P_AO_2. It can be calculated from the following equation.

$$G_{fb} = \frac{(dP_AO_2/d\dot{V}_A) \text{ open}}{(dP_AO_2/d\dot{V}_A) \text{ closed}} - 1$$

where the output or controlled variable is considered to be local alveolar oxygen tension (P_AO_2) and the disturbing input is considered to be local alveolar ventilation ($\dot{V}_A$). The derivative refers to the change of the controlled variable that results from a small change of the disturbing input. The subscripts refer to the state of the feedback loop. An open loop condition indicates that local $\dot{Q}$ control by P_AO_2 due to hypoxic pulmonary vasoconstriction is absent and thereby opens the feedback loop. Under closed loop conditions, local $\dot{Q}$ control by P_AO_2 is in operation; the addition of this relation therefore completes the feedback loop. If the local $\dot{Q}$ control by P_AO_2 were completely ineffective, it would make no difference whether the feedback loop was open or closed, therefore the value of the two derivatives would be equal and G_{fb} would be zero. On the other hand, if the feedback loop operated perfectly so that P_AO_2 would remain unchanged despite a change of $\dot{V}_A$, then ($dP_AO_2/d\dot{V}_A$)closed would be zero and G_{fb} would increase without bound.

The numerical methods used to calculate G_{fb} have been described in detail elsewhere (5), so only an outline of the procedure will be described here. The general approach is as follows. First, the initial conditions for gas exchange variables are set. Then, the disturbing input and the output or controlled variable are selected from the gas exchange variables. The effects of local $\dot{Q}$ control by P_AO_2 on pulmonary gas exchange are incorporated into each lung compartment. This effect is achieved by causing compartmental blood flow to vary with any

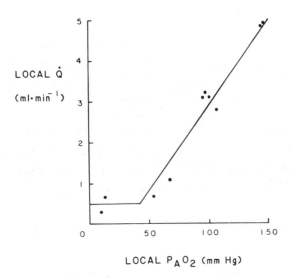

Figure 3. Effect of alveolar oxygen tension (P_AO_2, mmHg, horizontal axis) on local pulmonary blood flow ($\dot{Q}$, ml/min, vertical axis) in a small group of lung lobules that comprises less than 1% of the lungs. Therefore, changes in the status of local gas exchange have no measureable effect on overall pulmonary gas exchange. Solid circles are the data points, the lines are fitted by eye.

change in local P_AO_2 from its value assigned under initial conditions. The changes of compartmental blood flow with local P_AO_2 are proportional to the changes measured in the coati mundi (Figure 3). Gas exchange is then calculated and values for these variables are stored. Throughout this paper we shall confine ourselves to considering pulmonary gas exchange under steady state conditions, although it possible to adapt this analysis to investigate the transient state (6). The disturbing input is then increased by ten percent and gas exchange recalculated and values of the disturbing input and controlled variable are stored. This process is repeated after decreasing the value of the disturbing input by ten percent. There are now three values of the disturbing input and three values of the controlled variable to which is fitted with a Lagrangian second degree polynomial. The resulting equation is then used to enumerate the first derivative with respect to the disturbing input at its initial value. This entire process is then repeated after excluding the effect of local $\dot{Q}$ control by P_AO_2 from operating in each lung compartment. The required derivative is then obtained under open loop conditions thus enabling the estimation of gain due to feedback.

III.   SINGLE LUNG UNIT

With the local $\dot{Q}$–P_AO_2 curve measured in the coati mundi (figure 3), we calculated G_{fb} for a single lung unit (Figure 4) using air as the inspired gas and normal mixed venous blood gas composition ($P_{\bar{v}}O_2$ of 40mmHg and $P_{\bar{v}}CO_2$ of 46 mmHg). Because of the nonlinear nature of the gas exchange relations, G_{fb} is dependent on the initial conditions and varies with the ventilation–perfusion ratio. The maximum value of G_{fb} is 0.87, and occurs at a $\dot{V}_A/\dot{Q}$ ratio of 0.4. G_{fb} of this value means that local $\dot{Q}$ reduces by nearly half the change of P_AO_2 that would have occurred if there had been no local $\dot{Q}$ control. This result indicates that local $\dot{Q}$ control is moderately effective at minimizing changes in P_AO_2.

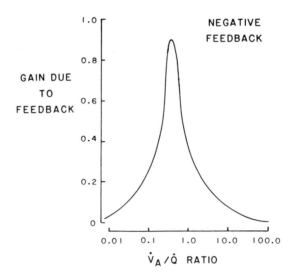

Figure 4. Gain due to feedback in a single lung unit. Gain due to feedback (G_{fb}) is plotted on the vertical axis, ventilation–perfusion ratio ($\dot{V}_A/\dot{Q}$) is plotted on the horizontal axis. The disturbing input is alveolar ventilation and the controlled variable is alveolar oxygen tension. However, in a single feedback loop, G_{fb} is identical to the open loop gain which is a measure of feedback efficiency widely used by engineers. In this circumstance, G_{fb} would be identical if the controlled variable was considered to be the end-capillary oxygen content or the ventilation–perfusion ratio (3,4).

By linearizing the oxygen and carbon dioxide dissociation curves, we were able to use an algebraic approach to analyze the factors involved in determining the this bell-shaped relation between G_{fb} and $\dot{V}_A/\dot{Q}$ (5). The shape of this curve is dependent primarily on the relation by which changes of $\dot{V}_A/\dot{Q}$ ratio alters P_AO_2. The shape of the local $\dot{Q}-P_AO_2$ response curve has little effect as long as it is monotonic. The $\dot{V}_A/\dot{Q}$ at which G_{fb} is maximal is dependent on the slope of the oxygen dissociation curve averaged over its operating range, and that the maximal value of G_{fb} is dependent not only on the slope of the local $\dot{Q}-P_AO_2$ response curve but also on the inspired–mixed venous oxygen tension difference. It is these two features that make oxygen, rather than carbon dioxide, alveolar gas tension well suited for local $\dot{Q}$ control. Oxygen has an Ostwald's partition coefficient of 0.36 so that it operates maximally on moderately low ventilation–perfusion ratios, whereas CO_2 has a higher partition coefficient of 11.2 so that it would operate maximally at high ventilation–perfusion ratios. The large P_I-P_v difference of 109 mmHg for O_2 contrasts with the smaller P_v-P_I of 46 mmHg for CO_2.

IV. MULTICOMPARTMENT LUNG

Von Euler's and Liljestrand's hypothesis was concerned with the ability of hypoxic pulmonary vasoconstriction to readjust the distribution of pulmonary blood flow. Therefore, it seemed pertinent to examine the effect of local $\dot{Q}$ control due to P_AO_2 on a lognormal distribution of ventilation–perfusion ratios arranged in parallel. With overall alveolar ventilation, pulmonary blood flow, oxygen uptake and carbon dioxide output were maintained constant, and G_{fb} were calculated for both arterial oxygen tension and arterial carbon dioxide tension as the controlled variable. A small change of the lognormal standard deviation of ventilation distribution is the disturbing input in both cases. Figure 5 presents a remarkable finding: G_{fb} varies with the degree of $\dot{V}_A/\dot{Q}$ dispersion. Indeed, at high degrees of $\dot{V}_A/\dot{Q}$ inequality, positive feedback behavior occurs. Positive feedback behavior indicates that in these limited circumstances, an increase in ventilation–perfusion inequality will result in a greater deterioration of arterial blood gas tensions due to the presence of hypoxic pulmonary vasoconstriction in contradiction to the von Euler–Liljestrand hypothesis.

Although positive feedback behavior is present, the gain is less than unity. Therefore, it does not represent an indicator of instability which is usually associated with positive feedback. Nevertheless, it is surprising because the lung is composed of 100 compartments in which local $\dot{Q}$ control operates in each compartment with a negative feedback effect. The reason for this result must be related to the parallel arrangement of compartments. Figure 6 compares two

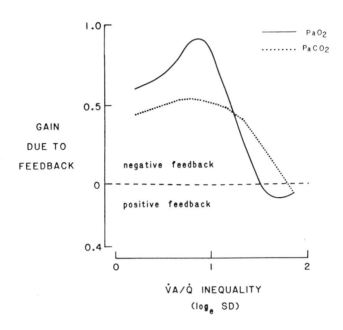

Figure 5. Gain due to feedback in a multicompartment lung when the controlled variable is the arterial blood oxygen tension (P_aO_2, continuous line) and when the controlled variable is arterial blood carbon dioxide tension (P_aCO_2, dotted line). The disturbing input is the degree of ventilation–perfusion inequality in both cases. To demonstrate the ability of local $\dot{Q}$ control by P_AO_2 to redistribute pulmonary blood flow, the overall ventilation and overall blood flow are held constant at 5.1 and 6.0 l/min, respectively. Mixed venous blood gas composition varied in order to maintain oxygen uptake and carbon dioxide output constant at 240 and 300 ml/min, respectively. Gain due to feedback (G_{fb}) is plotted on the vertical axis; the degree of ventilation–perfusion inequality, expressed as the lognormal standard deviation of the distribution of ventilation–perfusion ratios (log_e SD) is plotted on the horizontal axis . Note that local $\dot{Q}$ control by P_AO_2 affects the distribution of ventilation–perfusion ratios, therefore both oxygen and carbon dioxide exchange are affected.

distributions of $\dot{Q}$ with the magnitude of G_{fb}. With the narrow distribution of $\dot{Q}$, G_{fb} is maximal in compartments with relatively low ventilation–perfusion ratios and the preponderance of pulmonary blood flow is received by compartments with higher ventilation–perfusion ratios. Therefore, hypoxic pulmonary vasoconstriction acts to divert pulmonary blood flow from those compartments with low ventilation–perfusion ratios to compartments with a higher $\dot{V}_A/\dot{Q}$ ratios and consequently, higher end-capillary oxygen tensions. As a result, local $\dot{Q}$ control minimizes the deleterious effects of an increase in $\dot{V}_A/\dot{Q}$ inequality on P_aO_2. In contrast, with a broad distribution of $\dot{Q}$, G_{fb} is maximal in compartments with relatively high ventilation–perfusion ratios and the preponderance of pulmonary blood flow is received by compartments with low ventilation-perfusion ratios. Therefore, hypoxic pulmonary vasoconstriction acts to divert pulmonary blood flow from those compartments with higher ventilation–perfusion ratios to compartments with a lower $\dot{V}_A/\dot{Q}$ ratios. Consequently, local $\dot{Q}$ control magnifies the deleterious effects of an increase in $\dot{V}_A/\dot{Q}$ inequality on P_aO_2. Therefore, the positive feedback behavior can be attributed to the parallel arrangement of the network in which local $\dot{Q}$ control is operating, rather than a property of hypoxic pulmonary vasoconstriction itself.

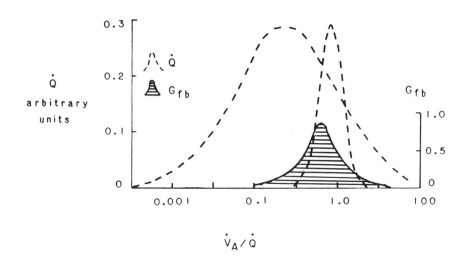

Figure 6. Comparison of distributions of pulmonary blood flow in an inhomogeneous lung with the gain due to feedback (G_{fb}) in a single lung unit. The left vertical axis is pulmonary blood flow ($\dot{Q}$, arbitary units), the right vertical axis is G_{fb}, and the horizontal axis is ventilation–perfusion ratio ($\dot{V}_A/\dot{Q}$) on a log scale.

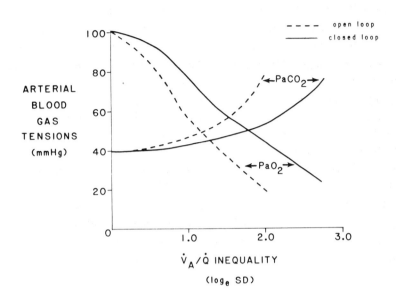

Figure 7. Effect of hypoxic pulmonary vasoconstriction on arterial blood gas tensions when a homogeneous lung is subjected to increasing ventilation-perfusion inequality. Arterial blood gas tensions (mmHg) are plotted on the vertical axis and the degree of ventilation–perfusion inequality assessed by the lognormal standard deviation of the distribution of ventilation–perfusion ratios (log$_e$*SD). The changes that occur in the absence of hypoxic pulmonary vasoconstriction are shown by the interrupted line (open loop) and the changes that occur in the presence of hypoxic pulmonary vasoconstriction are shown by the continuous line (closed loop).*

We have not been able to define a rigorous mathematical definition of the effects of local $\dot{Q}$ control on pulmonary gas exchange because of the nonlinear nature of the system. Nevertheless we have been able to develop a general statement or theorem that describes its effects in the presence of $\dot{V}_A/\dot{Q}$ inequality. The effects of local $\dot{Q}$ control on pulmonary gas exchange depend on (i) the magnitude of the gain due to feedback in a single lung unit, (ii) the proportion of blood flow received by compartments with $\dot{V}_A/\dot{Q}$ ratios where that gain is maximal, and (iii) the $\dot{V}_A/\dot{Q}$ ratios of compartments that receive the preponderance of pulmonary blood flow.

The term "gain due to feedback" means little to the clinician who would prefer to have the effects of hypoxic pulmonary vasoconstriction on pulmonary gas exchange in terms of arterial blood gas tensions. To this end, we recalculated the changes in arterial blood gas tensions that occur when ventilation-perfusion inequality is increased in a multicompartment lung model as calculated originally by West [7]. Overall alveolar ventilation, overall pulmonary blood flow, oxygen uptake and carbon dioxide output are held constant at 5.1 l/min, 6.0 l/min, 300 ml/min and 240 ml/min respectively. A progressive rise of P_aCO_2 and fall of P_aO_2 worsen with increasing degrees of ventilation–perfusion inequalilty (Figure 7). There are similar changes of mixed venous blood gas tensions, which are not shown here, until a limit is reached when $P_{\bar{v}}O_2$ falls to zero. We then incorporated local $\dot{Q}$ control by P_AO_2 in each of the 100 compartments and estimated the changes in pulmonary gas exchange. At any particular level of ventilation-perfusion inequality, the deterioration of the arterial blood gas tensions was moderately protected by hypoxic pulmonary vasoconstriction (Figure 7). Furthermore, the lung could withstand a greater degree of $\dot{V}_A/\dot{Q}$ inequality before mixed venous blood oxygen tension falls to zero.

It should be emphasized that this result is limited in scope for a number of reasons. First, it only describes the changes in arterial blood gas tensions from one initial condition: the homogeneous lung. For example, if the initial log_eSD was 1.5, the results would be quite different. Second, it is not easy to determine the way hypoxic pulmonary vasoconstriction exerts its effect on the distribution of ventilation-perfusion ratios. Figure 7 should not be considered as predictive because it only uses lognormal distributions and it assumes that the ventilation–perfusion inequality is based on a parallel arrangement of ventilation and perfusion between lung compartments. It has been postulated that in lung disease collateral ventilation between lung units may have a significant effect on pulmonary gas exchange. Recently, we have become interested in determining the effects of hypoxic pulmonary vasoconstriction on pulmonary gas exchange in these circumstances.

V. TYPE OF INHOMOGENEITY

The most extreme form of collateral ventilation occurs when inspired gas of one compartment is derived solely from the alveolar gas of another compartment. This serial ventilatory arrangement is markedly different from the parallel ventilatory arrangement where the inspirate for all compartments is obtained from the same source. The differences are very apparent from the symbol-arrow diagram (Figure 8). Figure 8 compares the working relations that operate in two compartments with a parallel ventilatory arrangement with the working relations that operate in two compartments with a series ventilatory arrangement.

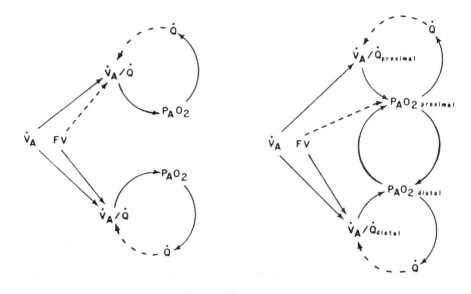

Figure 8. Symbol–arrow diagram of two compartment models, one with a parallel ventilatory arrangement (on the left) and the other with a series ventilatory arrangement (on the right). An explanation of the symbol–arrow diagram is given in the legend of Figure 2.

In the series ventilatory arrangement, the proximal compartment is the sole source of inspired gas to the distal compartment. In addition, expired gas from the distal compartment has to flow into the proximal compartment. Therefore, the alveolar oxygen tension of the proximal compartment is dependent on P_AO_2 and alveolar ventilation of the distal compartment. As a result of this interdependence of alveolar oxygen tensions, there is a positive feedback loop formed between the proximal and distal compartments with the series ventilatory arrangement that does not exist for the parallel ventilatory arrangement. Therefore, we anticipated that the effects of local $\dot{Q}$ control by P_AO_2 on pulmonary gas exchange will differ markedly in a two compartment model in which there is a series ventilatory arrangement compared with a two compartment model in which there is a parallel ventilatory arrangement.

To investigate this possibility we incorporated hypoxic pulmonary vasoconstriction into the two compartment models of Wagner and Evans because it enables us to compare series and parallel models that are equivalent in their gas exchange function (8). Figure 9 shows the results of these comparisions. In the

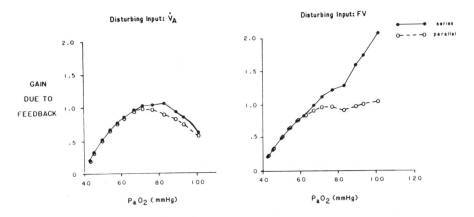

Figure 9. Gain due to feedback in a two compartment lung unit. The disturbing input is a change in the distribution of alveolar ventilation (FV) and the controlled variable is arterial blood oxygen tension. The initial overall $\dot{V}_A/\dot{Q}$ for each model is unity. The inspired gas is air, the mixed venous blood gas composition is held constant with $P_{\bar{v}}O_2$ and $P_{\bar{v}}CO_2$ of 40 and 46 mmHg respectively. On the horizontal axis is plotted the arterial oxygen tension (P_aO_2 of each pair of equivalent models. On the vertical axis is the gain due to feedback (G_{fb}) of the models with a series ventilatory arrangement and the G_{fb} of models with a parallel ventilatory arrangement.

left hand panel is the gain due to feedback when change in overall alveolar ventilation is used as the disturbing input and arterial oxygen tension is the controlled variable. Mixed venous blood gas composition is held constant and overall pulmonary blood flow was unconstrained. In the right hand panel is the gain due to feedback obtained under similar circumstances except that the disturbing input is changes in the distribution of ventilation between the two compartments (FV in figure 8). For the series ventilatory arrangement, FV is the fraction of overall alveolar ventilation to the distal compartment. The alveolar ventilation of the proximal compartment is the overall alveolar ventilation. For the parallel ventilatory arrangement, FV is the fraction of overall alveolar ventilation to one of the compartments, the fraction of overall alveolar ventilation to the other compartment is (1 − FV). Gain due to feedback tends to vary with the increasing degrees of ventilation-perfusion inequality which is indicated by the decreasing value of the arterial oxygen tension for each pair of series models and their parallel equivalent. For both disturbing inputs, gain due to feedback is greater for the series ventilatory arrangement than for the parallel ventilatory arrangement. This result indicates that hypoxic pulmonary vasoconstriction operates with much greater effectiveness in a series than in a parallel ventilatory arrangement. It is another example of how the effects of hypoxic pulmonary vasoconstriction on pulmonary gas exchange is dependent on the nature of the network in which it operating.

VI.   SUMMARY

1. Hypoxic pulmonary vasoconstriction can considered as the controlling mechanism in a feedback system that regulates local ventilation–perfusion ratios.

2. In a single homogeneous lung unit, the gain due to feedback varies with the ventilation–perfusion ratio. Under normal conditions this negative feedback loop is moderately effective at regulating ventilation–perfusion ratios and has a maximal gain due to feedback of 0.87 at a ventilation–perfusion ratio of 0.4. This result assumes that the relation between local pulmonary blood flow and alveolar oxygen tension in the coati mundi and human are similar.

3. In an inhomogeneous lung unit, the effect of hypoxic pulmonary vasoconstriction on pulmonary gas exchange depends not only on the extent of inhomgeneity, but also on the type of inhomogeneity.

REFERENCES

1.   Euler US von and Lilejestrand G. (1946) *Acta Physiol Scand* **12**:301.
2.   Grant BJB, Davies EE, Jones H and Hughes JMB. (1976)*J Appl Physiol* **40**:216.
3.   Riggs DS. (1967)*Advan Enzyme Regulation* **5**:357.
4.   Riggs DS. (1970) *In* **Control Theory and Physiological Feedback Mechanisms**. Williams & Wilkins:Baltimore, MD.
5.   Grant BJB. (1982) *J Appl Physiol* **53**:110.
6.   Grant BJB and Schneider AM. (1983) *J Appl Physiol* **54**:445.
7.   West JB. (1969) *Respir Physiol* **7**:88.
8.   Wagner PD and Evans JW. (1977) *Respir Physiol* **31**:117.

Endothelial Function

The Pulmonary Endothelium: Summary

Historically, vascular endothelium was viewed as a static barrier, the properties of which determined relationships between transvascular fluid and protein flux and the transmural pressure gradients. Edema was viewed as the simple consequence of breaching the endothelial barrier, and therefore edema has been the hallmark of endothelial injury.

As a result of extensive research, greatly enhanced by the development of techniques for culturing vascular endothelial cells *in vitro*, it is now clear that endothelium (and endothelial cells) are much more active players in a host of normal and pathologic scenarios than previously supposed. Even the barrier function of endothelium may be more complex and interesting than inferred by Starling in his classic studies of fluid balance. And myriad functions of endothelium not directly related to its role as a barrier between blood and interstitium can affect functions of other cells proximate to and distant from the endothelium itself. Several fascinating possibilities are summarized in the several chapters in this section—processing of mediators, effects on the coagulation system, immunological properties, to name a few.

Many functions of endothelium seem (it would be more surprising if this were not the case) to be related to the endothelial surface. Perhaps a modern revision of the notion of endothelium as a barrier would be the endothelium as an interface, a concept which would include barrier properties but also emphasize the processing of bioactive substances at the endothelial luminal surface, immunological functions related to the endothelial surface, antithrombotic functions of endothelium, and influences of endothelial cells and molecules. The concept of endothelium as an interface could also include transducing functions; that is, the role of endothelial cells in moderating behaviour of vascular smooth muscle and perhaps other cells separated from the blood by the endothelial layer.

An expanded concept of endothelial structure and function requires a redefinition of endothelial injury and such a redefinition is not easily made. Edema is a consequence of endothelial injury, but likely a late consequence and, at least in many circumstances, perhaps not the consequence of greatest import to organ or organism function. Injurious stimuli undoubtedly cause a profusion of alterations in endothelial structure and function too subtle to cause edema. Whether any alteration in endothelial structure or function should be thought of as injury is not clear. On the one hand, such subtle alterations may precede endothelial cell destruction (and edema), but on the other hand, these structural and functional subtleties may be transient or, more to the point, may play a homeostatic role. It makes good teleological sense to conclude that responses of endothelial cells are designed to restore the endothelium to a normal state or to contribute to recovery of the organ or organism, and that it is only when the responses get out of hand that "injury" results.

Vascular endothelium is a dynamic and fascinating organ peculiarly situated to influence functions of other cells and even to integrate organ function at a higher level. Studies like those described in the excellent chapters in this section elucidate endothelial structure and function (and relationships between the two) and hold the promise of further insights into how endothelium acts to effect, transduce and mediate functions of whole organisms.

UNA S. RYAN

Pulmonary Endothelial Cells[1]

UNA S. RYAN
Department of Medicine
University of Miami School of
Medicine
Miami, Florida 33101

I   INTRODUCTION

    To discuss the state of the art of endothelial cells of the pulmonary circulation is to consider dynamic concepts, both in terms of our evolving understanding of endothelium but also in terms of the multiplicity of signals arriving at the endothelial surface. Current knowledge of pulmonary endothelial cells includes details of their structure, barrier properties, metabolic functions and responses to injury, all subjects addressed in the component chapters of this section (1-4). Many of the previously recognized properties of the endothelium, especially those involving exchange of gases, permeability characteristics and efficient processing, require maintenance of its special morphology: an extremely extensive, very thin monolayer, and are compromised if the monolayer is disrupted. It is now evident that modulations of endothelial cell activities and structures, that fall far short of frank disruption of the monolayer or of the cells themselves, can result in markedly altered properties (5). It may now be appropriate to consider some of the sensitive responses of endothelial cells to stimuli as "activation" phenomena and to begin to examine for such concepts as signal transduction and stimulus-secretion coupling at the endothelial surface.

    Constant developments in the field now allow an emerging view of pulmonary endothelium as a dynamic regulator, target, transducer and effector system.

[1]The work was supported by grants HL 21568, HL 33064 and Council for Tobacco Research 814.

351

II.   CONSTITUTIVE FUNCTIONS
          OF PULMONARY ENDOTHELIAL CELLS

Like Shakespeare's "Ages of Man" the unfolding story of pulmonary endothelium has seen its coming of age from being considered a more-or-less inert barrier with fixed permeability characteristics to being recognized as a metabolically active surface strategically placed to determine the composition of systemic arterial blood. We now know that endothelial cells are capable of metabolizing a wide range of vasoactive peptides, biogenic amines, adenine nucleotides and prostaglandins. Furthermore, many of the enzymes, receptors and transporters responsible for these metabolic processes, and their ultrastructural sites, are known (6).

Many metabolic activities of endothelium first recognized *in vivo* have been verified using endothelial cells in culture,(*e.g.* ref. 7); others have first been noted using cells in culture (*e.g.* ref. 8). The ease and convenience with which pulmonary endothelial cells can now be maintained in culture (9) is both a blessing and a bane. It has meant that cellular and molecular analytical techniques can be effectively applied to studies of pulmonary endothelium, but some endothelial cell properties must await verification *in vivo* before they can be ascribed as physiologically relevant functions.

By and large, most of the functions of endothelium involving processing of vasoactive substances can be considered constant properties. For example, the conversion of angiotenisin I to angiotensin II and degradation of bradykinin by angiotensin converting enzyme, seems to be a property shared by all endothelial cells to one degree or another and can be presumed to occur constantly as bloodborne substrates interact with endothelial cell-bound enzyme (10). Thus, a composite view of normal pulmonary endothelium depicts an intact monolayer, composed of metabolically active cells whose surfaces possess the requisite molecules to process substrates constantly delivered by flowing blood, to maintain a non-thrombogenic and immunologically privileged surface and to maintain a permeability barrier.

Quite clearly the constitutive properties of endothelium are lost when the monolayer or component cells are destroyed.

III.   ACTIVE RESPONSES TO INJURY

However, it is now becoming clear that endothelial cells also possess the ability to respond to injurious stimuli in ways that alter their hemostatic and immunologic potential (for review, see ref. 5). To cite a few examples: the levels of PGI_2 and thromboxanes released by pulmonary endothelial cells are greatly amplified by incubation of the cells with substances such as bradykinin,

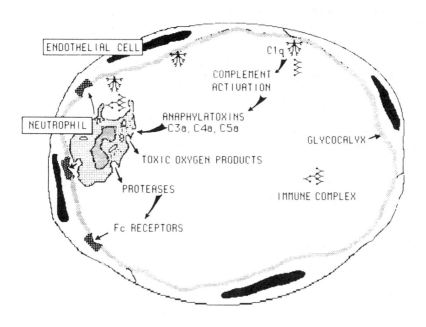

*Figure 1. Hypothetical sequence of events in inflammatory damage to
pulmonary endothelium in ovalbumin induced anaphylaxis. As antigen enters the
blood stream immune complexes would be formed. Those bearing Clq would bind
to endothelium, thereby inducing complement activation. Released
anaphylatoxins, including C5a, would attract neutrophils to the endothelial surface.
At the surface neutrophils would engulf bound immune complexes resulting in
release of neutrophil proteases and reactive oxygen metabolites. This would induce
further injury by unmasking latent Fc receptors, thus allowing binding of further
immune complexes and enhanced neutrophil mediated damage to endothelium.*

trypsin, thrombin or ionophore A23187 (11,12). Class II antigens are not
expressed constitutively by endothelial cells but become induced after exposure to
gamma interferon or tumor necrosis factor (13, 14). Endothelial cells do not
express receptors for the Fc portion of IgG nor for the C3b component of
complement unless the cells have been injured by virus infection, exposure to
white cell lysates, proteases, endotoxin or antibodies to endothelial surface
enzymes in the presence of complement, or have been stimulated by phagocytosis
of particulate material (5,6). Endothelial cells, normally actively antithrombogenic, can become markedly procoagulant after exposure to endotoxin or inter-
leukin 1 (15,16,17). Thus, episodic modulations in response to quite low levels

of injurious stimuli may transform the hemostatic and immunologic potential of endothelial cells. These alterations may involve ultrastructural changes in the endothelial glycocalyx or surface coat (5, 6) and are not simply the result of lysis or absence of the endothelial layer but may be regarded as activation responses of the endothelial cells to specific stimuli. Although the structural and functional modifications may be subtle, the outcome in terms of the pulmonary circulation, may be dramatic. The pulmonary endothelium is not simply a passive victim but can be regarded as an active participant in the events leading to vascular occlusion and damage (18).

IV.   MECHANISMS OF INFLAMMATORY DAMAGE

A few years ago, in an attempt to understand the sequence of events leading to pulmonary vascular obstruction and damage in the inflammatory response, a hypothetical pathway from initial initiating stimulus to resulting vascular injury (Fig. 1) was proposed on the basis of observations of aggregate anaphylaxis in guinea pigs (18).

Data are now available for many of the steps in the hypothetical sequence. Recently, Zhang *et al.* (8) have demonstrated that Clq (Fig. 2) binds to pulmonary endothelial cells by a specific, dose-dependent, saturable, reversible, receptor-mediated process (Fig. 3).

Furthermore, the binding of Clq is via the collagen like domain of the molecule not via the globular Fc binding head regions (Table 1).

TABLE I. Comparision of binding of ^{125}I-Clq and ^{125}I-Clq heads, both adjusted to 1.8 X 10^4 ct/min, to receptors on bovine endothelial cells (3.0 X 10^5) after incubation for 15 min at 0° C.

Experiment number	Percentage of total binding	
	Native Clq	Clq heads
1	74	-4
2	40	2
3	46	-3

(from ref. 8)

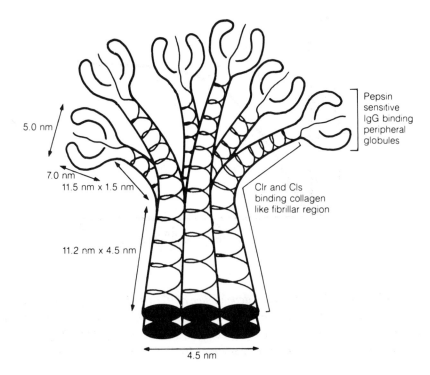

Figure 2. Clq is a 460,000 MW Glycoprotein that occurs both free in the circulation and as a subunit of the macromolecular first component of complement, Cl (from "Complement System," by GN Douglas, Behring Diagnostics, 1984)

Thus, receptors for the collagenous tail of Clq on pulmonary endothelial cells would have the effect of binding Clq-bearing immune complexes to the endothelial surface, and would provide a means by which the Fc segment of many classes of immune globulins and their complexes could bind to endothelium.

Bound immune complexes would have the effect of activating complement via the classical pathway. Anaphylatoxins, especially C5a, have a chemotactic effect attracting neutrophils to the endothelial surface. Marginated neutrophils would be expected to engulf bound immune complexes and in so doing would become activated. Products of activated neutrophils have a number of effects on endothelial cells. They result in the unmasking of latent Fc and C3b receptors on the endothelial surface (19) thus creating conditions for binding of a wide variety of immune complexes. Neutrophils have been reported to cause detachment of endothelial cells (20), an effect that would result in exposure of subendothelial basal lamina, a thrombogenic surface. In addition, activated

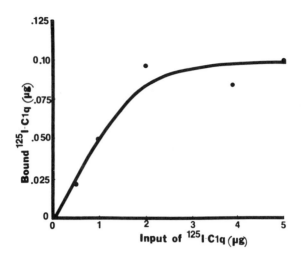

Figure 3. Concentration dependence of ^{125}I-Clq binding to bovine lung endothelial cells. Duplicate samples containing increasing quantities of ^{125}I-Clq in the presence or absence of 20 times the concentration of unlabeled Clq were incubated with 7×10^5 cells at an ionic stength of 10-15 for 15 min at 0 °C (from ref 8).

neutrophils have been shown to cause endothelial killing (21) by a mechanism likely to involve hydroxyl radical formation. (Fig. 4).

The source of iron necessary for conversion of neutrophil generated H_2O_2 to hydroxyl ion, via the Fenton reaction, has been shown to be the target endothelial cell rather than the neutrophil (22). Thus endothelial cells contribute actively to the interplay of events which may ultimately lead to their own demise.

Once the inflammatory pathways are activated a number of blood cell types may interact intimately with endothelium. In addition to neutrophils, platelets and platelet products are likely to play an active role. Platelet activating factor (PAF) has a number of interesting effects on pulmonary endothelial cells in culture (23).

Upon reaching confluency, endothelial cells form a characteristic "cobblestone" monolayer (9). One hour after addition of 1 nM platelet-activating factor to the growth medium, endothelial cells undergo a dramatic shape change from their normal polygonal morphology to a more elongated spindle-shaped form. More pronounced effects are evident in the presence of 0.1 nM phorbol-12-myristate-13-acetate (PMA), a potent activator of C kinase. The metabolic responses of endothelial cells (evaluated by measuring the activity of beta-adrenergic receptor-coupled adenylate cyclase in a crude membrane fraction and by

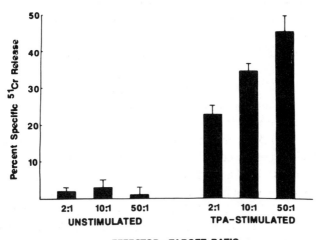

Figure 4. Bovine pulmonary artery endothelial cell killing by unstimulated and TPA (100 mg/ml)-stimulated human neutrophils. The values shown are the averages ± the differences between the individual values and the averages in a single experiment. In this experiment, the spontaneous release value was 7250 ± 920 cpm and the total release value was 38,900 ± 2810 cpm. The experiment was carried out three times with similar results. [from ref. 21].

assay of prostacyclin and thromboxane production by cultured endothelial cells) are blunted by PAF (23). Adenylate cyclase from control membranes was activated by isoproterenol in a dose-dependent manner (EC_{50}= 30 nM) from 0.8 to 5.5 pmol cAMP/min per mg of protein. If the membranes were isolated after preincubation of endothelial cells with 1 nM PAF or 0.1 nM PMA the adenylate cyclase activity was decreased by 70% and 90% respectively, and in both cases affinity for isoproterenol was lowered 3-fold (EC_{50}= 100nM) (Fig. 5). These data suggest that PAF interaction with endothelial cells leads to an apparent beta-adrenergic receptor desensitization probably acting via a phosphorylation mechanism involving C kinase. Incubation of endothelial cells for 30 min with 0.1 - 1.0 nM PAF caused inhibition of both prostacyclin and thromboxane production (55% and 75% respectively) indicating that PAF acts at a level common to both pathways of arachidonate metabolism. Similar results were obtained using PMA (0.1 nM) but not with phorbol-12,13-didecanoate, an inactive analog of PMA. Taken together these data indicate that C kinase is involved in PAF-induced alteration in receptor sensitivity at the plasma membrane level as well as in intracellular enzymes responsible for prostacyclin and thromboxane synthesis by endothelial cells. This downregulation of metabolic activity is accompanied by concomittant, dose-dependent shape changes.

In a separate set of studies (24), response to PAF was examined by loading confluent monolayers of pulmonary artery endothelial cells grown on quartz coverslips with the fluorescent calcium indicator FURA 2 and using a dual wavelength excitation fluorimeter. The coverslips were placed in Pucks saline, pH 7.4, in a cuvette so that the monolayer of cells was at 60° to the incident light. In the presence of 1 mM external calcium, PAF (10^{-8} M) gave a rapid increase in intracellular calcium with a dead time of 3 seconds and peaked within 10 seconds. Ca^{++} concentration reached a steady state within 12 seconds and remained stable for approximately 2 minutes but well above the basal level. The minimally effective dose for PAF was 10^{-11} M. 10^{-11} M PAF caused a much sharper increase in Ca^{++} concentration with shorter duration and returned back to the basal level within 30 seconds. Subsequent addition of 10^{-10} M PAF did not cause any additional increase in intracellular Ca^{++} concentration, suggesting that there is an apparent desensitization of the PAF receptors. Addition of ionomycin also caused a very rapid increase in calcium concentration with a well-defined peak, then a return to a new elevated steady state level. Subsequent addition of Mn^{++} (manganese chloride,

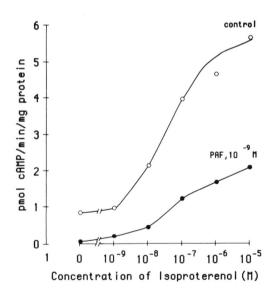

Figure 5. Decrease in adenylate cyclase activity in response to isoproterenol by endothelial membranes pretreated with 10^{-9} M platelet activating factor.

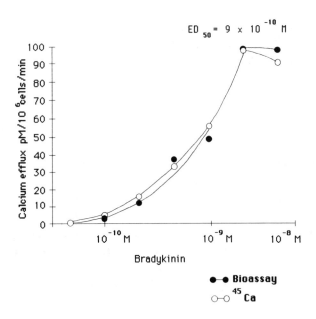

Figure 6. Effect of bradykinin on calcium efflux from pulmonary endothelium.

0.5 mM) caused rapid decrease of elevated Ca^{++} concentration back to the basal level. 1mM $MgCl_2$ decreased the effect of PAF on endothelial intracellular calcium. The thromboxane agonist U46619 added at the same concentration as PAF caused much less effect.

    Thus, the influence of PAF on endothelial morphology and metabolism may be a direct consequence of elevated intracellular calcium. The underlying role of Ca^{++} movements in signal transduction during the activation processes of endothelial cells may prove a fruitful area for study.

    A variety of agonists, including a number of platelet products, cause the release of endothelium dependent factors that affect vascular smooth muscle (25, 26, 27). Thus, conversation between blood-borne signals and vascular smooth muscle cells is largely determined by the intervening endothelial layer. In the presence of endothelium, platelet substances such as serotonin and ADP result in the production of endothelium dependent relaxing factors (EDRF), while in the absence of endothelium cause contraction of smooth muscle. Thus whether vasodilation or vasospasm occur can depend on the degree of damage to endothelial cells. The release of EDRF is closely dependent on calcium; the dose response for

EDRF release from pulmonary endothelial cells as measured by bioassay on rat aortic strips is virtually identical to the dose response for calcium efflux of the same cells (Fig. 6; 28), indicating a profound role for calcium in endothelial cell stimulus-secretion coupling.

V.   CONCLUSIONS AND FUTURE DIRECTIONS

Techniques for the study of endothelial activation by video time lapse microscopy are being developed (29-31). These studies indicate that activated endothelial cells migrate at faster rates and divide more rapidly than control endothelial cells. It is tempting to speculate that endothelial activation involves altered intracellular Ca^{++} levels and altered adenylate cyclase levels. It will be interesting to determine if these prove to be fundamental parameters accompanying alterations in endothelial cell behavior and kinetics, and to determine how seemingly minor cellular and molecular adjustments such as these contribute to the overall role of endothelial cells in determining the status of the pulmonary circulation.

ACKNOWLEDGMENTS

It is a pleasure to acknowledge the collaboration of Drs. Ward, Varani, Gannon, Schultz, Zhang, Grigorian, and Johns, and the contributions of all members of my laboratory.

REFERENCES

1.   Brigham KL. (1987) *In* The Pulmonary Circulation in Health and Disease (JA Will, CA Dawson, EK Weir, CK Buckner, eds.), Academic Press:New York, N.Y.
2.   Schneeberger EE. (1987) *In* The Pulmonary Circulation in Health and Disease (JA Will, CA Dawson, EK Weir, CK Buckner, eds.), Academic Press:New York, N.Y.
3.   Stimler-Gerard NP. (1987) *In* The Pulmonary Circulation in Health and Disease (JA Will, CA Dawson, EK Weir, CK Buckner, eds.), Academic Press:New York, N.Y.
4.   Crutchley DJ. (1987) *In* The Pulmonary Circulation in Health and Disease (JA Will, CA Dawson, EK Weir, CK Buckner, eds.), Academic Press:New York, N.Y.
5.   Ryan US. (1986) *Fed Proc* **45**:101.

6. Ryan US. (1986) *Ann Rev Physiol* **48**:263.

7. Ryan US, Ryan JW, Whitaker C and Chiu A. (1976) *Tissue & Cell* **8**:125.

8. Zhang SC, Schultz DR and Ryan US. (1986) *Tissue & Cell* **18**:13.

9. Ryan US. (1986) J Tissue Cult Methods (ed. Una S. Ryan) Vol. 10, Tissue Cult Assoc:Gaithersburg, MD.

10. Ryan US. (1985) *In* Handbook of Physiology : The Respiratory System 1. (AP Fishman and AB Fisher, eds.), Amer Physiol Soc:Bethesda, MD.

11. Crutchley DJ, Ryan JW, Ryan US and Fisher GH. (1983) *Biochem Biophys Acta* **751**:99.

12. Weksler BB, Ley CW, Jaffe EA. (1978) *J Clin Invest* **62**: 923.

13. Pober JS, Gimbrone MA, Cotran R, Reiss C, Burakoff S, Fiers W and Aults K. (1983) *J Exp Med* **157**:1339.

14. Pober JF, Bevilacqua MP, Mendrick DL, Lapierre LA, Fiers W, and Gimbrone Jr, MA. (1986) *J Immunol* **136**:1680.

15. Colucci M, Balconi G, Lorenzet R, *et al.* (1983) *J Clin Invest* **71**:1893.

16. Bevilacqua MP, Pober SJ, Majeau GR, Cotran RS, and Gimbrone MA. (1984) *J Exp Med* **160**:618.

17. Crutchley DJ, Conanan LB, and Ryan US. (1985) *Fed Proc* **44**:1844.

18. Ryan US and Ryan JW. (1983) *In* Clinics in Medicine. (PA Ward ed), WB Saunders:New York, Volume 3.

19. Ryan US, Schultz DR and Ryan JW. (1981) *Science* **214**:557 .

20. Harlan JM, Killen PD, Harber LA, Strike, GE, and Wright DG. (1981) *J Clin Invest* **68**:1394.

21. Varani J, Fligiel SEG, Till GO, Ryan US and Ward PA. (1985) *J Am Path* **53**:656.

22. Gannon DE, Varani J, Till GO, Ryan US, Simon RH, and Ward PA. (1986) *Lab Invest* (submitted) .

23. Grigorian GYu and Ryan US. (1986) FASEB summer conference, VT.

24. Grigorian GYu, Watson B and Ryan US. (1986) (submitted) (abstract).

25. Furchgott RF, Zawadzki JV, and Cherry PD. (1980) *Nature* **286**:373.

26. Vanhoutte PM and Houston DS. (1985) *Circulation* **72**:728.

27. Rubanyi GM and Vanhoutte PM. (1985) *J Physiol* **364**:45.

28. Johns A, Ryan US and Van Breemen C. (1986) (submitted)

29. Ryan US and Mayfield LJ. (1986) *J Tissue Cult Methods* **10**:55.

30. Mayfield LJ, Ryan US. (1986) 14th International Conference of European Society for Microcirculation, Linkoping, Sweden, June 8-14 (abstract).

31. Ryan US, Mayfield LJ and Goodwin JD. (1986) 4th International Symposium on the Biology of the Vascular Endothelial Cell, Noordwijkerhout, The Netherlands, August 19-23 (abstract).

Mechanisms of Lung Endothelial Injury[1]

KENNETH L. BRIGHAM[2]
Center for Lung Research
Department of Medicine
Vanderbilt University School of
Medicine
Nashville, Tennessee 37232

I. INTRODUCTION

Endothelial cells individually and the barrier which they form in aggregate are initial sites of injury in diseases of the systemic and pulmonary circulations. In the lungs, a functional breach of the microvascular endothelial barrier permits the pulmonary edema typical of the adult respiratory distress syndrome (ARDS) to occur. Endothelial injury may alter other vital functions of blood vessels as well (1).

The term, "injury", bears some definition. The term is often used in a morphological sense, but whether or not structural alterations in cells are evident may be simply a consequence of the sensitivity of the methods rather than a qualitative criterion. On the other hand, it seems inappropriate and probably wrong to interpret any alteration in cell function as injury. To the contrary, many, perhaps most, cellular responses are homeostatic, aimed at avoiding "injury".

[1] *Supported by grant number HL 19153 (SCOR in Pulmonary Vascular Diseases) from the National Heart Lung and Blood Institute and by grants from the Upjohn Company, the John and Laura Cooke Fund for Lung Research and The Bernard Werthan, Sr. Fund for Lung Research.*

[2] *Dr. Brigham is Joe and Morris Werthan Professor of Investigative Medicine.*

Also, "injury" is almost certainly not a single event; that bias will be obvious in this chapter. Injury is more properly viewed as a process in which many cellular events occur in some causally related sequence, the ultimate consequence of which is "injury".

Although much of the work related to mechanisms of endothelial injury concentrates on inflammation, particularly interactions between polymorphonuclear leukocytes and endothelial cells, it is not yet clear that neutrophils initiate endothelial injury *in vivo*. At least some insults which cause lung endothelial injury *in vivo* also injure lung endothelial cells *in vitro* in the absence of neutrophils.

II.   DIRECT INJURY OF LUNG ENDOTHELIUM

Alterations in endothelial cells devoid of the myriad other cells which might influence endothelial responses can only be studied in *in vitro* preparations. Several interventions which cause diffuse lung injury *in vivo* also injure lung endothelial cells *in vitro* and some of the mechanisms involved in this direct injury are being elucidated.

A.   Oxidant Mechanisms

Cells produce toxic metabolites of oxygen as a consequence of normal metabolism. Cells also contain several biochemical systems which metabolize or scavenge potentially toxic oxygen metabolites (2). Under some circumstances intracellular generation of reactive oxygen metabolites can be driven to exceed cellular protective mechanisms and result in cell injury.

Pulmonary oxygen toxicity in intact animal models is characterized by damage to lung endothelium (3). When endothelial cells grown in tissue culture are exposed to high ambient concentrations of oxygen, evidence of cell injury evolves over a time course similar to that for the *in vivo* situation. There is evidence that this hyperoxic injury results from the generation of toxic metabolites of oxygen within endothelial cells. If the antioxidant enzyme superoxide dismutase is provided to the interior of endothelial cells in culture, the cells are protected from oxygen toxicity whereas addition of the same enzyme to the exterior of the cells offers little protection (5).

Intracellular generation of oxygen metabolites has also been postulated as a mechanism of ischemia-reperfusion injury in the heart (5) and the intestine (6). Such injury is prevented by inhibitors of xanthine oxidase. The notion is that during ischemia, there is conversion of xanthine dehydrogenase to xanthine oxidase and accumulation of substrate for the oxidase enzyme. With reperfusion (reoxygenation) xanthine converts its substrates to uric acid, generating superoxide in the process (5). Some recent data suggest that xanthine dehydrogenase/xanthine oxidase may be preferentially concentrated in several organs, including the lungs (7).

Gram negative bacterial sepsis is a common clinical setting in which diffuse lung injury occurs. Endotoxins from such bacteria can injure several types of vascular endothelium in *in vitro* preparations.

When exposed to *E. coli* endotoxin, bovine pulmonary artery intimal explants show morphological evidence of injury within an hour of endotoxin exposure; these changes are accompanied by increased diffusional permeability of the explants to small hydrophilic solutes (8). Bovine and ovine pulmonary artery endothelial cells in culture are also injured by endotoxin exposure; evidence of injury includes morphological alterations, increased hydraulic conductance and diffusional permeability of endothelial monolayers (8), production of prostanoids, including prostacyclin and prostaglandin E_2 (8), detachment of cells from the culture dish (9) and release of intracellular contents (8,9). Endotoxin toxicity for endothelial cells in culture is enhanced by the presence of serum (8,9) and is unaffected by a number of drugs including corticosteroids and nonsteroidal antiinflammatory agents (9).

We have preliminary data indicating that the direct effects of endotoxin on bovine pulmonary endothelial cells in culture may involve intracellular generation of toxic metabolites of oxygen (10). Endotoxin induced cytotoxicity is prevented in a dose related manner by either the freely permeable hydroxyl radical scavenger, dimethyl sulfoxide (DMSO) or by the xanthine oxidase inhibitor, allopurinol. Additionally, endotoxin exposure causes release of the lipid peroxidation products, conjugated dienes (11), from endothelial cells in culture, suggesting oxidant injury. Endotoxin stimulates reduction of the redox dye, nitroblue tetrazolium (NBT) within endothelial cells in culture. Endotoxin exposure also induces increased concentrations of the mitochondrial associated antioxidant enzyme, mangano superoxide dismutase (12), suggesting that the cells have undergone oxidant stress. These findings, coupled with published data demonstrating that antioxidant enzymes added to the exterior of endothelial cells do not protect against endotoxin induced injury, implicate an intracellular source for toxic oxygen metabolites which may mediate cellular injury.

Several insults which cause lung endothelial injury in vivo also injure endothelial cells *in vitro* in the absence of any other cell type. For some of these insults, intracellular generation of toxic oxygen metabolites appears to be a mechanism of injury.

B.   Proteolytic injury

The consequences of release or activation of proteolytic enzymes for cells depend on relative concentrations of proteinases and antiproteinases in the local environment. This proteinase/antiproteinase balance can be altered either by increased proteinase activity or decreased antiproteinase activity and there is evidence for both in some forms of diffuse lung injury. Increased proteolytic activity has been detected in bronchoalveolar lavage fluid from patients with diffuse lung injury (13). Antiproteinases are inactivated by exposure to reactive oxygen metabolites and such inactivated antiproteinases have also been detected in bronchoalveolar lavage fluids from patients with diffuse lung injury (13).

Direct exposure of endothelial cells *in vitro* to proteinases alters the cells. Such alterations include changes in morphology, stimulation of prostacyclin production (14), unmasking of surface receptors (15), endothelial cell aggregation (16) and, under some circumstances, cell membrane injury (17).

Recent studies suggest that the direct injury of endothelial cells in culture by endotoxin may involve proteolytic mechanisms. We tested the effects of several antiproteinases added to the culture medium on responses to endotoxin exposure in bovine pulmonary endothelial cells (18). We found that several chloromethyl ketone derivatives and a proteinase substrate all effectively inhibited endotoxin induced cytotoxicity and prostacyclin production. These effects were related to the concentrations of the inhibitors. The cytoprotective effects were less in the absence of serum so that it is not yet clear whether the source of proteinase in these experiments was serum or whether cell associated proteinases were involved as well. In any case, these studies raise the possibility that proteolysis is involved in the injury of endothelial cells in the absence of neutrophils, usually presumed to be the primary source of destructive proteinases.

C.   Cyclic Nucleotide Metabolism and Endothelial Injury

Drugs which affect cyclic nucleotide metabolism can protect the lungs from injury. This phenomenon has been demonstrated in intact animals (19) and in isolated perfused lung preparations (20).

Effects of endotoxin on lung endothelial cells in culture are inhibited by drugs which act to increase intracellular concentrations of cyclic AMP (Hussein *et al.*, in preparation). We found that the phosphodiesterase inhibitor, methyl isobutylxanthine added to endothelial cell cultures prevented endotoxin induced release of lactate dehydrogenase and generation of prostacyclin; effects were related to the concentration of the drug. We found similar effects of dibutyryl cyclic AMP (a form of the substance which enters cells). Although proof that the mechanisms of endotoxin injury of endothelial cells involves alterations in cyclic nucleotide metabolism will require further biochemical studies, these preliminary data indicate that possibility.

III . LEUKOCYTE-ENDOTHELIAL INTERACTIONS

Leukocytes, especially neutrophils, appear to be important in the process of injury of vascular endothelium (21). Neutrophils sequester in microvessels, closely adherent to endothelial cells, in several models of lung injury (21, 22). Activated neutrophils can release proteinases and generate toxic oxygen metabolites, both of which can injure endothelial cells (23). Elimination of neutrophils from the blood or perfusate attenuates lung injury in several experimental models (24). Interventions which cause intravascular complement activation (and thus neutrophil activation) can result in lung endothelial injury (25, 26).

In *in vitro* endothelial preparations, exposure of endothelium to neutrophils in the presence of complement activated serum does not necessarily cause injury of endothelial cells or alterations in permeability of the endothelial layer (27). Neutrophils can be stimulated to injure endothelial cells in culture by phorbol esters, potent stimulators of neutrophil free radical generation, and, under those conditions, the injury appears to be free radical mediated (28). However, the relationship of these experiments to *in vivo* situations is not clear.

Recent studies indicated that neutrophils may be "primed" by very low concentrations of endotoxin so that, when subsequently stimulated, these cells can initiate injury of normal endothelial cells in culture (17). The mechanism of this response appears to involve neutrophil proteinases.

In addition, some forms of endothelial injury appear to be enhanced by the presence of neutrophils. For example, exposure of endothelial cells in culture to sublethal doses of hyperoxia renders the cells more susceptible to injury by complement stimulated neutrophils (29). We have recently shown that unstimulated neutrophils dramatically enhance endotoxin induced endothelial cytotoxicity and production of both prostacyclin and prostaglandin E_2 (31).

It seems apparent that interactions of leukocytes, especially neutrophils, with endothelium can be crucial events in the process of endothelial injury. Under some experimental circumstances, neutrophils appear capable of initiating injury of endothelial cells. However, it remains unclear whether the process of injury *in vivo* is initiated by interactions of leukocytes with microvascular endothelium. An alternative hypothesis is that the process is initiated by alterations in endothelial cells which changes the nature of leukocyte endothelial interactions to the detriment of the endothelium.

REFERENCES

1. Fishman AP (ed.). (1982) Endothelium. *Ann NY Acad Sci* **401**:1.
2. Freeman BA and Crapo JD. (1982) *Lab Invest* **47**:412.
3. Newman JH, Loyd J, English D, Ogletree M, Fulkerson W and Brigham KL. (1983) *J Appl Physiol* **54**:1379.
4. Freeman BA, Young SL and Crapo JD. (1983) *J Biol Chem* **258**:12534.
5. McCord JM. (1984) *N Engl J Med* **312**:159.
6. Granger DN, McCord JM, Parks DA, Hollwarth ME. (in press) *Gastroenterology*.
7. Jarasch ED, Bruder G and Heid HW. (1986) *Acta Physiol Scand* **548**:39.
8. Meyrick B, Ryan US and Brigham KL. (1986) *Am J Pathol* **122**:140.
9. Harlan JM, Harker LA, Reidy MA, Gadjusek CM, Schwartz SM and Striker GE. (1983) *Lab Invest* **48**:269.
10. Brigham KL and Meyrick B. (1986) *Amer Rev Resp Dis* **133**(5):913.
11. Ward PA, Till GO, Hatherill JR, Annesley TM and Kunkel RG. (1985) *J Clin Invest* **76**:517.
12. Shiki Y, Meyrick B, Brigham KL and Burr IM. (in press) *Am J Physiol*.
13. Cochrane CC, Spragg RG, Revak S, Cohen AB and McGuire WW. (1983) *Amer Rev Resp Dis* **127**:25.
14. Weksler BB, Ley CW and Jaffe EA. (1978) *J Clin Invest* **62**:923.
15. Ryan US, Schultz DR and Ryan JW. (1981) *Science* **214**:557.
16. Brigham KL, Meyrick B and Ryan US. (1984) *Tiss Cell* **16**:167.
17. Smedly LA, Tonnesen MG, Sandhaus RA, Haslett C, Guthrie LA, Johnston RB, Henson PM and Werthan GS. (1986) *J Clin Invest* **77**(4):1233.
18. Tumen JJ, Meyrick B, Berry LC and Brigham KL. (1986) *Amer Rev Resp Dis* **133**(4):A261.
19. Foy T, Marion J, Brigham KL and Harris TR. (1979) *J Appl Physiol* **46**:146.
20. Mizus I, Summer W, Farrukh I, Michael JR and Gurtner GH. (1985) *Amer Rev Resp Dis* **131**:256.
21. Brigham KL and Meyrick B. (1984) *Circ Res* **54**:623.
22. Meyrick B and Brigham KL. (1983) *Lab Invest* **48**:458.
23. Klebanoff SJ. (1975) *Sem Hematol* **12**:117.
24. Repine JE. (1985)*In* **The Pulmonary Circulation and Acute Lung Injury** (SI Said ed), Future Publishing Co:Mount Kisco, New York.
25. Ward PA, Till GO, Hatherill, JR, Annesley TM and Kunkel RG. (1985) *J Clin Invest* **76**:517.
26. Meyrick B and Brigham KL. (1984) *Am J Pathol* **114**:32.

27. Meyrick B, Hoffman L and Brigham KL. (1984) *Tiss Cell* **16**:1.
28. Shasby DM, Shasby SS and Peach MJ. (1983) *Amer Rev Resp Dis* **127**:72.
29. Suttorp N and Simon LM. (1982) *J Clin Invest* **70**:342.
30. Givens CD, Brigham KL and Meyrick B. (1986) *Amer Rev Resp Dis* **133**(4):A262.

Regulation of Transport and Permeability Properties of Pulmonary Endothelium[1]

EVELINE E. SCHNEEBERGER
Department of Pathology
Massachusetts General Hospital
Boston, MA, 02114

I. INTRODUCTION

The pulmonary capillary network is uniquely adapted to subserve one of the primary functions of the lung, namely that of gas exchange. It provides not only a vast capillary network but also forms an exceedingly thin cellular barrier to the diffusion of gases. In man the total surface area of the pulmonary capillary network is estimated to be approximately 70 m^2 (1) and in some regions the capillary endothelial cell cytoplasm is as little as 100 nm in thickness (1). The pulmonary endothelium is also of key importance in regulating the permeability and transport of substances across the air—blood barrier (2). It is the structural basis for this regulatory function that will be discussed.

Pulmonary microvascular endothelial cells are continuous and nonfenestrated. They are joined by tight junctions of varying complexity (3,4) and contain within their cytoplasm nonrandomly distributed plasmalemmal and coated vesicles (5). Their luminal surface is covered by a glycocalyx, composed of glycoproteins and glycolipids, which is focally interrupted by thin membranes covering the luminal opening of plasmalemmal vesicles. All these structures act in concert to regulate the passage of water and solutes across the pulmonary endothelium. The premise of the present discussion will be that tight junctions

[1] Supported by NIH Grant HL 25822.

and transcytotic vesicles form the permeable regions of the endothelium, but that it is the luminal glycocalyx which performs the sieving functions of the endothelium.

II.   TIGHT JUNCTIONS

Tight junctions, first described by Farquhar and Palade (6), bridge the gap between adjacent cells. Owing to their continuous, gasket-like structure near the apex of cells, they are strategically placed to regulate the permeability of the paracellular pathway. Tight junctions form not only a permeability barrier, but also function to maintain compositional and functional polarity in epithelial cells (7). Recent evidence suggests that this is the case in endothelial cells as well (8). Because pulmonary microvascular endothelial cells in situ are not readily accessible to electrophysiological measurements and endothelial cells do not readily form tight junctions under presently available *in vitro* culture conditions, little is known about the resistance properties of their tight junctions. In amphibian capillaries the paracellular pathway is of low resistance (0.9 - 3.0 W cm^2; 9). Freeze fracture studies, however, have elucidated the structure of tight junctions and it is possible to make some predictions with regard to their permeability properties on the basis of freeze fracture replicas (10).

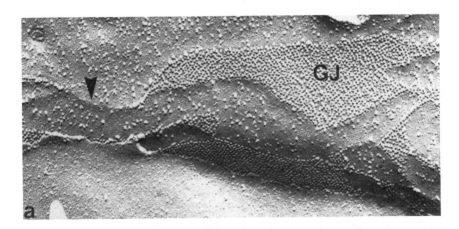

Figure 1a. Freeze fracture replica of an intercellular junction in an intra-acinar artery. The tight junction consists of rows of particles in shallow grooves on the E face (arrow) and low, particle-poor ridges on the P face (arrow head). Numerous large gap junctions (GJ) are present within the network of the tight junctions. Magnification x 72,500.

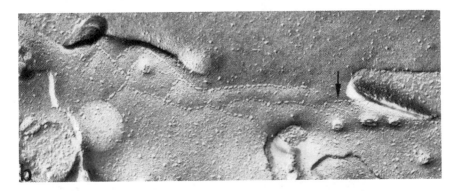

1b. Freeze fracture replica of a tight junction between pulmonary capillary endothelial cells. The tight junction consists of 2-3 rows of particles present in shallow grooves on the E face (arrow). Mag. x 75,000.

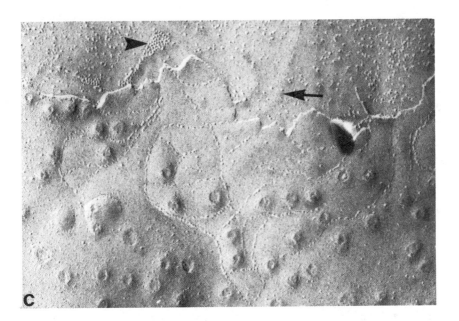

1c. Freeze fracture replica of a tight junction in an intra-acinar vein. The tight junction consists of several rows of particles in shallow grooves on the E face (small arrow) and faintly perceptible, particle-poor ridges on the P face. (large arrow). A rare, small gap junction (arrow head) is present. Mag. x 75,000.

To examine by freeze fracture the structure of tight junctions in the various segments of the intra-acinar pulmonary vascular network (3,4), the lungs of rats were perfused by the intra-arterial instillation of fixative while at the same time occluding the venous outflow (11). This resulted in the displacement of all the formed elements from the arterial to the venous side of the pulmonary circulation and permitted the use of erythrocytes as markers for the venous segments.

In intra-acinar arteries tight junctions consisted of 2 - 6 continuous, interconnected rows of particles in grooves on the E face and complementary, particle-poor ridges on the P face (Fig. 1a). Of particular interest, however, was the presence of a large number of gap junctions intercalated within the meshwork of the tight junctions suggesting the presence of extensive metabolic and electrotonic communication between endothelial cells in this part of the pulmonary vascular bed.

By contrast, tight junctions between pulmonary capillary endothelial cells consisted of only 1 to 3 interconnected rows of tight junction particles in shallow grooves on the E face and particle-poor ridges on the P face (Fig. 1b). No gap junctions were seen between endothelial cells in this segment of the pulmonary circulation.

In intra-acinar veins tight junctions consisted of 1 - 5 rows of particles on the E face and virtually particle-free, low ridges on the P face (Fig. 1c). In the venular segments occasional discontinuities were noted and in the larger segments a few, small gap junctions were observed.

It has been suggested that the rows of tight junction particles act as resistors to an electrical current passed across a cell monolayer (10). It is, therefore, reasonable to suggest that the venular segment of the pulmonary capillary bed is the most permeable. In view of the complexity of pulmonary arterial tight junctions and the presence of numerous gap junctions, it is unlikely that data derived from permeability studies carried out on pulmonary arterial endothelial cells in culture can be used to deduce the permeability properties of pulmonary capillary endothelial cells. Further studies will be required to establish the precise size and charge restrictions imposed on solutes passing through the endothelial, paracellular pathway in the various segments of the pulmonary vascular network.

Studies in a variety of tissues and cells in culture suggest an important role for calcium, cAMP, and cytoskeletal elements in the regulation of tight structure and function (see ref. 7 for a recent review). Whereas further studies are required to establish the precise role of cytoskeletal elements, it is possible that they are involved in the movement of proteins involved in junction formation. Attempts to isolate and characterize tight junctions biochemically have been difficult. Stevenson and Goodenough have identified by SDS gel chromatography in membrane preparations from mouse liver two major polypeptide bands with molecular weights of 37,000 and 48,000, respectively (12). Monoclonal antibodies raised to these proteins have been shown to localize immuno-cytochemically to the region of the tight junctions in tissues from a variety of species. (Goodenough, personal communication). However, further studies are required to precisely establish the mechanisms involved in the formation of tight junctions and the regulation of their function. Whereas physiological studies suggest that the paracellular pathway with its contained tight junctions regulate the passage of water and small water-soluble solutes (13) across epithelial and presumably endothelial cell monolayers, pinocytotic vesicles are thought to be involved in the transcellular transport of macromolecules (14).

III.   ENDOTHELIAL VESICLES

Both coated and noncoated vesicles are non-randomly distributed in pulmonary endothelial cells. In rat pulmonary capillary endothelial cells, noncoated transcytotic vesicles measure 65 and 60 nm in diameter on the thick and thin side, respectively. Because of the extreme attenuation of the endothelial cytoplasm, the numerical density of vesicles is greater on the thin (354 ± 21 vesicles/μm^3) than on the thick (255 ± 13 vesicles/μm^3) side.

Early in fetal development of the lung few pinocytotic vesicles are present. With fetal maturation there is a 10-fold increase in their numerical density (5). Unlike the differentiation of pulmonary epithelial cells (16), there is no difference in the rate of differentiation of pulmonary endothelial cells between upper and lower lobes. Interestingly, the numerical density of coated vesicles, the structures involved in receptor-mediated uptake, remains constant throughout gestation.

The precise mechanism whereby vesicles transport macromolecules across the endothelium remains unresolved. Whether this occurs by translocation, the formation of transient vesicle fusions, or by the formation of chains of vesicles continues to be a matter of controversy (17). A further intriguing observation has recently been reported (18,20). When endothelial cells are rapidly frozen and then processed by freeze substitution a remarkable reduction in the number of pinocytotic vesicles is observed. It is not clear at present whether data obtained by conventional fixation or by the newer rapid freezing techniques more accurately reflect the structure *in vivo* of endothelial cells.

Tight junctions and pinocytotic vesicles appear to represent the permeable regions of the endothelium and, in fact, these structures are particularly leaky when the vascular bed is perfused with protein-free solutions (21). As discussed below, experimental evidence suggests that it is the interaction of circulating proteins with the endothelial glycocalyx which contributes to maintaining normal vascular permeability (21).

IV.   GLYCOCALYX

Many years ago Drinker (22) and later Danielli (23) made the interesting observation that non-protein containing colloids are far less effective than protein containing colloids in preventing the formation of edema in perfused tissues. This so-called 'protein effect' was re-examined by Michel and his colleagues in a series of elegant studies in single perfused frog capillaries (24,26). They showed that perfusion of these capillaries with protein-free solutions resulted in a five-fold increase in hydraulic conductivity and in leakage of small solutes and macromolecules from such preparations. As little as 1.10 mg/ml of bovine serum albumin was sufficient to reverse these changes. The culmination of these studies was the formulation by Curry and Michel of their fiber matrix model of capillary permeability (27). In this model they suggested that channels through the endothelium are lined and covered by a network of fibrous glycoproteins, the interstices of which determine the molecular sieving properties of the capillary wall. The interaction of plasma proteins with the glycocalyx would order the latter in such a way as to tighten its meshwork thereby creating a barrier to the passage of water and hydrophilic solutes.

To examine this phenomenon in a mammalian species, we modified the bloodless fluorocarbon exchange transfused rat model originally described by Geyer (28). In brief, because of their remarkable gas carrying capacity fluorocarbon emulsions are effective blood substitutes affording a means of partially or completely removing circulating proteins in the live animal. For this purpose a fluorocarbon emulsion (Oxypherol ET, Alpha Therapeutic Co., Los Angeles, CA) was used. The emulsion contained 20% perfluorotributylamine and hydroxyethyl starch as an oncotic agent. When the composition of the emulsion is meticulously controlled it is possible to remove 99% of an animal's circulating blood without producing pulmonary edema (15). Following a complete exchange transfusion with fluorocarbon emulsion, there was no effect on the numerical density of endothelial vesicles. However, when such animals were given an intravenous dose of ferritin, a macromolecule readily visualized in the electron microscope, there was a five-fold increase in the number of vesicles containing ferritin and a ten-fold increase in the number of ferritin particles present in the basement membrane of pulmonary capillaries. This effect was completely reversible. The administration of 60 mg/ml of lyophilized rat serum protein, as a substitute for the hydroxyethyl starch in the fluorocarbon emulsion, reduced ferritin transport to baseline levels. In summary, these experiments validated the bloodless rat model and confirmed, in part, the observations of Michel and his colleagues.

In a subsequent study (29) the Curry and Michel fiber matrix model was tested by administering a single 1 ml bolus of fluorocarbon emulsion containing 60 mg/ml of lyophilized rat serum protein to a completely exchange transfused rat, followed by an intravenous injection of native ferritin as a macromolecular tracer. The strategy in this experiment was to insert circulating proteins solely into the meshwork of the glycocalyx and then to test whether this had an effect on the transport of ferritin across the endothelium. Immunocytochemical methods were used to localize the administered rat albumin and gamma globulin. As can be seen in Fig. 2, immediately after the administration of lyophilized rat serum protein, these proteins were confined solely to the meshwork of the glycocalyx. In such rats the permeability of the underlying endothelium to ferritin was identical to that of control animals (Table I).

That this was not due to an artifact introduced through the use of fluorocarbon was shown in control experiments in which in a normal, nonperfused control rat, a dense layer of reaction product was seen on the surface of the endothelium. This layer of adsorbed proteins in the region of the glycocalyx was more clearly seen when lungs were briefly perfused with Hanks' balanced salt solution to remove the luminal contents of the vessel (Fig. 2b). These observations provide direct support for the fiber matrix model. It should be noted, however, that lyophilized rat serum protein and not pure albumin or gamma

TABLE I. Transport of ferritin to basement membrane before and after protein replenishment in rats exchange transfused with fluorocarbon emulsion.

| | | | Particles/BM Area x 10^8/cm^2 | |
Group	Exposure of endothelium to protein (min)	Final circulating [protein](mg/μl)	Thick	Thin
1	0	0.4	35.1 ±11.7	17.0 ±49
2	3.5	16.9	5.3 ± 1.0	2.4 ±10
3	---	59.0	3.8 ± 1.1	2.2 ±10

Rats in group 1 were completely exchange transfused and not replenished with protein. Rats in group 2 received 1 ml of emulsion containing 60 mg of lyophilized rat serum protein after having been completely depleted of circulating proteins. Rats in group 3 are non-exchange transfused controls. Adapted from Schneeberger et al. 1984.

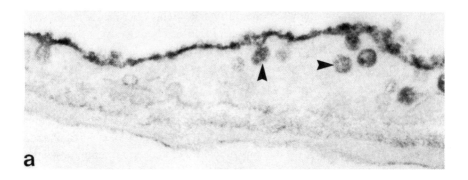

Figure 2a. Pulmonary capillary from a rat exchange transfused with fluorocarbon emulsion to a circulating protein concentration of <0.6 mg/ml. One ml of fluorocarbon emulsion containing 60 mg of lyophilized rat serum protein was administered intravenously 3.5 minutes before sacrifice. The distribution of rat albumin was localized by immunoperoxidase techniques. The reaction product is limited to the glycocalyx (arrows) and a few luminal vesicles (arrow heads). The permeability of this capillary to intravenously injected native ferritin was indistinguishable from that of normal control rats. Mag. x 62,500.

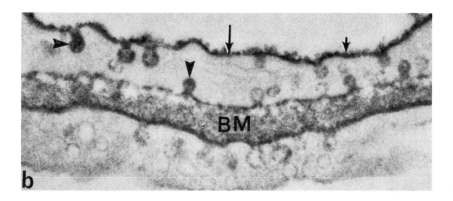

2b. Pulmonary capillary from a rat lung briefly perfused with Hanks' balanced salt solution to remove the luminal contents. The distribution of rat albumin was localized by immunoperoxidase techniques. Reaction product is limited to the glycocalyx (arrows), endothelial vesicles (arrow heads) and the basement membrane (BM). Mag. x 62,500.

globulin was administered. This is of interest in view of the observations of Rippe and his colleagues who have observed that, in contrast to frog capillaries, mammalian capillaries have a requirement for some as yet unidentified factor in serum which is necessary to maintain a normal state of impermeability (30). That is, albumin alone reduced the hydraulic conductivity of the rat hindlimb vascular bed to control levels, but whole serum was required to reduce albumin clearance to control values.

The bloodless rat model has also been used to examine the distribution of negative charge on pulmonary endothelium (31). Simionescu et al. have reported that the density of the negative charge on the luminal surface of pulmonary capillary endothelium is greater on the thick than the thin side of the capillary, and that the diaphragms at the entrance of endothelial vesicles do not bind cationized ferritin, suggesting that they do not bear a net negative charge (32). The latter observations could not be confirmed by others (33). We hypothesized that circulating proteins, adsorbed to the glycocalyx, might mask the expression of the negative charge. Rats were. therefore, subjected to a graded removal of circulating proteins by exchange transfusion with fluorocarbon emulsion; immediately before fixing the lungs, a dose of cationized ferritin was administered intravenously. Following the gradual removal of circulatingproteins, there was a concommittant increase in the extent of binding of cationized ferritin to the luminal plasma membrane as well as to vesicle diaphragms (Table II).

These results suggested that the intrinsic negative charge of the endo-thelial glycocalyx is masked *in vivo* by the presence of adsorbed circulating proteins. Recent studies suggest that components of the pulmonary interstitiumand basement membrane may govern the preferential flow of negatively charged as opposed to neutral dextrans into lung lymph (34). The interaction of solutes of varying charge with components of the interstitium remains, however, to be clarified.

TABLE II. Binding of cationized ferritin (CF) to luminal plasma membrane (LPM) and vesicle diaphragms (VD).

Group	Protein concentration (mg/ml)	% LPM binding CF		%VD binding CF	
		Thick	Thin	Thick	Thin
Control	60.6	7.5	6.0	7.5	5.0
Experimental	0.6	89.0	82.0	76.0	73.0

V.   SUMMARY

The studies summarized above indicate that tight junctions in the pulmonary vascular bed vary considerably in complexity and permeability depending on which vascular segment is examined. The presence of large numbers of gap junctions between intra-acinar pulmonary arterial endothelial cells suggests the presence of extensive metabolic and electrotonic coupling. Pinocytotic vesicles are largely responsible for macromolecular transport across pulmonary endothelium. However, the interaction of circulating proteins with the glycocalyx inhibits vesicular transport of tracer macromolecules and renders the underlying endothelium less permeable. Finally, the interaction of circulating proteins with the glycocalyx masks its intrinsic negative charge.

ACKNOWLEDGEMENT

The word processing skills of Mrs. Ruth Manozzi are gratefully acknowledged.

REFERENCES

1.   Weibel ER. (1963) **Morphometry of the human lung.** Academic Press:New York, NY.
2.   Schneeberger EE. (1978) *Fed Proc* **37**:2471.
3.   Schneeberger EE and Karnovsky MJ. (1976) *Circ Res* **38**:404.
4.   Schneeberger EE. (1981) *Circ Res* **49**:1102.
5.   Schneeberger EE. (1983) *Microvasc Res* **25**:40.
6.   Farquhar MG and Palade GE. (1965) *J Cell Biol* **26**:375.
7.   Schneeberger EE and Lynch RD. (1984) *Circ Res* **55**:723.
8.   Muller WA, Mendrick DL and Gimbrone MA. (1985) *J Cell Biol* **101**:143a.
9.   Crone C and Christensen C. (1981) *J Gen Physiol* **77**:349.
10.   Claude P. (1978) *J Membr Biol* **39**:219.
11.   Meyrick B and Reid LM. (1979) *Anat Rec* **193**:71.
12.   Stevenson BR and Goodenough DA. (1984) *J Cell Biol* **98**:1209.
13.   Pappenheimer JR, Renkin EM and Borrero LM. (1951) *Am J Physiol* **167**:13.
14.   Palade GE. (1960) *Anat Rec* **136**:254.
15.   Schneeberger EE and Neary BA. (1982) *Am J Physiol* **242**:H890.
16.   Schneeberger EE, Walters DV and Olver RE. (1978) *J Cell Sci* **32**:307.

17. Schneeberger EE. (1987) *In* **The Pulmonary Endothelium in Health and Disease.** (U Ryan ed), Marcel Dekker:New York, NY. In press.
18. Casley-Smit JR. (1985) *In* **Endothelial Vesicles.** (F Hammersen and DH Lewis, eds), Karger:Basel.
19. Robinson JM, Hoover RL and Karnovsky MJ. (1984) *J Cell Biol* **99**:287a.
20. Wagner RC and Andrews SB. (1985) *J Ultrastruct Res* **90**:172.
21. Michel CC. (1985) *In* **Frontiers in Physiological Research.** (DG Garlick and PI Korner, eds), Australian Academy of Science. Cambridge University Press.
22. Drinker CK. (1927) *J Physiol (London)* **63**:249.
23. Danielli JF. (1946) *J Physiol (London)* **98**:109.
24. Levick JR and Michel CC. (1973)*Quart J Exp Physiol* **58**:87.
25. Mason JE, Curry FE and Michel CC. (1977) *Microvasc Res* **13**:185.
26. Clough G and Michel CC. (1981) *J Physiol (London)* **315**:127.
27. Curry FE and Michel CC. (1980) *Microvasc Res* **20**:96.
28. Geyer RP. (1975) *Fed Proc* **34**:1499.
29. Schneeberger EE and Hamelin M. (1984) *J Physiol* **247**:H206.
30. Haraldsson B and Rippe B. (1985) *Acta Physiol Scand* **123**:427.
31. Schneeberger EE. In preparation.
32. Simionescu D and Simionescu M. (1983) *Microvasc Res* **25**:85.
33. Pietra GG, Sampson P, Lanken PN, Hansen-Flaschen J and Fishman AP. (1983) *Lab Invest* **49**:54.
34. Pietra GG, Fishman AP, Lanken PN, Sampson P and Hansen-Flaschen J. (1982) *Ann NY Acad Sci* **401**:241.

Interactions of Anaphylatoxins with Endothelium[1]

NORMA P. STIMLER-GERARD
*Pulmonary Unit, Department of
Medicine,
Beth Israel Hospital, and
The Thorndike Laboratory of
Harvard Medical School
Boston, MA 02215*

I.   INTRODUCTION

Activation of complement and generation of the anaphylatoxin peptides, C3a and C5a, has long been associated with inflammatory reactions (1-5). Recent advances have provided a good understanding of the molecular nature of these peptides (6-11), and as a result, we now have a firm basis for investigating their physiologic actions in complex experimental systems. As inflammatory agents, the anaphylatoxins are among the most potent mediators yet characterized for causing increases in vascular permeability, requiring as little as femtomole quantities of C5a to produce a measureable reaction in human skin (12). A number of observations of anaphylatoxin-induced permeability changes in the lung have been documented in several experimental models, and inroads have been made into understanding a neutrophil-dependent mechanism for this action. Many questions remain unanswered, however, including the ability of the anaphylatoxins

[1]*Supported in part by NIH Grant 36162. Dr. Stimler-Gerard is the recipient of National Institutes of Health Research Career Development Award HL 01777.*

to directly modify endothelial cell function or stimulate mediator release. From another perspective, the ability of endothelial cells to modify anaphylatoxin activity is also virtually unknown. The purpose of this report is to evaluate current literature on the topic and to summarize existing evidence relevant to potential mechanism(s) of anaphylatoxin action on the pulmonary endothelium.

II.   C5a-INDUCED PERMEABILITY CHANGES: A NEUTROPHIL-
        DEPENDENT MECHANISM

The action of serum carboxypeptidase on anaphylatoxins generated *in vivo* results in rapid conversion of both C3a and C5a to their des arginine forms (13). C3a is completely inactivated by this process, while the activity of C5a is only modified to a variable extent, depending upon the species (14). Thus, investigators of acute injury resulting from *in vivo* complement activation have generally considered C5a (or C5a$_{des \ Arg}$) as the only important anaphylatoxin contributing to the reactions observed.

In the rat, a model was developed for studies of pulmonary inflammatory reactions mediated by complement activation using intratracheal instillation of pre-formed immune complexes (15). The degree of injury produced was estimated by determining the extravasation of ^{125}I-labelled plasma protein (rat albumin) in the lung six hours after administration of immune complexes. This measure of vascular permeability was significantly elevated in immune complex-treated animals compared with controls, and the degree of injury correlated well with the ability of the immune complexes to fix complement in rat serum *in vitro*. The morphologic changes also included a massive influx of polymorphonuclear leukocytes and a severe hemorrhagic reaction in the lungs of these animals. Depletion of either complement or neutrophils prior to administration of the immune complexes afforded protection from both the permeability changes and pulmonary hemorrhage. Further, no influx of neutrophils in the lungs was observed in complement-depleted animals (16). These investigators concluded that both neutrophils and complement are necessary to enhance pulmonary vascular permeability in this type of inflammation. Further, since C5a is known to be the major neutrophil-stimulating complement component present in activated serum (17,18), it was reasoned that this peptide was the required complement fragment to produce the effect.

Desai *et al.* (19) examined the ability of chemotactic agents to promote increases in vascular permeability in hamster lung. These investigators studied the accumulation of ^{111}In-labelled neutrophils and ^{125}I-labelled albumin following intratracheal administration of human C5fr (functionally purified C5a) or the synthetic bacterial chemotactic peptide, formyl-methionyl-leucyl-phenylalanine (fMLP). Surprisingly, they found no significant elevation in ^{125}I-labelled albumin in the lungs with 600 or 1000 ED_{50} units of C5fr at time points from 5 min to 4 hr. Neutrophil accumulation, however, progressed from 1.5 times the control at 20 and 60 min to slightly more than two times that of saline-treated animals at 4 hours. Administration of 1000 ED_{50} units of fMLP produced no change in the vascular permeability index during the first 20 min, but, unlike C5fr, the synthetic peptide increased vascular permeability to 1.5- 2 times that of the controls by 60 min to 4 hr after administration. Neutrophil accumulation was elevated to 2 - 2.5 times normal. These data indicate that activation and extravasation of neutrophils in the lung is possible without concurrent vascular permeability changes, suggesting that the chemotactic stimulus is not sufficient to produce pulmonary inflammation.

These investigators also examined the inflammatory potential of intact C5 (19). Intratracheal administration of a quantity of this protein capable of generating only 250 - 500 ED_{50} units of C5a-dependent chemotactic activity resulted in dramatic changes in both vascular permeability and neutrophil accumulation after 4 hours (2-and 4-fold increases, respectively, in vascular permeability and neutrophil accumulation), although no elevation in these parameters was noted by 60 min. Thus C5 can be activated in the lung parenchyma to generate chemotactic and vascular permeability enhancing activity. In addition, the data suggest that increases in vascular permeability may require the presence of another C5-derived peptide distinct from $C5a_{des\ Arg}$, the putative component of the chemotactically active C5fr used in these studies.

We studied the the ability of the anaphylatoxin peptides, C3a and C5a, to produce acute pulmonary injury in the guinea pig. Both these peptides had previously been characterized as proinflammatory products of complement

TABLE I. Changes in vascular permeability observed 20 min after intrabronchial administration of anaphylatoxins in guinea pigs.

Treatment	(n)	Permeability	% of Control
Saline	(7)	0.28±0.097	100
Porcine C5a des Arg	(5)	0.49±0.076	175
Porcine C3a	(5)	0.45±0.087	161

Animals were treated with 15 µg/kg porcine $C5a_{des\ Arg}$ or 200 µg/kg porcine C3a. Permeability was calculated from the ratio of ^{125}I-BSA in lungs to ^{125}I-BSA in 1 ml blood (mean ± S.E.). (Data from ref. 24)

activation in other systems (3,20,21), stimulating increases in cutaneous vascular permeability (22,23), and smooth muscle contraction (23) in addition to the neutrophil stimulating activity unique to C5a (18). We therefore initiated investigations into the acute injury caused by purified preparations of these peptides,with the expectation that there may be a difference in the degree or pattern of the injury produced (30). Intrabronchial instillation of C3a, C5a or $C5a_{des\ Arg}$ isolated from complement-activated porcine serum in quantities which corresponded to the expected anaphylatoxin levels in 2-5 ml of blood, resulted in significant elevations in extravascular ^{125}I-labelled albumin within 20 min (Table I). C3a caused an increase in vascular permeability similar in magnitude to that produced by C5a, yet this peptide has been shown to be inactive as a chemotaxin for neutrophils *in vitro* (7). Both peptides also produced acute respiratory distress and morphologic evidence for smooth muscle contraction in both airways and blood vessels, and formation of aggregates of platelets and neutrophils (24). At this short time interval, no influx of neutrophils was noted.

Shaw and coworkers studied the pulmonary inflammation induced by human $C5a_{des\ Arg}$ in the rabbit (25). As in rats, hamsters and guinea pigs, this anaphylatoxin produced acute pulmonary inflammation characterized by intra-alveolar accumulation of neutrophils, erythrocytes, edema fluid and endothelial cell damage adjacent to or in the vicinity of neutrophils. Depletion of circulating neutrophils or adsorption of the anaphylatoxin with immobilized antibody against the peptide protected the animals from such injury, indicating a requirement for both elements in this species as well.

A difference in the degree of inflammation produced by C5a and $C5a_{desArg}$ was noted by Larsen *et al.* (26). These investigators found, as we had observed in the guinea pig (24), that the des-arginine form of the peptide caused considerably more injury that intact C5a. Henson *et al.* (27), suggested an explanation for this phenomenon based on the increased avidity of neutrophil receptors for C5a compared with $C5a_{des\ Arg}$. These cells may effectively remove this peptide from circulation by degradation following internalization of the C5a-receptor complex (28). Thus, $C5a_{des\ Arg}$, with a lower affinity for neutrophil receptors, has an increased opportunity to interact with other cells.

In an examination of this scenario, the *in vivo* clearance and tissue distribution of ^{125}I-labelled C5a and $C5a_{des\ Arg}$ were studied following intravenous injection in rabbits (29). Both peptides are rapidly cleared from the blood, with more than 50% of the radiolabel removed within the first 2 minutes after injection. Clearance of C5a was more rapid than $C5a_{des\ Arg}$ by a small but reproducible amount. The degree of neutropenia caused by C5a was much greater than for $C5a_{des\ Arg}$, suggesting preferential uptake of this peptide by PMNs. At early times most of the radiolabel appeared in the lung followed by a decline within 4 hours. This was followed by a transient appearance in the kidney beginning 30 min after injection. Accumulation in the spleen was also evident, remaining fairly constant for the duration of the experiment. When animals were first depleted of neutrophils with nitrogen mustard, the accumulation in the lung was not altered, indicating a PMN-independent mechanism for pulmonary sequestration of the anaphylatoxin. No radiolabel appeared in the spleen and accumulation in the kidney was considerably slower. Clearance was shown to operate through a receptor-dependent mechanism since pretreatment with cobra venom factor (which should block receptor sites by saturating them with endogenously formed C5a) led to suppression of the rate of clearance of radiolabelled peptides by 40-65%. Attempts to demonstrate binding to vascular endothelial cells or another target cell in the lung by autoradiography produced equivocal results.

Studies of the vascular permeability enhancing effects of C5a in rabbit skin showed little effect if the peptide was injected alone (30,31). When the peptide was injected in combination with vasodilating prostaglandins, including PGE_1, PGE_2 or PGI_2, the vascular permeability was markedly potentiated and the response was blocked by prior depletion of circulating neutrophils (30). Thus, these data indicated that inflammatory edema resulting from extravascular activation of complement is dependent on the concomitant effects of a leukocyte/endothelial cell interaction triggered by C5a, and the generation of a vasodilating prostaglandin.

Henson et al. (32) similarly observed a marked enhancement in pulmonary vascular permeability when cobra venom factor-induced complement activation was accompanied by infusion of PGE_2. Subsequently, Larsen et al. (26) examined the effects of brief periods of hypoxia prior to intravenous infusion of C5a or cobra venom factor. Hypoxia is known to stimulate prostaglandin synthesis (33), and as was observed in rabbit skin, lung injury was also significantly potentiated. These investigators noted a 5-fold increase in albumin and 10-fold increase in neutrophils in the bronchoalveolar lavage fluid. Meclofenamate treatment suppressed the effect of the combination of hypoxia and cobra venom factor, confirming the production of prostaglandins in these reactions.

Thus, these data support a mechanism of complement-induced increases in vascular permeability mediated through the action of C5a on neutrophils. In the rabbit, at least, there appears to be an additional requirement for vasodilating prostaglandins. The initial reports of inflammatory responses in this species initiated by intratracheal instillation of C5a alone may be explained by prostaglandin formation due to the trauma delivered during surgical preparation of the animal (34). Indeed, it is possible that prostaglandins or other vasodilating substances are necessary to promote C5a-induced increases in vascular permeability in other species as well, but that such a requirement has not been shown because of difficulties in preventing endogenous release.

Till *et al.* (35), in studies of the effects of intravascular complement activation with cobra venom factor in the rat, confirmed previous findings with respect to the role of neutrophils and C5a in promoting vascular injury. They further showed that pretreatment with an antihistamine afforded only a small degree of protection ($\approx$15%), whereas depletion of neutrophils reduced leakage of plasma protein by $\approx$70%. Pretreatment of these animals with catalase and/or superoxide dismutase afforded a similar degree of protection as neutrophil depletion indicating that the effect of these cells is mediated by formation of toxic oxygen metabolites.

Thus, the weight of evidence strongly favors the concept that complement-induced endothelial cell injury depends upon C5a-mediated stimulation of neutrophils. These stimulated neutrophils adhere to the pulmonary capillary endothelial cell layer, producing superoxide anion and hydrogen peroxide, thereby disrupting the adjacent endothelial cells and leading to the observed permeability changes. (Concurrent production of vasodilating substances may be required in some species as well.)

III.   NEUTROPHIL-INDEPENDENT PERMEABILITY CHANGES

While the mechanism described above appears to be effective for the types of pulmonary injury included in these studies, it may be an oversimplification to suggest that it is the exclusive mechanism by which complement anaphylatoxins can produce vascular permeability changes in the lung. Our findings with C3a, for example, are somewhat more difficult to explain. As shown by the data in Table I, intratracheal instillation of this peptide clearly results in an increase in vascular permeability within 20 min, to an extent similar to that reached by C5a (24). The neutrophil stimulating properties of C3a, however, are still unsettled, with several laboratories reporting an absence of chemotactic activity *in vitro* (7,36), while others report chemotaxis (37), binding (38), and lysosomal enzyme release with this peptide (39). It is possible that C3a is chemotactic for neutrophils, at least *in vivo*, and evidence supporting such activity has been reported (40). Alternatively, C3a may act directly on the endothelial cells (41), or on another cell type distinct from the neutrophil which also has the ability to cause endothelial cell damage. C3a is reported to act on a number of other cell types in the lung, including macrophages (42) and platelets (43,44); however, such mechanisms for C3a-induced increases in pulmonary vascular permeability have not been explored.

A potentially different complement-dependent mechanism for increasing pulmonary vascular permeability was observed by chance in an immunologic attempt to modulate the activity of angiotensin converting enzyme (ACE) *in vivo*. A carboxyl dipeptidase localized on the luminal side of endothelial cells, this enzyme rapidly converts angiotensin I to angiotensin II and inactivates bradykinin (45-47). Caldwell *et al.* (48) injected goat antibody specific for purified rabbit ACE into rabbits and observed severe pulmonary injury and a rapidly lethal response. The injury was apparently not due to the anticatalytic activity of the antibody *per se*, since peptide inhibitors are not lethal, but appeared to be immunologic in origin. Rats treated with antibody directed against the rabbit enzyme which cross-reacts *in vitro* did not undergo a similar rapidly lethal reaction (48). Rats treated with antibody against rat ACE, however, developed pulmonary injury as did rabbits. These animals responded in a dose-dependent fashion to anti-ACE antibody with increasing pulmonary vascular permeability, and the effect was blocked by prior complement depletion (49). Further investigations by Caldwell *et al.* (51) cast some doubt on the role of complement in this response. These investigators showed a similar degree of pulmonary injury in animals treated with Fab fragments of the antibody as was observed with intact IgG. Since the Fab fragments are not capable of activating compelement *in vitro*, it appeared that another mechanism was in effect. *In vitro* studies showed that purified, solubilized ACE is capable of activating C1 directly and that anti-ACE IgG potentiates the activity. Fab fragments, however, had no such effect.

Camussi *et al.* (52) may have shed some light on the mechanism of this injury. They showed that rabbits depleted of neutrophils were not protected from injury by anti-ACE antibody, and that significant quantities of platelet-activating factor were released upon immune stimulation. They postulated that C5a generated by activation of complement may be the critical stimulus, since this anaphylatoxin is capable of stimulating PAF release from other cells (53,54). Thus, another potential mechanism of complement anaphylatoxin-induced increases in pulmonary vascular permeability results from primary immunologic response on the endothelial cells which activates complement followed by anaphylatoxin-dependent stimulation of PAF release.

IV.   STUDIES WITH ENDOTHELIAL CELLS IN CULTURE

Denney and Johnson (62) first provided evidence for uptake of C3a by cultured human umbilical vein endothelial cells. Using ^{125}I-labelled C3a, they showed that these cells bind the peptide in a time- and concentration-dependent manner. This uptake was not associated with binding to a specific receptor, however, since binding of radiolabelled ligand was not affected by excess unlabelled peptide. In addition, the binding sites were not saturated at 10^{-6} M C3a, and prolonged incubation of the peptide with the cells resulted in a decrease in the spasmogenic activity of the material. These findings may reflect an interaction of the peptide with angiotensin converting enzyme on the surface of the endothelial cells. Pharmacologic evidence that angiotensin converting enzyme may inactivate C5a in guinea pigs was provided by Lim *et al.* (56). These investigators reported that the vascular permeability changes caused by intradermal injection of C5a in these animals was significantly enhanced if they were pretreated with captopril, a potent inhibitor of ACE (57). It was not clear in these studies, however, whether the results were mediated by an effect of the drug on angiotensin converting enzyme or serum carboxypeptidase, or both, since the respective activities of these peptidases were not assessed.

We recently showed that purified rabbit lung angiotensin converting enzyme is capable of degrading C3a *in vitro* (58). Incubation of 3 nmoles of porcine C3a with 70 mIU angiotensin converting enzyme for 2 hr at 37°C resulted in quantitative removal of the carboxyl-terminal dipeptide, Ala-Arg (Table II). In addition, preliminary studies of binding of C3a to frozen sections of guinea pig lung showed uptake of ^{125}I-C3a as a function of time, but net ligand bound decreased rapidly (Figure 1). When captopril was included in the incubation buffer, the extent of binding was not as great at early time points, but the peptide appeared to remain bound to sites in the tissue and was not inactivated. We do not yet know whether this specific binding of C3a to guinea pig lung tissues in the presence of captopril reflects receptor sites that promote physiologic changes in the tissue, since the spasmogenically inactive $C3a_{des\ Arg}$ blocks binding of ^{125}I-C3a as well as the intact peptide. The possibility that $C3a_{des\ Arg}$ has biologic activities

TABLE II. Amino acid analysis of residues released from C3a and C5a by angiotensin converting enzyme

Experiment[*]	C3a[+]	C5a[+]
1	Ala, Arg	Gly, Arg
	(0.63)(0.74)	(0)(0)
2	Ala, Arg	Gly, Arg
	(0.86)(0.80)	(0)(0)

[*]Exp. 1: 3.24 nmoles C3a or C5a + 70 mIU ACE, 2.5 hr, 37°C.
   Exp. 2: 3.24 nmoles C3a or C5a + 70 mIU ACE, 4 hr, 37°C.
[+]Values in parentheses reflect residues released above control without ACE; expressed as mol/mol, determined by acid hydrolysis of digests resolved on C18 Sep Pak cartridges. (Data from ref. 58)

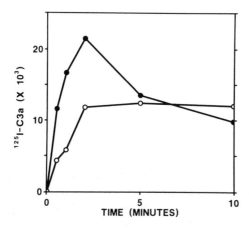

Figure 1. Effect of captopril on the specific binding of ^{125}I-labelled C3a by guinea pig lung tissues. Frozen sections, 10 μm thick, containing 20-25 μg protein, were incubated at 4°C with 1 μM ^{125}I-C3a with (°) or without (•) 10 μM captopril. Specific binding was determined by subtracting ^{125}I-cpm bound in the presence of 100-fold excess unlabelled C3a. Each point is the mean of four determinations.

in the lung has not been well studied. Regardless, these data support a potential role for clearance of the anaphylatoxins, especially C3a, by angiotensin converting enzyme present on the endothelial cell surface.

Additional evidence supporting a neutrophil-dependent mechanism for C5a-induced endothelial cell injury, gleaned from experiments performed *in vivo*, has been provided by several *in vitro* investigations. Sacks *et al.* (59), developed an *in vitro* model of this process using ^{51}Cr-labelled human umbilical vein cells in culture. In this system, neutrophils activated with complement induced endothelial cell damage as assessed by the release of isotope. Complement-activated serum or purified C5a alone had no significant effect, nor did neutrophils treated with heat-inactivated serum or C3a. Injury appeared to require close contact of the endothelial cells with neutrophils, since cytochalasin B treatment (which blocks adherence of the PMNs) prevented ^{51}Cr release. In addition, evidence was provided for mediation of the effect by toxic oxygen metabolites since superoxide dismutase and catalase afforded protection. Similar findings have been reported *in vivo* (35).

Tonnensen *et al.* (60) made similar observations using assays of neutrophil adherence to endothelial cells with ^{51}Cr-labelled neutrophils. They found dose-dependent increases in the adherence of neutrophils using purified C5a,

C5a$_{des\ Arg}$, or fMLP in concentrations ranging from 10^{-10} to 10^{-6} M. The binding was rapid, occurring within two minutes, and diminished upon removal of the chemotactic stimulus. Incubation of the chemotactic factors with endothelial cells followed by washing failed to increase subsequent adherence, indicating that the effect is specific for neutrophils.

V.   LIPID MEDIATOR RELEASE FROM ENDOTHELIAL CELLS

An additional, potentially useful approach to evaluating a role for the anaphylatoxin peptides on endothelial cells may be through studies of the lipid metabolites released. Camussi et al. (52) provided evidence for release of platelet-activating factor from endothelial cells in vivo following infusion of anti-ACE antibody. The authors suggested that this reaction might be a direct effect of C5a since it was not blocked by neutrophil depletion and the anaphylatoxin is capable of inducing PAF release from other cells (53-54).

Additional experiments show that endothelial cells in culture release PAF when stimulated with thrombin (61). However, incubation with zymosan-activated plasma containing C5a$_{des\ Arg}$ produced no such effect (62). Unfortunately, a negative experiment in this case may not be very meaningful since it is well known that endothelial cells can lose certain receptors in culture (63).

VI.   SUMMARY

Clearly, we have a great deal to learn about the interactions of the complement anaphylatoxins with the pulmonary endothelium. The action of C5a-stimulated neutrophils appears to be a well accepted mechanism for enhancing vascular permeability. Whether C3a acts by a similar mechanism is not altogether clear, although one might predict it to be the case. In addition, there appears to be a catabolic role of the endothelium for these peptides, as there is with angiotensin I and bradykinin. The release of mediators by these peptides is almost totally unknown.

REFERENCES

1.   Friedberger EZ. (1910) Immunitætsforsch Exp Ther 4:636.
2.   Schultz WH. (1910) J Pharmacol Exp Therap 2:221.
3.   Osler AG, Randall GH, Hill BM and Ovary Z. (1959) J Exp Med 110:311.

4. Hahn F and Oberdorf AZ. (1950) *Immunitætsforsch Exp Ther* **107**:528.
5. Lepow IH, Dias da Silva W, Eisele JW. (1968) *In* **Biochemistry of the acute allergic reactions** (KF Austen and EL Becker, eds) Blackwell:Oxford.
6. Jacobs JW, Rubin JS, Hugli TE, Bogardt RA, Mariz IK, Daniels JS, Doughaday WH and Bradshaw RA. (1978) *Biochem* **17**:5031.
7. Fernandez HN and Hugli TE. (1978) *J Biol Chem* **253**:6955.
8. Gerard C and Hugli TE. (1979) *J Biol Chem* **254**:6346.
9. Huber R, Scholze H and Diesenhofer J. (1980) *Hoppe-Zeyler's Z Physiol Chem* **361**:1389.
10. Muto Y, Fukumoto Y and Arata Y. (1985) *Biochem* **24**:6650.
11. Hoeprich PD and Hugli TE. (1986) *Biochem* In press.
12. Vallota EH and Muller-Eberhard HJ. (1973) *J Exp Med* **137**:1109.
13. Bokisch VA and Muller-Eberhard HJ. (1970) *J Clin Invest* **49**:2427.
14. Gerard C and Hugli TE. (1981) *Proc Natl Acad Sci USA* **78**:1833.
15. Scherzer H and Ward PA. (1978) *Am Rev J Immunol* **121**:947.
16. Scherzer H and Ward PA. (1978) *Am Rev Respir Dis* **117**:551.
17. Shi HS, Snyderman R, Friedman E, Mellors A and Mayer MM. (1968) *Science* **162**:361.
18. Ward PA and Newman LJ. (1969) *J Immunol* **102**:93.
19. Desai U, Kreutzer DL, Showell H, Arroyave CV and Ward PA. (1979) *Am J Pathol* **96**:71.
20. Dias da Silva W and Lepow IH. (1967) *J Exp Med* **125**:921.
21. Jenson JA. (1967) *Science* **155**:1122.
22. Lepow IH, Willims-Kretschmer K, Kilpatrick RA and Rosen FS. (1970) *Am J Pathol* **61**:13.
23. Cochrane CG and Muller-Eberhard HJ. (1968) *J Exp Med* **127**:371.
24. Stimler NP, Hugli TE and Bloor CM. (1980) *Am J Pathol* **100**:327.
25. Shaw JO, Henson PM, Henson J and Webster RO. (1980) *Lab Invest* **42**:547.
26. Larsen GL, Webster RO, Worthen GS, Gumbay RS and Henson PM. (1985) *J Clin Invest* **75**:902.
27. Henson PM, McCarthy K, Larsen GL, Webster RO, Giclas PC, Dreisen RB, King TE and Shaw JO. (1979) *Am J Pathol* **97**:93.
28. Chenoweth DE and Hugli TE. (1980) *J Immunol* **124**:1517.
29. Webster RO, Larsen GL and Henson PM. (1982) *J Clin Invest* **70**:1177.
30. Jose PJ, Forrest MJ and Williams TJ. (1981) *J Immunol* **127**:2376.
31. Williams TJ and Jose PJ. (1981) *J Exp Med* **153**:136.
32. Henson PM, Larsen GL, Webster RO, Mitchell BC, Goins AJ, Henson JE. (1982) *Ann NY Acad Sci* **384**:287.
33. Said SI, Yoshida T, Kitamura S and Vreim C. (1974) *Science* **185**:1181.

34. Webster RO, Larsen GL, Mitchell BC, Goins AJ and Henson PM. (1982) *Am Rev Respir Dis* **125**:335.
35. Till GO, Johnson KJ, Kunkel R and Ward PA. (1982) *J Clin Invest* **69**:1126.
36. Van Epps DE and Chenoweth DE. (1984) *J Immunol* **132**:2862.
37. Damerau B, Grunefeld E and Vogt W. (1978) *Naunyn-Schmiedeberg's Arch Pharmacol* **305**:181.
38. Glovsky MM, Hugli TE, Ishizaka T, Lichtenstein LM and Erickson BW. (1979) *J Clin Invest* **64**:804.
39. Showell HJ, Glovsky MM and Ward PA. (1982) *Int Archs Allergy Appl Immunol* **67**:227.
40. Damerau B, Hollerhage HG and Vogt W. (1978) *Naunyn-Schmiedeberg's Arch Pharmacol* **302**:45.
41. Bjork J, Hugli TE and Smedegard G. (1985) *J Immunol* **134**:1115.
42. Hartung HP, Bitte-Suerman D and Hadding U. (1983) *J Immunol* **130**:1345.
43. Grossklaus CHR, Damerau B, Lemgo E and Vogt W. (1976) *Naunyn-Schmiedeberg's Arch Pharmacol* **295**:71.
44. Polley MJM and Nachman RL. (1983) *J Exp Med* **158**:603.
45. Ryan JW, Roblero J and Stewart JW. (1970) *Adv Exp Med Biol* **8**:263.
46. Dorer FE, Ryan JW and Stewart JM. (1974) *Biochem J* **141**:915.
47. Soffer RL. (1976) *Ann Rev Biochem* **45**:73.
48. Caldwell PRB, Wigger HJ, Das M and Soffer RL. (1976) *Febs Lett* **63**:82.
49. Conroy JM, Hoffman H, Kirk ES, Hirzel HO, Sonnenblick EH and Soffer RL. (1976) *J Biol Chem* **251**:4828.
50. McCormick JR, Thrall RS, Kerlin A and Ward PA. (1980) *Clin Immunobiol Immunopath* **15**:444.
51. Caldwell PRB, Wigger HJ, Fernandez LT, D'Alisa RM, Tse-Eng D, Butler VP and Gigli I. (1981) *Am J Pathol* **105**:54.
52. Camussi G, Pawlowski I, Bussolino F, Caldwell PRB, Brentjens J and Andres G. (1983) *J Immunol* **131**:1802.
53. Lynch JM, Lotner GZ, Betz SJ and Henson PM. (1979) *J Immunol* **123**:1219.
54. Camussi G, Tetta C, Bussolino F, Caligaris-Cappio F, Masera C and Segoloni G. (1981) *Int Archs Allergy Appl Immunol* **64**:25.
55. Denney JB and Johnson AR. (1979) *Immunol* **36**:169.
56. Lim HW, Kamide R and Gigli I. (1985) *Brit J Derm* **112**:43.
57. Ondetti MA and Cushman DW. (1982) *Ann Rev Biochem* **51**:283.

58. Stimler NP, Hendricks CL, Ozols JB and Gerard C. (1985) *Fed Proc* **44**:1267.

59. Sacks T, Moldow CF, Craddock PR, Bowers TK and Jacobs HS. (1978) *J Clin Invest* **61**:1161.

60. Tonnesen MG, Smedly LA and Henson PM. (1984) *J Clin Invest* **74**:1581.

61. Prescott SM, Zimmerman GA and McIntyre TM. (1984) *Proc Natl Acad Sci USA.* **81**:3534.

62. Zimmerman GA, McIntyre TM, Prescott SM. (1985)*Circulation* **72**:718.

63. Ryan US, Mortara M and Whitaker C. (1980) *Tissue and Cell* **12**:1161.

Hemostatic Potential
of the Pulmonary Endothelium

DAVID J. CRUTCHLEY[1]
Research Division
Miami Heart Institute
Miami Beach, Florida 33140

I.   INTRODUCTION

Vascular endothelium comes into direct contact with the blood, and so is strategically located to affect blood fluidity. In turn, the endothelium may itself be affected by blood coagulation, not only as a consequence of vascular occlusion but also more directly by vasoactive substances released by platelets and leukocytes associated with the clot.

It has long been appreciated that intact, healthy vascular endothelium does not support blood clotting, an observation which originally led to the assumption that endothelium is an inert layer separating the blood from subendothelial tissues. However, healthy endothelium merely fulfills an important requirement for an effective hemostatic system, *i.e.*, that it should be quiescent under normal conditions. In fact, endothelium is now known to produce and express a complex array of hemostatic factors, which can both promote and inhibit the coagulation process. Under normal conditions, the antithrombogenic factors predominate.

[1]*The author's work was supported in part by Grant HL 25864 from the National Heart, Lung and Blood Institute, and by a generous grant from the Lucille P. Markey Charitable Bequest.*

The pulmonary vascular bed is unique in at least three respects. First, it receives the entire cardiac output. Second, it performs the vital functions of gas exchange and hormone processing. Third, the pulmonary vascular bed has an enormous endothelial cell content. In view of this, one might expect the hemostatic potential of the pulmonary endothelium to be especially well regulated.

Most of the detailed biochemical studies on endothelial hemostatic factors have been carried out using cells derived from nonpulmonary origins, especially human umbilical veins and bovine aortas. Recent studies, carried out in collaboration with Dr. Una S. Ryan of the University of Miami School of Medicine, suggest that pulmonary endothelial cells also possess a potent and complex hemostatic system. Nevertheless, many questions remain unanswered, including those of whether the hemostatic potential of the pulmonary endothelium varies according to its location in the vascular bed. Presumably, such questions will be answered when pulmonary capillary cells become routinely available in culture.

II. STIMULATION OF ENDOTHELIAL PROCOAGULANT ACTIVITY BY ENDOTOXIN

Recent studies show that endothelial cells derived from human umbilical veins and bovine aortas acquire procoagulant activity when exposed to agents such as bacterial endotoxin, thrombin, and interleukin-1 (1-3). The activity is due to the increased synthesis and expression of thromboplastin (tissue factor; Factor III), a 45-50 kDa glycoprotein complexed with phospholipid. Thromboplastin is a key procoagulant factor since it can initiate blood coagulation via both the extrinsic and intrinsic pathways (4,5). Thus, it potentiates the Factor VIIa-mediated cleavage of Factor X to Factor Xa (extrinsic pathway), and of Factor IX to Factor IXa (intrinsic pathway). Initiation of Factor IX activation appears to be the primary role for thromboplastin in endothelial cells (6). In the presence of Factor VIII, Factor IXa further activates Factor X. Factor Xa, formed via either pathway, then converts prothrombin to thrombin in a reaction which requires Factor V. Thrombin is a pivotal coagulant enzyme: it converts soluble fibrinogen to insoluble fibrin, activates platelets, and inhibits vessel wall fibrinolytic activity (7,8). Thrombin-induced platelet activation leads not only to the formation of platelet clumps but also to increased Factor Xa binding and Factor V activity on the platelet surface (9), thereby amplifying the coagulant potential.

The endothelial surface provides all of the factors necessary for these procoagulant mechanisms to proceed. Thus, endothelial cells not only express thromboplastin activity, but also possess specific binding sites for Factors VII, IX

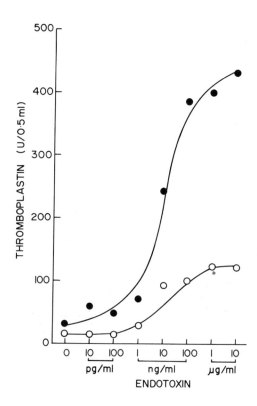

Figure 1. Stimulation of thromboplastin activity in bovine pulmonary endothelial cells by endotoxin. Confluent cells were incubated for 6 h with serum-free medium containing endotoxin at the concentrations shown. Thromboplastin activity in cell sonicates was then measured by a specific chromogenic assay for Factor Xa (•) or by a plasma coagulation assay (°). Activity was calculated by reference to a standard thromboplastin preparation, and is expressed in units/0.5 ml endothelial sonicate.

and X (10,11), and synthesize factor V (12). Factors IX and X bound to the endothelial cell surface can be readily activated to Factors IXa and Xa, respectively, and prothrombin can be activated on the endothelial surface by Factor Xa (6,13,14).

In keeping with results obtained with non-pulmonary endothelial cells, we find that bovine pulmonary arterial endothelial cells express increased thromboplastin activity following incubation with very low concentrations (10 ng/ml or higher) of endotoxin (Figure 1). The induction process is relatively slow, requiring 4-6 hours to appear and 24 hours to reach maximum. Endotoxin-stimulated levels of thromboplastin activity reach 20-fold basal levels.

Endothelial thromboplastin activity can be measured by its ability to generate Factor Xa in a Factor VII-, Factor X-supplemented assay (15). In this assay, endothelial cell sonicates are mixed with a low concentration (less than 0.1%) of bovine plasma, as a source of factor VII, and with purified bovine Factor X. The resulting formation of Factor Xa is assessed by the cleavage of a specific chromogenic substrate, N-benzoyl-Ileu-Glu-Gly-Arg-p-nitroanilide (Kab1 S-2222). Assay specificity is provided by treating the plasma with 10 mM diisopropyl-fluorophosphate (DFP), which inactivates Factor VIIa and abolishes endothelial thromboplastin activity. The level of endothelial thromboplastin activity is calculated by reference to a standard thromboplastin preparation.

Endothelial thromboplastin activity can also be measured by a recalcified plasma coagulation assay. In this assay, endothelial cell sonicates are mixed with bovine plasma, calcium, and phospholipids. Once again, assay specificity is attained by DFP treatment of the plasma, and the level of endothelial thrombo-plastin activity is calculated by reference to a standard thromboplastin preparation.

Surprisingly, levels of endothelial thromboplastin activity are considerably lower when assessed by the coagulation assay, relative to the chromogenic assay (Figure 1). Thus, it appears that most of the potential procoagulant activity of thromboplastin in bovine pulmonary endothelial cells is masked by anticoagulant factors which inhibit blood clot formation. Such factors do not prevent the generation of Factor Xa, or inhibit its ability to cleave a low molecular weight chromogenic substrate. Although the precise identity of the putative anticoagulant species in bovine pulmonary endothelial cells is not yet established, studies on endothelial cells derived from other sources indicate that at least three proteins would be candidates for such a role. These are: α2-macro-globulin, heparin-like proteoglycans, and thrombomodulin.

α2-Macroglobulin is a large (800 kDa) protein which is present in the plasma. Immunofluorescence studies suggest that α2-macroglobulin may be associated with vascular endothelial cells, including those derived from bovine pulmonary arteries (16,17), although these results have been challenged (18). In addition, it is not clear whether endothelial cells actively synthesize α2-macro-globulin or merely take it up from the plasma. α2-Macroglobulin is a non-specific protease inhibitor, which appears to function by "trapping" the protease within a cage-like structure (19). Once trapped, the protease is denied access to its natural, high-molecular mass substrate, although smaller substrates can still be efficiently cleaved (20). α2-Macroglobulin, if present functionally in bovine pulmonary endothelial cells, could explain the apparent discrepancy between the chromogenic and coagulation assays: Factor Xa, produced as a result of endothelial thromboplastin activity and subsequently bound by $\alpha2$-macroglobulin, would not be able to cleave prothrombin but could readily liberate 4-nitroaniline from a chromogenic substrate.

Several studies have also indicated that endothelial cells produce heparin sulfate and other proteoglycans, which function as anticoagulants in a manner analogous to that of heparin (21,22). Thus, they bind to the plasma protein, antithrombin III, and dramatically enhance its ability to inactivate Factor Xa and thrombin (23).

The full anticoagulant potential of endothelial heparin-like species would not be realized under the conditions of the chromogenic assay, where levels of plasma (and therefore of antithrombin III) are low; it should, however, be realized under the conditions of the coagulation assay, where large amounts of antithrombin III would be supplied by the plasma. The presence of functional heparin-like species in bovine pulmonary endothelial cells could therefore provide an additional explanation for the apparent discrepancy between the two assays.

The third candidate for the role of endothelial anticoagulant factor is thrombomodulin. This 75 kDa glycoprotein is localized on endothelium and catalyzes thrombin-mediated activation of protein C (24). Activated protein C, in turn, has several important anticoagulant effects: it inhibits blood clotting, principally by proteolytic inactivation of Factor V (25), amd stimulates endothelial fibrinolytic activity, principally by proteolytic inactivation of a fibrinolytic inhibitor (26). Thrombomodulin may also exhibit direct thrombin-inhibitory effects (27), although this has been challenged (28). Once again, the small amount of plasma (and therefore, of protein C) in the chromogenic assay suggests that the full anticoagulant potential of endothelial thrombomodulin would not be expressed in this assay.

In summary, bovine pulmomary endothelial cells under resting conditions express little or no procoagulant activity. Although exposure to low concentrations of endotoxin induces the expression of thromboplastin, its procoagulant potential appears to be largely masked by anticoagulant factors.

III.   SUPPRESSION OF ENDOTHELIAL FIBRINOLYTIC ACTIVITY BY ENDOTOXIN

In contrast to their lack of procoagulant activity, resting bovine pulmonary endothelial cells possess marked fibrinolytic activity. This appears to be due primarily to their ability to synthesize and secrete plasminogen activators.

These are narrow-spectrum serum proteases which cleave the plasma protein, plasminogen, to yield the broad-spectrum protease, plasmin. This in turn converts insoluble fibrin into soluble fibrinopeptides, thereby effecting clot dissolution.

Plasminogen activators may be divided into two distinct classes: tissue-plasminogen activators (tPA) and urokinases. The former bind to fibrin, a reaction which dramatically enhances their ability to activate plasminogen (29). Urokinases, on the other hand, have little affinity for fibrin, and can activate plasminogen in its absence. These observations suggest that tPA may be the more important enzyme in physiological fibrinolysis. However, more recent studies show that urokinase is produced as a single-chain pro-enzyme (pro-urokinase) (30). Unlike urokinase, plasminogen activation by pro-urokinase appears to exhibit considerable fibrin-specificity (31). Thus, it is likely that both tPA and urokinase have physiological relevance to the fibrinolytic system, a suggestion which is reinforced by the finding that endothelial cells appear to produce both types of plasminogen activator (32-34). Multiple forms of plasminogen activator are also produced by bovine pulmonary endothelial cells: studies utilizing SDS-polyacrylamide gel electrophoresis show that these cells produce primarily a 45 kDa urokinase, and release both urokinase and high-molecular weight plasminogen activators (35). These latter species may consist of complexes between tpA and a stable inhibitor; the complexes are dissociated sufficiently by SDS to exhibit fibrinolytic activity (33).

Endotoxin dramatically suppresses the fibrinolytic activity of bovine pulmomary arterial endothelial cells (Figure 2). Like the thromboplastin-stimulating effects of endotoxin, the fibrinolytic suppressive effects are slow in onset, requiring 6 hours to appear, and are seen with low concentrations (1 ng/ml or higher) of endotoxin.

Gel electrophoresis studies indicate that endotoxin has no effect on the type or amount of plasminogen activators produced by these cells. Thus, it appears that endotoxin exerts its fibrinolytic-suppressive effects by inducing the synthesis or expression of a fibrinolytic inhibitor. Direct evidence for this is two-fold: first, conditioned medium from endotoxin-treated cells directly inhibits urokinase and tPA, but not plasmin; second, fibrinolytically inactive complexes between [125I]-labelled urokinase amd the endotoxin-induced inhibitor can be obtained by gel filtration techniques. The endotoxin induced inhibitor has an approximate molecular mass of 50 kDa, and is relatively labile (35). The latter property distinguishes it from the unusually stable plasminogen activator inhibitor reported in bovine aortic endothelial cells (36), and raises the interesting question of whether systemic and pulmonary endothelial cells differ qualitatively with respect to their fibrinolytic systems.

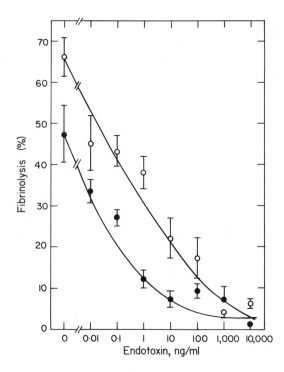

Figure 2. Suppression of fibrinolytic activity in bovine pulmonary endothelial cells by endotoxin. Confluent cells were incubated for 6 h with serum-free medium containing endotoxin at the concentrations shown. Fibrinolytic activity in cell sonicates (•) and conditioned media (°) was then measured by a plasminogen-supplemented (^{125}I) fibrin plate assay. Values are means ± SE of 5 experiments.

IV. SUMMARY

From the above considerations, it is apparent that the hemostatic potential of the pulmonary endothelium results from a complex balance, not only between active factors which have opposing biological actions (for example, thromboplastin and plasminogen activator), but also between active factors and specific inhibitors (for example, plasminogen activator and plasminogen-activator inhibitor).

This point is particularly well emphasized by the effects of bacterial endotoxin on bovine pulmonary arterial endothelial cells. Thus, our studies show that quiescent pulmonary endothelial cells, like endothelial cells derived from other sources, show little or no procoagulant activity but do possess an active fibrinolytic system. When exposed to low concentrations of endotoxin, these cells show increased thromboplastin activity, although its procoagulant potential appears to be largely masked by anticoagulant factors such as macroglobulin, heparin-like proteoglycans, and thrombomodulin.

Concomitant with the increase in thromboplastin activity, endotoxin causes an inhibition of fibrinolytic activity in these cells. Such effects are not due to decreased production of plasminogen activators but rather to the increased synthesis or expression of a specific plasminogen activator-inhibitor.

Since endotoxins are found in the outer walls of Gram-negative bacteria, it is likely that the pulmonary endothelium will be exposed continuously to these substances during severe Gram-negative sepsis. The dual effects of endotoxin on procoagulant and fibrinolytic activity would tend to render the endothelial surface more thrombogenic, and may contribute to the disseminated intravascular coagulation and fibrin deposition often seen in the lungs of patients with severe sepsis or the adult respiratory distress syndrome.

REFERENCES

1. Colucci M, Balconi G, Lorenzet R, Pietra A, Locati D, Donati MB and Semeraro N. (1983) *J Clin Invest* **71**:1893.
2. Brox JH, Osterud B, Bjorklid E and Fenton JW. (1984) *Brit J Hæmatol* **57**:239.
3. Bevilacqua MP, Pober JS, Majeau GR, Cotran RS and Gimbrone MA. (1984) *J Exp Med* **160**:618.
4. Nemerson Y and Pitlick FA. (1972) *Prog Hemostas Thromb.* **1**:1.
5. Osterud B and Rapaport SI. (1977) *Proc Natl Acad Sci USA* **74**:5260.
6. Stern DM, Nawroth P, Handley D and Kisiel W. (1985) *Proc Natl Acad Sci USA* **82**:2523.
7. Loskutoff DJ. (1979) *J Clin Invest* **64**: 329.
8. Gelehrter TD and Sznycer-Laszuk R. (1986) *J Clin Invest* **77**:165.
9. Miletich JP, Jackson CM and Majerus PW. (1977) *Proc Natl Acad Sci USA* **74**:4033.
10. Rodgers GM, Broze GJ and Shuman MA. (1984) *Blood* **63**:434.
11. Heimark RL and Schwartz SM. (1983) *Biochem Biophys Res Comm* **111**:723.
12. Cerveny TJ, Fass DN and Mann KG. (1984) *Blood* **63**:1467.
13. Stern DM, Drillings M, Kisiel W, Nawroth PP, Nossel HL and LaGamma K. (1984) *Proc Natl Acad Sci USA.* **81**:913.

14. Rodgers GM and Shuman MA. (1983) *Proc Natl Acad Sci USA* 80:7001.
15. Crutchley DJ. (1986) *J Tissue Culture Methods* In press.
16. Becker CG and Harpel PC. (1976) *J Exp Med* 144: 1.
17. Ryan US, Clements E, Habliston D and Ryan JW. (1978) *Tissue and Cell* 10: 535.
18. Marymen F, Van der Schueren B, Van Leuven F, Cassiman JJ and Van den Berghe H. (1982) *Haemostasis* 11:210.
19. Feldman SR, Gonias SL and Pizzo SV. (1985) *Proc Natl Acad Sci USA* 82:5700.
20. Downing MR, Bloom JW and Mann KG. (1978) *Biochemistry* 17:2649.
21. Colburn P and Buonassisi V. (1982) *Biochem Biophys Res Comm* 104:220.
22. Marcum JA, McKenney JB and Rosenberg RD. (1984) *J Clin Invest* 74:341.
23. Griffith MJ. (1982) *J Biol Chem* 257:7360.
24. Esmon NL, Owen WG and Esmon CT. (1982) *J Biol Chem* 257:859.
25. Walker FJ, Sexton PW and Exmon CT. (1979) *Biochim Biophys Acta* 571:333.
26. Sakata Y, Curriden S, Lawrence D, Griffin JH and Loskutoff DJ. (1985) *Proc Natl Acad Sci USA* 82:1121.
27. Esmon CT, Esmon NL and Harris KW. (1982) *J Biol Chem* 257:7944.
28. Maruyama I, Salem HH, Ishii H and Majerus PW. (1985) *J Clin Invest* 75:987.
29. Hoylaerts M, Rijken DC, Lijnen HR and Collen D. (1982) *J Biol Chem* 257:912.
30. Wun T-C, Ossowski L and Reich E. (1982) *J Biol Chem* 237:7262.
31. Gurewich V, Pannell R, Louie S, Kelley P, Suddith RL and Greenlee R. (1984) *J Clin Invest* 73:1731.
32. Levin EG and Loskutoff DJ. (1982) *J Cell Biol* 94:631.
33. Levin EG. (1983) *Proc Natl Acad Sci USA* 80:6804.
34. Booyse FM, Osikowicz G, Feder S and Scheinbuks J. (1984) *J Biol Chem* 259:7198.
35. Crutchley DJ and Conanan LB. (1986) *J Biol Chem* 261:154.
36. Loskutoff DJ, van Mourik JA, Erickson LA and Lawrence D. (1983) *Proc Natl Acad Sci USA* 80:2956.

Mechanisms of Pulmonary Hypertension

Mechanisms of Pulmonary Hypertension, 1986: Introduction

An understanding of the pathophysiologic mechanisms which cause pulmonary hypertension is crucial to a logical approach to the prevention and treatment of this condition. However, despite an immense amount of research during the last forty years, the underlying mechanisms remain uncertain in virtually all forms of pulmonary hypertension, as indicated below.

The etiologies of the different subsets of primary pulmonary hypertension (plexogenic, veno-occlusive and thrombotic) remain unresolved. Similarly, the occurence of plexogenic pulmonary hypertension in a small percentage of patients with hepatic cirrhosis is unexplained. The ingestion of aminorex fumarate, an anorectic drug, in Europe between 1966 and 1968 led to the development of pulmonary hypertension in 1 to 2% of those exposed, but the pathologic process and the reasons for individual susceptibility are not apparent. The cause of the pulmonary hypertension which may occur in scleroderma and other collagen vascular diseases is unknown. A multitude of factors can contribute to the severity of the persistent pulmonary hypertension syndromes of the neonate, but no one etiologic factor has yet been demonstrated at the molecular or cellular level.

When right heart failure appears in patients with chronic obstructive airways disease, the pulmonary hypertension is usually attributed to parenchymal destruction and hypoxic pulmonary vasoconstriction. Unfortunately, the means by which hypoxia induces both vasoconstriction and chronic remodelling of the pulmonary vascular bed are still the subject of debate. Congenital heart disease causing left to right shunts and high pulmonary blood flow frequently results in pulmonary hypertension, associated with histologic changes in both endothelium and vascular smooth muscle. While shear-stress and platelet/endothelial interactions are important, the sequence of events which culminate in the Eisenmenger syndrome are poorly defined.

Questions remain even in thromboembolism and mitral stenosis, where the immediate causes of pulmonary hypertension appear obvious. It has been estimated that there are 430,000 survivors of symptomatic pulmonary embolism in the United States each year. A very small fraction of these develop chronic pulmonary hypertension, and the reason for their susceptibility is unknown. In mitral stenosis, when pulmonary capillary wedge pressure is elevated above 25 mmHg, most patients have a rise in pulmonary arterial pressure over and above the passive increase in wedge pressure. Although this reactive vasoconstriction has long been recognized, the mechanism responsible for inducing it is not understood.

There are other gaps in our knowledge of the pathophysiologic processes underlying different causes of pulmonary hypertension, but these examples are sufficient to indicate that further research is needed. The speakers and presenters of posters in the session on the Mechanisms of Pulmonary Hypertension describe the current status of this search for answers and provide new insights in many areas.

SIDNEY CASSIN   E. KENNETH WEIR

Mechanisms of Pulmonary Hypertension: An Overview

G.R. BARER
C.J. EMERY
D. BEE
R.A.WACH
Department of Medicine,
University of Sheffield,
Sheffield S10 2RX, England

I.   INTRODUCTION

Many questions but few answers pertain to pulmonary hypertension. Because pulmonary artery pressure, Ppa, can only be measured invasively, we lack wide population surveys and 24 hour profiles which cover rest, activity, sleep, anxiety. Pulmonary hypertension has been defined as a mean resting pressure >20 mmHg. However, rats exposed to 12% O_2 for only 2 hours daily for 4 weeks develop right ventricular hypertrophy and polycythaemia (1). Thus daily fluctuations may be important. The influence of hypoxia, hypercapnia and certain vasoactive substances differs in pulmonary and systemic vessels. Moreover, it is not suspected that disordered sodium metabolism, renal ischaemia or sympathetic overactivity are associated with pulmonary hypertension as they are with systemic hypertension.

At what level does pulmonary hypertension become harmful? Mean pulmonary artery pressure is 50-60 mmHg in the full-term fetus. Levels of 28 mmHg are found in healthy residents of the high Andes and still higher levels are found in healthy rats exposed chronically to hypoxia in the laboratory. Yet these levels are associated with a poor prognosis in adult patients with chronic obstructive airways disease, COAD. Many believe that this degree of overload

The Pulmonary Circulation
in Health and Disease

leads to right heart failure. Yet in obstructive airways disease the right ventricle sustains a normal or even elevated cardiac output against this level of Ppa (2). In pulmonary hypertension the right ventricle hypertrophies and its fibres increase in size to become similar to those of the left ventricle as they were in the fetus. Why should the right ventricle fail if it has only returned to fetal conditions where the two ventricles are of similar size and eject against similar pressures? Perhaps up to a point the right ventricle hypertrophies and sustains its output against a greater load through increased filling pressure according to Starling's Law. Does the hypertrophied heart of COAD really behave differently from the enlarged right ventricle of high altitude residents and hypoxic rats? It may be that when right ventricular hypertrophy develops in adult life there is insufficient development of capillaries to maintain adequate diffusion of O_2. These arguments do not apply to cases of primary pulmonary hypertension and congenital pulmonary hypertension where systemic levels of Ppa may be found. Some physicians do not think that pulmonary hypertension, per se, is a killing factor in hypoxic lung disease (2). The correlation of Ppa with prognosis may mean that pulmonary hypertension has consequences other than pressure overload which might be lethal. Pulmonary hypertension is associated with disordered endothelial metabolism and hormone balance and reflexes from the region affect renal function and fluid balance. Oedema may have causes other than right heart failure. Pulmonary hypertension impairs gas exchange from ventilation/perfusion mismatch, shunts, high flow, low cardiac output or œdema around microvessels. Thus respiratory failure may be equally important to cardiac failure.

Both mechanisms causing pulmonary hypertension and mechanisms initiated by raised pressure will be addressed. Progress in understanding will depend heavily on animal studies because controlled and repeated measurements are difficult in man and we cannot study the early stages of disease. Many animal "models" have been developed (3). It is necessary to study chronic states because, in established pulmonary hypertension, structural changes in vessel walls, changes in blood viscosity, coagulation problems and destruction of vessels can be major contributors to the raised pressure, in addition to primary factors such as vasoconstriction, back pressure or high flow. The pulmonary hypertension of chronic hypoxia illustrates principles common to several forms of pulmonary hypertension. Rats exposed to 10% O_2 develop a high Ppa in 2 weeks (Table I) and have been used to study structural, rheological, hæmodynamic and biochemical changes in the pulmonary vasculature and its reactivity to vasoactive agents.

TABLE I.   Properties of the pulmonary circulation in chronically hypoxic* and control rats (means ± SEM)

Measurement	Chronically hypoxic rats	Control rats	p value
Mean pulmonary artery pressure (mmHg)	35.8 ±2	15.8 ± 0.6	<0.001
Arterial compliance ml/mmHg	$6.1 \times 10^{-3} \pm 0.2$	$8.7 \times 10^{-3} \pm 0.2$	<0.01
Lung vascular volume (ml)	0.179 ± 0.01	0.199 ± 0.06	NS
Length left pulmonary artery (arbitrary units)	2.53 ± 1	2.25 ± 0.06	<0.05
% of thick-walled peripheral vessels[†]	22.5 ± 0.9	11.5 ± 0.5	<0.001
Number of arterioles in crosssection of lungs	185.6 ± 9.9	168.7 ± 12	NS
% medial thickness of arterioles as % of external diameter	7.3	0	

* 2 or more weeks in 10% O_2

† muscular vessels as % total arterioles and venules <50 μm diameter in alveolar region. Data from references 3,4,5.

II.   STRUCTURAL FACTORS

Structural factors which contribute to pulmonary hypertension include encroachment on the lumen of vessels by newly formed muscle, intimal proliferation, destruction of vessels, occlusion by thrombi or cells, and stiffening of larger vessels by new connective tissue. Some features of chronically hypoxic rats are shown in Table I. When they breathed air so that hypoxic vasoconstriction was eliminated, Ppa was 36 mmHg compared with 16 mmHg in control rats (3). Radiographs of pulmonary arteries filled with Barium-gelatine showed that vessels down to 1mm external diameter were narrower than those of controls when filled at the same pressure but attained similar diameters when filled at a higher pressure (4). They were, therefore, stiffer, attributable to deposition of new elastic tissue. The length of main arteries from hilum to periphery was increased. Lengthening of arteries might be causally related to the development of longitudinal muscle which is common in pulmonary hypertension. In chronically hypoxic rats arterioles surrounded by alveolar ducts and alveoli were narrowed ≈14% by internal development of new muscle. These changes affect vascular resistance, oscillatory pressure and flow characteristics, and their transmission to capillaries. They occurred rapidly, within two or three weeks in hypoxic rats, but resolved very slowly on return to normoxia. P_{pa} was still raised after six weeks recovery but normal after twenty weeks. At this time residual changes in arterioles were still detectable (4). We await exploration of the stimuli to growth and resolution. Slow resolution is also observed in Highlanders returning to sea-level and impedes improvement by O_2 therapy in COAD. In chronically hypoxic rats there was no evidence for vascular destruction. The count of arterioles in the alveolar region (< 50 μm diameter) was undiminished and the volume of the whole vascular bed, measured with [125] I-labelled albumen, was similar to controls (5). However, destruction of damaged vessels may occur in other types of pulmonary hypertension. In severe hypoxia endothelial blebs developed in alveolar capillaries together with alveolar wall œdema, both of which would affect resistance (6).

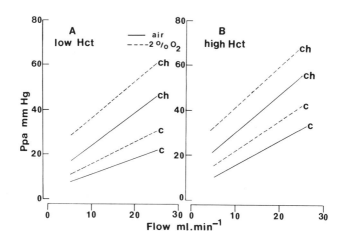

Fig. 1. Effect of polycythœmia on pulmonary vascular resistance. Mean regression lines relating pulmonary artery pressure, P_{pa}, to flow in isolated lungs of control, C, and chronically hypoxic, CH (3 weeks 10% O_2) rats. A) 9 C and 8 CH lungs perfused with low hœmatocrit (Hct, 34 ±0.3%) blood during normoxia (ventilation with air + 5% CO_2) and hypoxia (ventilation with 2% O_2, 5% CO_2). B) 9 C and 10 CH lungs perfused with high Hct blood (52 ±2.3%) during normoxia and hypoxia. Unpublished.

III. RHEOLOGICAL FACTORS

Rheological factors in pulmonary hypertension include polycythaemia in COAD, changes in platelets and other coagulation disorders. Increased blood viscosity due to a raised hæmatocrit (Hct) contributes substantially to the raised Ppa of chronically hypoxic rats (7,8). We measured pressure/flow (P/$\dot{Q}$) relations in isolated control and chronically hypoxic rat lungs perfused either with their own or each other's blood at normal temperature and pH. Figure 1A shows P/$\dot{Q}$ lines for both groups perfused with low Hct blood during both hypoxia and normoxia. Figure 1B shows similar lines during perfusion with high Hct blood; each line is steeper than during perfusion with normal blood; there is higher resistance. In both groups there was a significant relation between Ppa and Hct, such that Ppa rose 7.5 mmHg for a 15% rise in Hct. In man with COAD it is contested as to whether polycythæmia contributes to pulmonary hypertension as opposed to hypervolæmia which coexists. Recently Empey and colleagues performed erythropheresis in ten patients with COAD, which achieved an isovolæmic fall in Hct. There was a significant fall in Ppa and symptomatic improvement (9).

Platelets have been implicated in several forms of pulmonary hypertension. In chronically hypoxic rats the platelet count decreased significantly after 7 days hypoxia and remained low. Mean platelet volume increased, a change

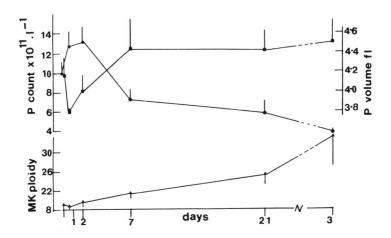

Fig. 2. Changes in platelets, p, and megakaryocytes, MK, in rats caused by exposure to hypoxia (10% O_2). Means ± SEM, from above down: platelet count;platelet volume; megakaryocyte ploidy. Dr. B. Metcalfe, unpublished.

associated in other circumstances with increased production of thromboxane B_2 (10,11). There was DNA synthesis in megakaryocytes such that their ploidy increased (Fig. 2). Evidence that platelets are formed by fragmentation of megakaryocytes in the pulmonary circulation is gaining credence (12). The story is fragmentary but adds up to a prediction that hypoxia activates platelets. Kentera *et al.* (13) also observed thrombocytopenia in chronically hypoxic rats, which they attributed to sequestration in the tissues.

Changes in the coagulation cascade and fibrinolysis are primary causes of some forms of pulmonary hypertension and secondary factors in others. Pulmonary endothelial damage from sheer stress, toxins, or hypoxia leads to platelet and neutrophil activation, release of complement, O_2 free radicals, prostanoids and leucotrienes. There ensue thrombosis, vasoconstriction, damage to membranes and ground substance, formation of œdema and pulmonary hypertension. Complex cascades and interactions which involve cellular and chemical elements are coming to light as a result of studies on models of the adult respiratory distress syndrome (14). Interventions provide hope that the cycle of vascular damage leading to some forms of pulmonary hypertension may one day be interrupted.

IV.   HÆMODYNAMIC FACTORS

Hæmodynamic factors in pulmonary hypertension include increased vascular resistance, flow or impedance, the development of Starling resistors in the circuit and decreased compliance. The impedance spectrum and the fraction of cardiac work employed in overcoming oscillatory components of pressure and flow have been studied during acute experimental elevation of Ppa, but we have little information as to their role in chronic pulmonary hypertension. Resistance is increased, and compliance decreased in established pulmonary hypertension. Reuben *et al.* (15) showed that acute rises in Ppa in dogs caused reciprocal changes in resistance and compliance, which maintained a constant time constant for the pulmonary circulation so that pulsations in capillary flow were unaltered; in some patients with pulmonary hypertension this relationship broke down.

Hæmodynamic changes associated with pulmonary hypertension in chronically hypoxic rats were studied under controlled conditions in isolated blood-perfused lungs. Fig. 1A shows altered pressure/flow (P/$\dot{Q}$) relations in the lung in chronically hypoxic rats. Compared with control rats, the pressures were higher at all flow rates and the line was steeper, not due to a reduction in the vascular bed (Table I). The extrapolated intercept on the pressure axis was also increased. In control rats, hypoxia caused an increase in slope but in chronically hypoxic rats

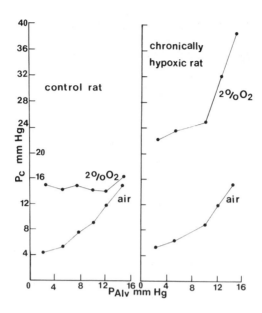

Fig. 3. Relationship between alveolar pressure, Palv and critical closing pressure, Pc (intercept on pressure axis of pressure/flow line) in a control rat, left, and a chronically hypoxic rat, right (10% O_2, 3 weeks) during normoxia (air + 5% CO_2) and hypoxia (2% O_2, 5% CO_2). Unpublished.

it caused a parallel movement of the $P/\dot{Q}$ line. An increased slope is attributable to narrowing of vessels while a parallel shift suggests the development of a Starling resistor in the circuit. The title Starling resistor is given to small vessels which collapse due to external pressure or high muscle tone in their walls. Then this "surrounding pressure" exceeds left atrial pressure, and it forms the effective downstream pressure for flow.

In patients with chronic bronchitis during exercise, Harris and colleagues showed shifts in the $P/\dot{Q}$ line similar to those shown in Fig.1 for chronically hypoxic rats (16). By occlusion of one pulmonary artery they obtained pressures at two flow rates during rest and exercise. During exercise in normal subjects and patients with mitral stenosis, $P/\dot{Q}$ points lay on a continuation of the line at rest. However, shifts in the points away from the normal line occurred in normal subjects when they breathed against an expiratory resistance. It was thought that, due to airflow obstruction, the bronchitic patients might have a raised alveolar pressure, Palv, during exercise which was transmitted to arteries to cause a rise in Ppa. Thus Palv may contribute to pulmonary hypertension in COAD.

The effect of alveolar pressure might be influenced by the presence, in both COAD and hypoxic rats, of muscular arterioles in a state of tone in the alveolar region. We measured P/$\dot{Q}$ lines in isolated blood-perfused lungs of control and chronically hypoxic rats at several alveolar pressures during both normoxia and hypoxia; Palv was always greater than left atrial pressure (17). There were differences between control and hypoxic rats which suggested that vasoconstriction due to hypoxia had moved to a more peripheral site in the latter, probably to newly muscularised arterioles. In normoxia an increase in Palv had caused a parallel shift in the P/$\dot{Q}$ line equivalent to ΔPalv in both groups, which suggested that Palv had caused a Starling resistor. In hypoxia, a similar rise in Palv caused a parallel shift in the P/$\dot{Q}$ line > ΔPalv in hypoxic rats but much < ΔPalv in control rats. Our interpretation was that in control rats, in whom arterioles in the alveolar region are non-muscular, hypoxia caused a Starling resistor due to increased muscle tone to develop in upstream extra-alveolar vessels; when Palv was raised it opened up this extra-alveolar resistor and the P/$\dot{Q}$ line moved by the small pressure difference between the upstream and alveolar resistors. By contrast, in chronically hypoxic rats, we suggest that hypoxia caused increased tone in muscular arterioles in the alveolar region. A rise in Palv was transmitted to and somehow enhanced tone in these arterioles so that the Starling resistor remained in alveolar vessels and the P/$\dot{Q}$ line moved by an amount $\geq$ Palv. Figure 3 illustrates this point. Alveolar pressure is plotted against the extrapolated intercept of the P/$\dot{Q}$ line on the pressure axis; this intercept is a measure of pressure surrounding any Starling resistor (also called the critical closing pressure). The intercept increases with Palv in both rats in normoxia and in the chronically hypoxic rat in hypoxia; in the control rat the intercept is unaffected by Palv until the latter exceeds 12 mmHg when we presume it "opens up" an upstream Starling resistor. Development of new muscle in pulmonary hypertension may alter vascular responses.

In chronically hypoxic rats, arterial compliance was significantly less than in control rats (5, Table I). This change would affect the impedance spectrum, reflection waves and transmission of phasic flow and pressure to capillaries.

V. VASCULAR REACTIVITY AND BIOCHEMICAL CHANGES

Increased vascular reactivity and biochemical changes may be important in development and maintenance of pulmonary hypertension. Increased reactivity should be defined as a shift in the dose-response curve and a lower threshold dose. Factors which determine reactivity include properties of contractile proteins, excitation-contraction coupling, cell membrane properties, cell internal and external ionic environment, and the modifying effect of hormones and other

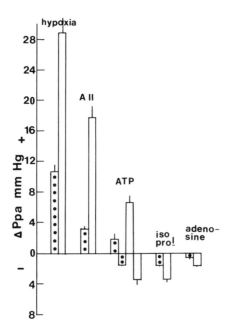

Fig. 4. Changed responses to pulmonary constrictor and dilator agents in chronically hypoxic (○) compared with control (•) rats. Increases or decreases in pulmonary artery pressure, Ppa, are shown ± SEM. From left to right: Ventilation with 2% O$_2$: angiotensin (0.5 μg); ATP (50 μg; note this has a constrictor followed by a dilator action); isoproterenol (1 μg); adenosine (50 μg). Data from reference 6.

vasoactive substances. The amount of smooth muscle in the wall will affect the response without altering the threshold. Increased changes in Ppa in response to dilator and constrictor agents have been detected in many types of pulmonary hypertension in man and animals. Dilator responses may be a measure of reversibility and may be undetectable in the normal pulmonary circulation because of low tone. In chronically hypoxic rat lungs we detected a shift in the dose-response curve to the pressor effects of angiotensin II and ATP; increased dilator effects of ATP, adenosine and isoproterenol suggested increased tone (5, Fig. 4). We also found greater increases in Ppa in response to a range of low O$_2$ tensions and enhancement of hypoxic vasoconstriction, which contrasted with the "blunted" hypoxic vasoconstriction found by McMurtry and colleagues in chronically hypoxic rats (18). This discrepancy may depend on a different balance of factors which affect reactivity and on the age and strain of rat. Like McMurtry's group we

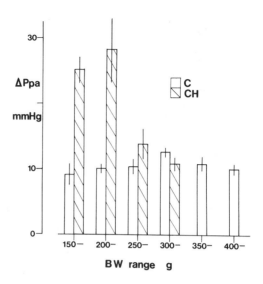

Fig. 5. Reactivity of pulmonary vessels to hypoxia in control, C, and chronically hypoxic, CH, rats (10% O_2, 3 weeks) of varying body weight, BW. Isolated blood-perfused lungs. Columns represent rise in pulmonary artery pressure, Ppa, during ventilation with 2% O_2. Data from reference 24.

found a blunted response after two days of hypoxia. After three weeks of hypoxia, control rats had similar responses over a wide age range, whereas chronically hypoxic rats had large responses when young which diminished with age (19, Fig. 5). Ou and colleagues found that exposure to hypoxia enhanced the response of one strain of rat but blunted another (20). Reactivity of muscle may determine the peaks which occur on exercise, when catecholamines may circulate and hypoxæmia increase. These episodes and sleep hypoxæmia may lead to progressive damage.

Vasoconstriction may be an initiating cause in pulmonary hypertension. Many vasoconstrictor substances are found in the lung or arrive from elsewhere in the blood. They differ in their longitudinal site of action on the vascular bed and many are processed by lung epithelium. It is necessary to find out the substances and concentrations to which different parts of the pulmonary circulation are exposed in different circumstances. For example, angiotensin II is formed from angiotensin I by angiotensin-converting enzyme (ACE) in the endothelium, perhaps mainly in capillaries. If this is so, angiotensin II is presented only to the pulmonary veins on which it may have little action. Indeed its action on pulmonary vessels, though large in isolated rat lungs, is small *in vivo* in several species in doses which can be tolerated (21); it seems unlikely that it can play a big role *in vivo*. For therapeutic reasons we need to know the site of action of dilators. Histamine H_1 vasoconstriction seems to be venous but a potent H_2 dilator action is revealed when tone is high. Bradykinin also has vasoconstrictor and dilator effects whose sites of action are unknown. Much more exploration is needed before we can begin to find out if any natural substances, for example, 5-hydroxytryptamine in Raynaud's phenomenon, can be implicated in vasoconstriction in patients. Many drugs and poisons affect the pulmonary vasculature directly or through release or hindered uptake of natural vasoactive substances. Several antidepressant and anorectic drugs which affect lung metabolism caused large acute rises in Ppa in cats (unpublished). Two, iprindole and chlorphentamine, chronically administered to rats, caused pulmonary hypertension [control Ppa 16 ±1, iprindole, 24 ±2, chlorphentermine, 20 ±1 mmHg, both p< 0.01 (Dr. J. Herget, unpublished)]. The effect of life-long administration of pulmonary vasoactive drugs must be considered.

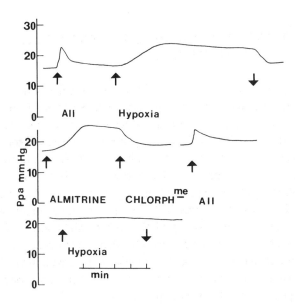

Fig. 6. Pulmonary vasoconstriction by Almitrine and hypoxia. Trace from isolated blood perfused rat lung (constant flow) ventilated with air + 5% CO_2. Changes in pulmonary artery pressure, Ppa, from above down caused by the following stimuli: angiotensin II (0.5 μg); hypoxia (2% O_2); Almitrine (50 μg); chlorpheniramine (2 mg) A II (0.5 μg); hypoxia. Unpublished.

Hypoxic vasoconstriction may initiate pulmonary hypertension in COAD. The mechanism remains elusive but new insight may come from the study of the respiratory stimulant drug Almitrine (Servier). It mimics the effect of hypoxia both on the carotid body and the pulmonary vasculature (22). In rats, its action, compared with that of other pulmonary vasoconstrictor substances, was relatively specifically inhibited by a fall in temperature, the Ca^{++} transport inhibitor verapamil and by chlorpheniramine (Dr. C.J. Emery, unpublished). In isolated blood-perfused rat lungs, the mean increase in Ppa at constant flow caused respectively by ventilation with 2% O_2 or by 50 µg Almitrine at 15°C was 3.7 ±0.9 (SEM) and 4.4 ± 1.8 mmHg; corresponding rises at 38°C were 12.3 ± 2.4 and 9.2 ± 2.0 mmHg. Figure 6 shows that chlorpheniramine given during vaso-constriction caused by Almitrine brought Ppa nearly down to the control line; a vasoconstrictor response to angiotensin II remained but hypoxic vasoconstriction was abolished. Verapamil abolished the response to hypoxia and Almitrine but the response to angiotensin II was untouched or enhanced (22 and Emery, unpublished).

VI.   PREVENTION AND DIMINUTION OF PULMONARY HYPERTENSION BY DRUGS.

It is for clinicians to decide as to whether this is desirable or possible, but we may get clues as to mechanisms of pulmonary hypertension from the numerous substances shown to minimise its development in animals. In hypoxic pulmonary hypertension these include methyl dopa, ß adrenoreceptor antagonists, a high sodium diet, heparin, Ca^{++} transport inhibitors, ACE inhibitors, ß amino-proprionitrile, and cyclooxygenase and lipoxygenase inhibitors (8, 23-28). In adult respiratory distress syndrome, anti-oxidants, O_2 scavengers, and the suppression of neutrophils and platelets play a role (14). There seems no common factor. Some cause vasodilation or reduce vasoconstriction, others inhibit growth factors, protein synthesis or erythropoiesis, restrict endothelial damage or the output of leucotrienes, or alter the renin-AII-aldosterone axis or bradykinin breakdown. It is conspicuous that no experiments so far indicate a role for the sympathetic nervous system in the genesis of pulmonary hypertension.

VII.   MECHANISMS PROVOKED BY PULMONARY HYPERTENSION

Foremost for discussion is the question as to whether hypertension due to hypoxia or other causes provokes right heart failure and whether this is the sole cause of œdema and hepatomegaly (29). Studies with radionuclide ventriculography in different circumstances should settle this point. We must look at hormonal and renal function changes which follow pulmonary hypertension and the disordered lung metabolism which accompanies it. The consequences of ACE reduction for angiotensin II production, aldosterone release, fluid balance and of bradykinin inactivation are still to be worked out. The role of the natriuretic factor, present in both atria, is not yet understood. The disturbances of renal function in hypoxic cor pulmonale in the presence of normal cardiac output were discovered in the 1950's and remain unexplained. A new prospect has emerged with the discovery that hypoxia, through stimulation of the carotid body, causes natriuresis or Na^+ retention according to its severity (30). Pulmonary hypertension affects gas exchange, and the consequences of hypoxia and hypercarbia, constant or intermittent, must affect many organs including the heart. The challenge to unravel these important questions is very great.

REFERENCES

1.   Moore-Gillon JC and Cameron IR. (1985) *Clin Sci* **69**:595.
2.   Finlay M, Middleton HC, Peake MD and Howard P. (1983) *Eur J Respir Dis* **64**:254.
3.   Herget J, Suggett AJ, Leach E and Barer, GR. (1978) *Thorax* **33**:468.
4.   Finlay M, Suggett AJ and Barer, GR. (1986) *Q J Exp Physiol* **71**:151.
5.   Emery CJ, Bee D and Barer, GR. (1981) *Clin Sci* **61**:569.
6.   Scott KWM, Barer GR, Leach E and Mungall IPF. (1978) *J Path* **126**:27.
7.   Barer GR, Bee D and Wach RA. (1983) *J Physiol* **336**:27.
8.   Kentera D, Susic D and Kanjuh V. (1985) *Prog Res Respir* **20**:26.
9.   Wallis PJW, Skehan JD, Newland AC, Wedzicha JA, Mills PG and Empey DW. (1986) *Clin Sci.* **70**:91.
10.   Metcalfe B, Warren C, Slater D, Trowbridge EA, Martin JF and Barer GR. (1984) *Clin Sci* **67**(Suppl. 9):76.
11.   Martin JF, Trowbridge EA, Salmon G and Plumb J. (1983) *Thrombosis Research* **32**:443.
12.   Trowbridge EA, Martin JF and Slater DN. (1982) *Thrombosis Research* **28**:461.
13.   Kentera D, Zdravkovic M, Rolovic Z and Susic D. (1985) *Respiration* **48**:159.
14.   Said SI (Editor). (1985) **The Pulmonary Circulation and Acute Lung Injury.** Futura:New York.

15.   Reuben SR, Gersch BJ, Swadling JP and Lee G de J. (1970)
       Cardiovascular Res 4:473.
16.   Harris P, Segal N and Bishop, JM. (1968) *Cardiovascular Res* 2:72.
17.   Wach RA, Emery CJ, Bee D and Barer, GR. (1986) *Cardiovascular Res*
       In press.
18.   McMurtry IF, Petrun MD and Reeves JT. (1978) *Amer J Physiol*
       235:H104.
19.   Bee D and Wach RA. (1984) *Resp Physiol* **56**:91.
20.   Ou LC, Sardella GL, Hill NS and Tenney SM. (1986) *Respiration
       Physiol* **64**:81.
21.   Suggett AJ, Mohammed FH and Barer GR. (1980) *Clin Exp Pharm &
       Physiol* **7**:263.
22.   Bee D, Gill GW, Emery CJ, Salmon GL, Evans TW and Barer GR.
       (1983) *Bull Europ Physiopath Respir* **19**:539.
23.   Suggett AJ and Herget J. (1977) *Clin Sci* **53**:397.
24.   Ostadal B, Ressl J, Urbanova D, Widimsky J, Prochazka J and Pelouch
       V. (1978) *Basic Res Cardiol* **73**:422.
25.   Kentera D, Susic D and Zdravkovic M. (1985) *Basic Res Cardiol* **80**:142.
26.   Stanbrook HS, Morris KG and McMurtry IF. (1984) *Amer Rev Respir
       Dis* **139**:81.
27.   Kerr JS, Riley D, Frank MM, Trelstad RL and Frankel HM. (1984)
       J Appl Physiol **57**:1760.
28.   Morganroth ML, Stenmark KR, Morris KG, Murphy RC, Mathias
       M, Reeves JTV and Oelkel NF. (1985) *Amer Rev Respir Dis* **131**:488.
29.   Howard P. (1983) *Brit Med J* **287**:1159.
30.   Honig A. (1983) *In* **Physiology of arterial chemoreceptors.** (H Acker and
       R O'Regan, eds) Elsevier North Holland Biomedical Press:Amsterdam.

Pulmonary Hypertension in the Presence of High Blood Flow

MARLENE RABINOVITCH[1]
Department of Cardiology,
The Hospital for Sick Children,
Toronto, Canada

I.   INTRODUCTION

In congenital heart defects producing high pulmonary blood flow, pulmonary hypertension is inevitably associated with the presence of structural changes in the vascular bed. This chapter describes the nature of these vascular changes, and discusses their association with heightened pulmonary vascular reactivity and with the development of fixed elevation in pulmonary vascular resistance. Recent studies are aimed at identifying and understanding the specific alterations in the cell biology of the vessel wall. The findings should lead to an improved ability to control the reactive pulmonary circulation and ultimately to retard the progression or induce the regression of even advanced vascular changes.

II.   NATURE OF THE PROBLEM

In congenital heart defects with increased pulmonary blood flow secondary to intra or extracardiac left to right shunts, severe elevation in pulmonary vascular resistance may develop causing reversal of the shunt, cyanosis and right heart

[1]*Supported by a Research Associate Award from the Heart and Stroke Foundation of Ontario (HSFO) and by an HSFO Term Grant.*

The Pulmonary Circulation
in Health and Disease

423

failure. This is believed to result from the progressive development of structural changes in the peripheral pulmonary arteries. Certain types of cardiac defects have a higher incidence and a more malignant form of this complication than others (1-5). For example, the transmission of high pulmonary artery pressure along with high flow in an unrestrictive ventricular septal defect is invariably associated with a higher incidence and more rapid progression of vascular changes than occurs with an atrial septal defect where there is only high flow. The combination of high pressure and flow with cyanosis and polycythemia as occurs with the combination of transposition and a ventricular septal defect usually signals extremely rapid progression of vascular changes; *i.e.,* within the first year of life, infants may develop fixed elevation in pulmonary vascular resistance (5-6).

III.   NATURE OF THE VASCULAR CHANGES

In an infant with a congenital heart defect and increased pulmonary blood flow, the earliest pulmonary vascular changes reflect altered growth and development of the arteries (7-9). Three progressively severe stages are seen (10-11) which correlate with the hemodynamic state (Figure 1).

A.   Grade A

There is abnormal extension of muscle into small peripheral arteries, or, in addition, a mild increase in wall thickness of the normally muscular arteries (less than 1.5 times normal). These patients have increased pulmonary blood flow but normal mean pulmonary arterial pressure. Meyrick and Reid have shown from ultrastructural studies of lung biopsy tissue that the basis for this change is a differentiation to smooth muscle of the precursor cells, the pericyte in the nonmuscular region of the artery, and the intermediate cell in the partially muscular region (12). Whether the stimulus for this change is stretching of cells due to a widened pulse pressure, and whether vasoactive mediators may be involved, is currently under study.

B.   Grade B

As in Grade A, there is increased extension of muscle, but, in addition, there is more severe medial hypertrophy of normally muscular arteries. When medial wall thickness is greater than 1.5 but less than 2 times normal (Grade B mild), mild pulmonary hypertension is usually present. When medial wall thickness equals or is more than twice normal (Grade B severe), pulmonary hypertension is always present and often with pressure values greater than half

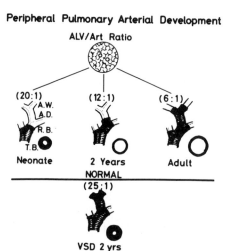

Figure 1. *Schema of normal peripheral pulmonary arterial development and abnormal development in a child with a ventricular septal defect and high pulmonary artery pressure and resistance at two years. Normally, muscle extends with age into arteries more peripheral within the acinus; the wall thickness of the normally muscular arteries decreases and there is a decreasing ratio of alveoli to arteries, indicating an increase in the number of arteries. In a child with a ventricular septal defect, abnormalities in all three features of normal growth and remodelling may be seen, i.e. "precocious" extension of muscle into peripheral arteries, medial hypertrophy of muscular arteries and a reduced concentration of arteries, i.e. increased alveolar arterial ratio. T.B.= artery accompanying a terminal bronchiolus; R.B.= artery accompanying a respiratory bronchiolus; A.D.= artery accompanying an alveolar duct; A.W.= artery accompanying an alveolar wall; ALV-Art= alveolar-arterial ratio. (Reproduced with permission;10.)*

systemic level. The medial thickness is due to hypertrophy as well as hyperplasia of preexisting smooth muscle cells and also an increase in the intercellular ground substance and elastin and collagen.

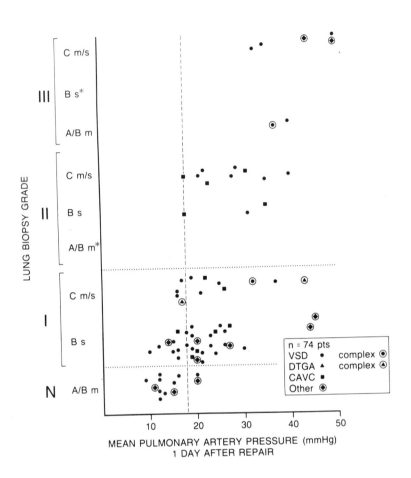

Figure 2. Lung biopsy grade is correlated with mean pulmonary arterial pressure recorded the day after surgical repair. The dashed vertical lines separate the normal from the abnormally elevated pressure values and the dotted horizontal lines separate the biopsy grades. Note that with the more severe Heath Edwards changes on lung biopsy tissue there is a trend toward a greater proportion of patients with elevated pulmonary arterial pressures and higher values. A, B, C, are morphometric grades: m = mild, s = severe. N, I, II, III are Heath-Edwards grades, N = normal, * = no patients in this group, VSD = ventricular septal defect, DTGA = D-transposition of the great arteries. CAVC = complete atrioventricular canal, complex = associated abnormality. (Reproduced with permission;11).

C.   Grade C

In addition to the findings of late Grade B, arterial concentration is reduced and usually arterial size also. Patients with these changes have elevation in pulmonary vascular resistance of greater than 3.5 u•m^2. When arterial number is less than half normal (Grade C mild), pulmonary vascular resistance values are often in excess of 6 u•m^2. The basis of Grade C is likely the failure of new vessels to grow normally, although some loss of arteries may also occur.

These features precede and are separate from the changes described qualitatively and graded by Heath and Edwards (13). Grades A and B are refinements of Grade I of the Heath and Edwards classification. Grade C is a separate change not previously addressed. It is frequently seen alone but is often present with Heath Edwards Grade II (cellular intimal hyperplasia) and almost invariably accompanies Grade III (fibrous intimal hyperplasia with elastosis and occlusion). Grade IV (dilatation complexes) and Grade V (angiomatoid formation) represent advanced irreversible changes, and Grade VI (fibrinoid necrosis) is endstage disease.

IV.   FUNCTIONAL SIGNIFICANCE OF THE VASCULAR CHANGES

Whether and to what extent abnormal growth and structural remodeling of the pulmonary vascular bed is permanent and results in functional impairment has been determined by correlating the morphologic features with postoperative hemodynamic studies. In lung biopsy tissue from patients with congenital heart defects, we have analyzed both the quantitative features of abnormal growth and remodeling of the pulmonary arteries, and the changes described by Heath and Edwards, and have correlated them with the hemodynamic behavior of the pulmonary circulation in the immediate post-operative period in the Intensive Care Unit (Figure 2) and one year later at the time of the routine cardiac catheter study (11; Figure 3). Patients with only medial hypertrophy, *i.e.* Grade B (severe) and Heath Edwards Grade I often have elevated pulmonary artery pressure values in the early post-operative period and frequently suffer "pulmonary hypertensive" crises. Both the presence and severity of pulmonary hypertension in the early post-operative period are increasingly predictable with increasingly advanced changes on lung biopsy, *i.e.* reduced artery number (grade C) and intimal hyperplasia (Heath Edwards II-III; 11). The regression of pulmonary hypertension is influenced both by the severity of pulmonary vascular changes and the age at repair. Patients operated within the first eight months of life have normal pulmonary hemodynamics one year after repair regardless of the severity of vascular changes in the lung biopsy sections. Patients with vascular abnormalities of only B severity

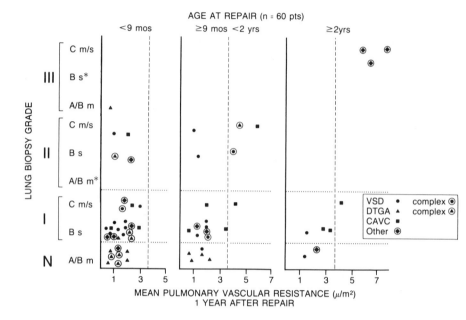

Figure 3. Graph correlating lung biopsy grade with pulmonary vascular resistance 1 year after cardiac repair. Patients who underwent repair within the first 8 months of the life, but not those operated upon later, had normal pulmonary vascular resistance regardless of the severity of their structural changes. Abbreviations as in Figure 2. (Reproduced with permission;11).

(Heath Edwards I), also have normal pulmonary hemodynamics at the one year followup catheter study. Those with more severe changes will have persistent elevation in pulmonary vascular resistance (11).

V.   DIAGNOSIS OF THE VASCULAR CHANGES

A.   Lung Biopsy

Quantitative techniques have been successfully applied to the analysis of lung biopsy tissue prepared by frozen section to help the surgeon decide between a palliative and a corrective procedure when preoperative hemodynamic data are borderline or difficult to obtain or interpret (14). The ability to predict from biopsy tissue whether even mild elevation in pulmonary vascular resistance will be present post-operatively is of increasing importance in the consideration for surgery of patients who require a Fontan type procedure, *i.e.* the placement of a right atrial to pulmonary arterial conduit (15). Patients with tricuspid atresia who have had previous systemic to pulmonary arterial shunts, and those with single ventricle and previous pulmonary arterial bands are particularly problematic. In the latter there may be incomplete regression of the vascular changes (16,17), particularly when the band was placed in later infancy. Also, it may be inaccurate to assess pulmonary artery pressure and resistance with a catheter partially occluding the pulmonary outflow. The same criticism can be applied to directing catheters through narrowed or tortuous shunts. While we have found lung biopsy definitely helpful in clinical decision-making, it must be ensured that the section is adequate. Specifically, several pre-acinar vessels must be included and the distal pathways traced from them (18).

B.   Wedge Angiography

Techniques of wedge angiography have been developed to assess preoperatively the structural state of the pulmonary vascular bed (Figure 4; 19,20). Changes that can be evaluated qualitatively, *i.e.* sparsity of arborization of the pulmonary tree, abrupt termination, tortuosity and narrowing of small arteries, and reduced background capillary filling, generally reflect advanced changes in the pre-acinar arteries of at least Heath-Edwards Grade III severity (19). We described a technique to quantitatively assess features on a pulmonary wedge angiogram (20) that allows prediction of both mild and severe vascular abnormalities. A balloon catheter is directed to the origin of the axial artery of the posterior basal segment of the lower lobe (the right lung is usually chosen). Contrast material is injected, and the injection is filmed on biplane cine. The rate of tapering of the arteries is evaluated by measuring the length of segment over which the lumen diameter narrows between 2.5 and 1.5 mm. The abruptness of tapering correlates in severity with the degree of abnormality in the intra-acinar arteries, assessed both morphometrically and by the Heath-Edwards classification (Figure 4). Decreased background filling and increased pulmonary circulation time are predictive of patients with more advanced changes. There are, however, some pitfalls in the interpretation of the wedge angiogram. An incomplete injection will give the impression of decreased background filling, and incomplete occlusion of the vessel by the balloon will make the circulation time falsely rapid. Previous placement of a pulmonary artery band will, owing to post-stenotic dilatation, give the false impression of "abrupt tapering." Some patients with advanced pulmonary vascular disease will not have abrupt tapering, because the intimal hyperplasia has extended

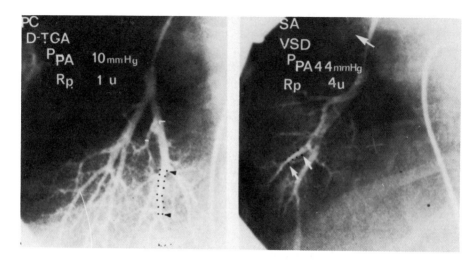

Figure 4. (Left) A wedge angiogram shows gradual tapering of the axial artery in a child with TGA and normal pulmonary artery pressure (PPA) and resistance (RP). Approximate segment length between 2.5 and 1.5 mm internal diameter is marked off (arrows). (Right) A wedge angiogram in a child with a VSD shows rapid tapering of the artery when there is increased pulmonary artery pressure and resistance. An approximate segment length between 2.5 and 1.5 mm internal diameter is marked off (arrows). Large arrow denotes takeoff to the right pulmonary artery. [Reproduced with permission from M. Rabinovitch and L. Reid. Cardiovascular Clinics (MA Engle ed) 11(2):149, 1981].

even into larger pre-acinar arteries narrowing the lumen uniformly. The same will be true of patients who have had severe vasoconstriction from birth and never much of a left to right shunt. These patients, however, will all have a decrease in background filling and a prolongation of the pulmonary circulation time.

VI.   CONTROL OF THE REACTIVE PULMONARY CIRCULATION

A major challenge in cardiology is to understand and control the reactive pulmonary circulation, as this can be particularly problematic in the early post-operative period after repair of a congenital heart defect with increased pulmonary blood flow. The "pulmonary hypertensive crises" (21) are thought to result from interaction of vascular endothelium with platelets and leukocytes that are post-cardiopulmonary bypass and may more easily release vasoactive substances (22), *e.g.* thromboxanes and leukotrienes. Various methods of managing "post-operative pulmonary hypertension" have been proposed. In our own Unit, we have benefited from continuous monitoring of pulmonary artery and left atrial pressures. To maintain the pulmonary artery pressure ≤ half systemic level, we institute hyperventilation (PaCO$_2$ 25-30 torr), and, if necessary, continue for several post-operative days. Thereafter, weaning from the ventilator can usually be accomplished slowly and with the help of intravenous vasodilators; specifically, we give nitroglycerin followed by phenoxybenzamine if there is evidence of left ventricular dysfunction; β agonists, salbutamol or isoproterenol are helpful if there is a component of pulmonary congestion. Almost all patients can be weaned from this therapy after one week.

There are, however, some patients who maintain a high level of pulmonary vascular resistence and are refractory to vasodilator therapy despite what appear to be relatively mild vascular changes on light microscopy (medial hypertrophy). In our most recent lung biopsy studies from patients with congenital heart defects and pulmonary hypertension, we are trying to learn more about the nature of altered endothelial–platelet and leukocyte and endothelial–smooth muscle interactions which may be relevant to the mechanism of heightened pulmonary vascular reactivity, and to the development of progressive pulmonary vascular disease.

VII.   ENDOTHELIAL DYSFUNCTION IN PULMONARY HYPERTENSION ASSOCIATED WITH HIGH FLOW

We have identified structural and functional changes in the pulmonary vascular endothelial cells. On scanning electron microscopy the endothelial surface of normal pulmonary arteries has a "corduroy-like" appearance in that the cells form narrow, even ridges. The endothelial surface of hypertensive pulmonary arteries has a "cable-like" appearance in that the cells form deep twisted ridges (23; Figure 5). The "hypertensive endothelium" might therefore be predisposed to interact "roughly" with marginating blood elements such as platelets and leukocytes, and this would facilitate release of vasoactive substances. On transmission electron microscopy, endothelial cells from hypertensive arteries have an increased volume proportion of rough endoplasmic reticulum and microfilament bundles suggesting heightened protein synthesis and metabolic activity, and an altered cytoskeleton (Figure 6).

Since endothelial cells produce von Willebrand Factor (vWF) and since altered endothelial-platelet interaction has been implicated as part of the mechanism, we applied immunocytochemical techniques to determine whether pulmonary endothelial cells from hypertensive arteries may be producing increased vWF. Using an immunoperoxidase stain, we found that "hypertensive" pulmonary

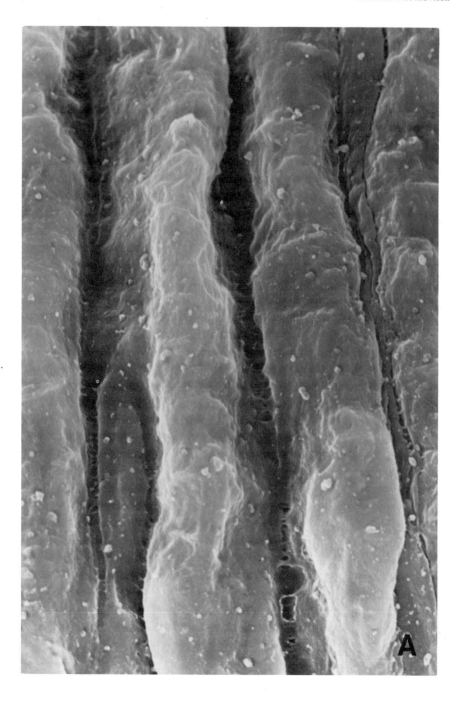

Figure 5A.

arteries stain densely for vWF, whereas nonhypertensive vessels do not (Figure 7). Moreover, most patients with pulmonary hypertension had elevated circulating components of the vWF molecule (24), as evidenced by increased antigenic (vW:Ag) and in some cases biologic (vW:rist) activity. Further multimeric analysis suggests that some of these patients have loss of the high molecular weight form of vWF, a feature which suggests a propensity for abnormal platelet aggregation and potential formation of platelet fibrin microthrombi.

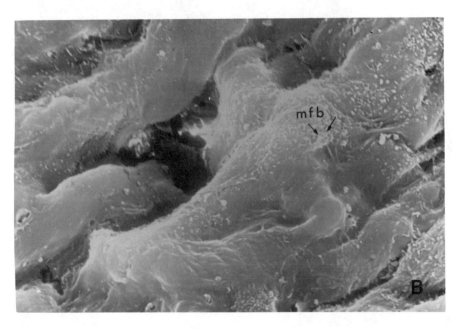

Figure 5. Scanning electron photomicrographs of pulmonary artery endothelial surfaces. A. Normal pulmonary artery shows "corduroy pattern", neat closely aligned ridges. B. Hypertensive pulmonary artery shows "cable" pattern, deep knotted ridges, and numerous microvilli (MV) (x 810).

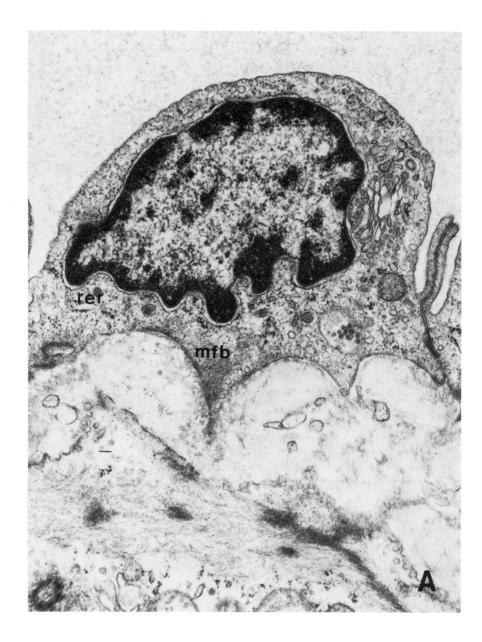

Figure 6. Transmission electron photomicrographs of pulmonary artery endothelial cells. Compared to normal endothelial cell in A, endothelial cell in B,

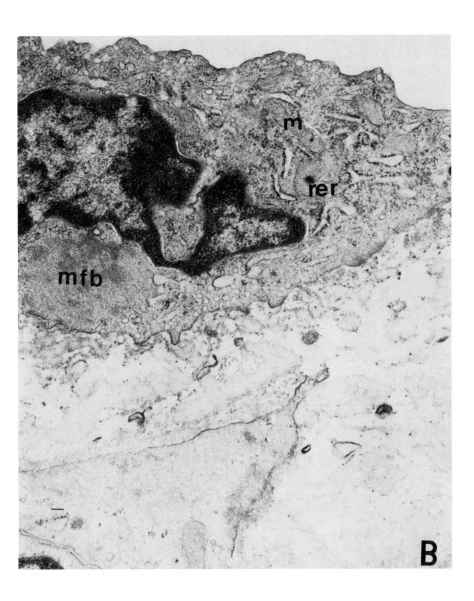

from hypertensive pulmonary artery shows increased rough endoplasmic reticulum (rer) and microfilament bundles (mfb); m = mitochondria (x 34,000).

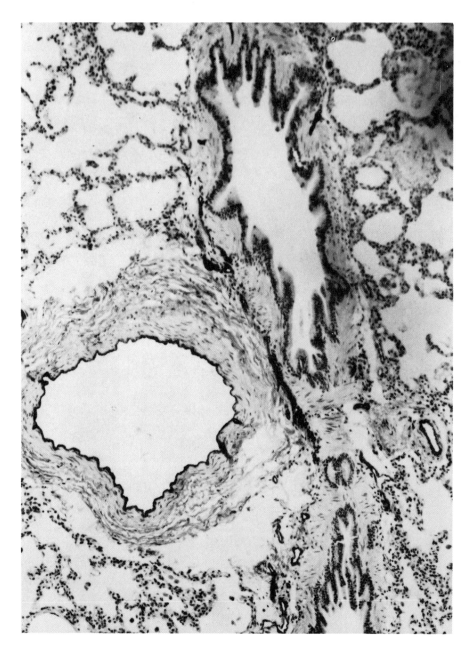

Figure 7. Lung biopsy section from a patient with pulmonary hypertension; thick walled pulmonary artery with endothelium and deeply positive immunoperoxidase stain for factor VIII (π). (Magnification x 160).

VIII. ABNORMAL ENDOTHELIAL-SMOOTH MUSCLE INTERACTION ASSOCIATED WITH INCREASED PULMONARY BLOOD FLOW

Further and most recent observations on lung biopsy tissue suggest to us that a process of degradation and increased synthesis of connective tissue proteins in the subendothelium and media may be important in the pathogenesis of pulmonary vascular disease, and may explain why some infants, with excessive elastin and collagen in the media of their arteries, may have fixed elevation in pulmonary vascular resistance despite only medial hypertrophy on light microscopy, or why others in whom the mechanism may not "turn off" after repair have rapidly progressive pulmonary vascular disease.

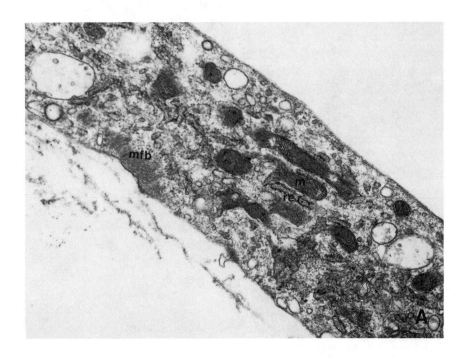

Figure 8. Electron photomicrographs from cells cultured on transducer; compared to A, cell from a stationary dome, cell from a dome that was pulsated 100 times/minute at high pressure, 100/60 mmHg for 48 hours, shows increased rough endoplasmic reticulum (rer) and microfilament bundles (mfb); m = mitochondria. (Magnification x 34,000).

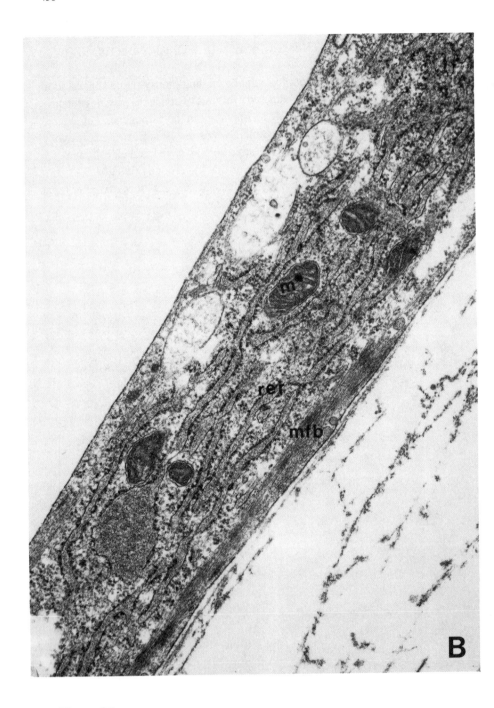

Figure 8B.

IX.   A WORKING HYPOTHESIS

Based upon our studies in human lung biopsy tissue, we have developed a working hypothesis concerning the pathogenesis of pulmonary vascular disease. In it, we suggest that a congenital heart defect with increased pulmonary blood flow secondary to a left to right shunt afflicts an abnormally high pulse pressure on the pulmonary vascular bed. This alters the endothelium of the vessels both structurally and functionally. Either due to abnormal interaction with blood elements or because of intrinsic changes in the endothelial cells, there is release of a protease into the subendothelium which allows induction of growth and differentiation of smooth muscle cell precursors to mature smooth muscle. This results in abnormal muscularization of normally nonmuscular peripheral arteries. In normally muscular arteries the protease released may be elastase, which brings endothelial and smooth muscle cells in close contact and this causes induction of smooth muscle hypertrophy and hyperplasia. The hypertrophied smooth muscle cells then produce increased connective tissue proteins, elastin, collagen and ground substance, which results in a decreased compliance of the vessel wall and progressive luminal occlusion.

X.   *IN VITRO* SYSTEMS

Newly developed techniques of harvesting pulmonary artery endothelial and smooth muscle cells from central pulmonary arteries (25) and from microvessels (26) will help greatly in testing this hypothesis and in answering basic questions related to endothelial-smooth muscle and endothelial-blood element (platelet, leukocyte) interactions. We have devised a system in which we are able to grow to confluence pulmonary artery endothelial cells harvested from newborn lamb microvessels on flexible membranes and then pulsate them at high pressure thus "mimicking" the condition of a congenital heart defect with increased pulmonary flow (27). We use the flexible polyvinyl-chloride membrane of a Hewlett-Packard transducer dome, attached to bellows stainless-steel tubing and a reciprocating generator pump. We have carried out experiments in which we have compared endothelial cells pulsated for 48 hours at high pressure (100/60 mmHg), low pressure (20/10 mmHg) and non-pulsated. Cells pulsated at high pressure had, on scanning electron microscopy, a more raised surface, with thickened intertwined filopodia. On transmission electron microscopy, there was an increase in microfilament bundles and in rough endoplasmic reticulum (Figure 8). These changes are similar to those on lung biopsy tissue from patients with congenital heart defects and increased flow and pressure. We are carrying out studies to determine the nature of the functional disturbances associated with these structural abnormalities. We have tried to determine whether pulsating endothelial cells enhances the release of the endothelial derived growth factor, *i.e.* acts as a smooth muscle mitogen. Preliminary studies have failed to demonstrate increased smooth muscle DNA synthesis (incorporation of ^{3}H-thymidine) when cultured in conditioned medium from endothelial cells pulsed at high pressure. Moreover, there was no increase in protein synthesis (^{14}C leucine incorporation) which might reflect the induction of smooth muscle hypertrophy. It is possible that an interaction with pulsated smooth muscle cells is important or that platelets are necessary. The latter hypotheses can be tested in this model. We have been successful in pulsating smooth muscle cells at high pressure on the membranes and can test the effect of endothelial conditioned medium on these cells. We have isolated ovine platelets with good functional activity and are in a position to determine whether they release growth factors when incubated with endothelial or smooth muscle cells pulsated at high pressure.

Other models of congenital heart disease with high pulmonary blood flow, *i.e.* the newborn lamb in which a ventricular septal defect has been created (28) will offer further opportunities to study the evolution of pulmonary vascular disease and to attempt to alter its course.

XI.   CONCLUSION

In the setting of a congenital heart defect with increased pulmonary flow and pressure, the ultrastructural changes reflecting heightened endothelial metabolic activity and the smooth muscle hypertrophy and hyperplasia probably represent an initial adaptation to the altered hemodynamics. The progressive thickening of the vascular wall probably reflects overzealous synthesis of connective tissue proteins by hypertrophied smooth muscle cells and perhaps endothelial cells as well. The decrease in pulmonary flow as the cross-sectional area of the vascular bed becomes reduced (decreased lumen and number of arteries), and the potential to compensate by right to left shunting allows the vascular disease to pass into a less rapidly progressive phase. Future progress in the control and treatment of pulmonary vascular disease will depend upon understanding the genetic control mechanisms which underly processes such as release of proteases, mitogens and synthesis of connective tissue proteins.

REFERENCES

1. Rudolph AM and Nadas AS. (1962) *N Engl J Med* **267**:968,1022.
2. Besterman E. (1961) *Br Heart J* **23**:587.
3. Reid JM, Stevenson JG, Coleman EN, Barclay RS, Welsh TM, Fyfe WM and Inal JA. (1964) *Br Heart J* **26**:600.
4. Newfeld EA, Sher M, Paul MH and Higashi N. (1977) *Am J Cardiol* **39**:721.
5. Newfeld EA, Paul MH, Muster AJ and Idriss FS. (1974) *Am J Cardiol* **34**:75.
6. Waldman JD, Paul MH, Newfeld EA, Muster AJ and Idriss FS. (1977) *Am J Cardiol* **39**:232.
7. Wagenvoort CA, Neufeld HN and Edwards JE. (1961) *Lab Invest* **10**:751.
8. Hislop A and Reid LM. (1973) *Thorax* **28**:129.
9. Hislop A, Haworth SG and Reid L. (1975) *Br Heart J* **37**:1014.
10. Rabinovitch M, Haworth SG, Castaneda AR, Nadas AS and Reid L. (1978) *Circulation* **58**:1107.
11. Rabinovitch M, Keane JF, Norwood WI, Castaneda AR and Reid L. (1984) *Circulation* **69**:655.
12. Meyrick B and Reid LM. (1980) *Am J Pathol* **101**:527.
13. Heath D and Edwards JE. (1958) *Circulation* **18**:533.
14. Rabinovitch M, Castaneda AR and Reid L. (1981) *Am J Cardiol* **47**:77.
15. Fontan F and Beaudet E. (1971) *Thorax* **26**:240.
16. Rabinovitch M, Sanders SP, Castaneda AR and Reid L. (1981) *Am J Cardiol* **47**:947 (abstr).
17. Juaneda E and Haworth SG. (1984) *Br Heart J* **52**:575.
18. Haworth SG. (1984) *Br Heart J* **52**:557.
19. Nihill MR and McNamara DG. (1978) *Circulation* **58**:1094.
20. Rabinovitch M, Keane JF, Fellows KE, Castaneda AR and Reid L. (1981) *Circulation* **63**:152.
21. Jones ODH, Shore DF, Rigby ML, Leijala M, Scallan J, Shinebourne EA and Lincoln JCR. (1981) *Circulation* **64**:11.
22. Addonizio VP Jr, Smith JB, Strauss JF III, Colman RW and Edmunds LM Jr. (1980) *J Thorac Cardiovasc Surg* **79**:91.
23. Rabinovitch M, Trusler GA, Williams WG, Rowe RD, Olley PM and Cutz E. (1983) *Circulation* **68**:111.
24. Rabinovitch M, Andrew M, Thom H, Williams WG, Trusler GA, Rowe RD, Olley PM and Wilson GJ. (1983) *Circulation* **68**:111(abstract).
25. Ryan US, Clements E, Habliston D and Ryan JW. (1978) *Tissue and Cell* **10**:535.

26. Ryan US, White LA, Lopez M and Ryan JW. (1982) *Tissue and Cell*
     14:597.

27. Rabinovitch M, Mullen M, Watchurst T and Spicer P. (1985) *Am Rev
     Resp Dis* **131**:A410.

28. Boucek MM, Chang R and Synorst DP. (1985) *Ped Res* **19**:887.

Persistent Pulmonary Hypertension Syndromes in the Newborn[1]

MICHAEL A. HEYMANN
JULIEN I.E. HOFFMAN
*From the Cardiovascular Research
Institute and Departments of Pediatrics,
Physiology, and Obstetrics,
Gynecology, and Reproductive
Sciences,
University of California,
San Francisco, California 94143*

I. INTRODUCTION

The syndrome of persistent pulmonary hypertension in the immediate newborn period, also sometimes called persistent fetal circulation syndrome, is characterized by failure of parts of the circulation to undergo the normal transition from the fetal to the postnatal state (1-3). The primary abnormality is continued maintenance of a high pulmonary vascular resistance (normal in the fetus) with consequent reduction below normal of pulmonary blood flow; in addition there may be persistence of right-to-left shunting through the ductus arteriosus or foramen ovale or both. Many factors are responsible for the physiologic and physical control of pulmonary vascular resistance and for its normal fall after birth. It is likely therefore that the syndrome of persistent pulmonary hypertension, due

[1]*This research was supported in part by U.S. Public Health Service
Program Project Grant HL 24056, and by BRSG Grant S07 RR05355 awarded by
the Biomedical Research Support Program, Division of Research Resources,
National Institutes of Health.*

to failure of normal regression of pulmonary vascular resistance, is caused by alterations in or failure of several mechanisms acting together rather than a single cause. The resultant syndrome, which invariably occurs in otherwise normal full term infants, leads to severe, often lethal, cardiorespiratory distress regardless of the etiology.

II.   PHYSIOLOGY

A.   Fetal circulation

In the fetus gas exchange occurs in the placenta and pulmonary blood flow is low, supplying only nutritional requirements for lung growth and perhaps, as in the adult, performing some metabolic or "para-endocrine" function. In near term fetal lambs (term 145 days gestation) pulmonary blood flow is about 35-50 ml/100g lung tissue, about 8 to 10% of the total (combined left and right ventricular) output of the heart (4). The right ventricle ejects about two-thirds of the total cardiac output of 450-500 ml/kg/min (5) but most of this flow is diverted away from the lungs, through the widely patent ductus arteriosus, to the descending thoracic aorta and towards the umbilical placental circulation for oxygenation. Fetal pulmonary arterial blood pressure increases progressively with advancing gestation and at term is about 50 mmHg (mean), exceeding mean aortic blood pressure by about 1-2 mmHg (6,7). Resting pulmonary vascular resistance is extremely high early in gestation and falls progressively over the last half of gestation, due most likely to new vessel growth and the increase in cross sectional area (8,9); however, baseline resistance still is very much higher than in the adult.

B.   Transitional circulation

After birth and the initiation of pulmonary ventilation, pulmonary vascular resistance falls rapidly associated with an 8-10 fold increase in pulmonary blood flow. In normal full term lambs pulmonary arterial blood pressure falls to near adult levels within 1-2 hours; in the human this takes longer and by 24 hours of age mean pulmonary arterial blood pressure may be only half systemic (10). After the initial rapid fall there is a slow progressive fall with adult levels reached within 2-6 weeks after birth depending on species (11). With the large increase in pulmonary blood flow, the increased pulmonary venous return into the left atrium leads to an increase in left atrial pressure and a reversal of the pressure difference between the left and right atria. The valve of the foramen ovale thus closes, preventing any significant right to left shunting of blood. In addition the ductus arteriosus constricts and closes functionally within several hours (12), thereby effectively separating the pulmonary and systemic circulations.

C.   Physics of flow through the pulmonary vascular bed

The physical factors that control flow through the pulmonary vasculature can be defined by applying the hydraulic equivalent of Ohm's law and the Poiseuille-Hagen relationship. The hydraulic equivalent of Ohm's law states that the resistance to flow equals the mean pressure fall between two points divided by flow. For the pulmonary vascular bed resistance (R_p) is the mean pressure fall from the pulmonary artery (Ppa) to the pulmonary vein (Ppv) divided by pulmonary blood flow (Q_p).

$$R_p = (Ppa - Ppv)/Q_p$$

Because we are interested in increased pulmonary arterial blood pressure, this can be rearranged to give:

$$Ppa = Ppv + Q_p \cdot R_p$$

From this it can be seen that an elevation of pulmonary arterial blood pressure may occur with an increase of pulmonary venous pressure, pulmonary blood flow, or pulmonary vascular resistance. However, these factors are not necessarily independent. For example, with an atrial septal defect, pulmonary blood flow may be increased but pulmonary arterial blood pressure remain normal. The increased pulmonary blood flow has caused pulmonary vascular resistance to fall by dilating and perhaps recruiting arteries; the product $Q \cdot R$ does not change and pulmonary arterial blood pressure does not rise. However, because there is no zone I in the newborn lung, and less of zone II than in the adult, there is less ability to recruit new lung vessels when pulmonary flow rises. Pulmonary arterial blood pressure is therefore likely to be higher than in the older infant with a similar increase in flow.

In newborns with persistent pulmonary hypertension the pulmonary flow is invariably decreased so that increased flow is not a cause for the syndrome. It may be more difficult to exclude a raised pulmonary venous pressure as the primary cause because congenital lesions such as cor triatriatum or pulmonary venous obstruction produce no characteristic physical findings.

In most newborns who have pulmonary hypertension, pulmonary vascular resistance is increased, and the factors involved in determining vascular resistance need to be considered. According to the Poiseuille formula for flow of a Newtonian fluid through a straight glass tube:

$$R = (8/p) \ (1/r^4) \ (h).$$

That is, resistance is the product of a constant (8/p), the length of the tube (1) divided by the fourth power of its internal radius (r^4), and the viscosity (h) of the liquid flowing through it. Strictly, many of the criteria for applying this relationship do not pertain to biologic systems. Blood is not a Newtonian fluid; arteries branch, curve,taper and are distensible; and flow is pulsatile. Nevertheless, the Poiseuille relationship does apply and is useful when considering the pathophysiologic variables involved in producing an increased pulmonary vascular resistance and pulmonary hypertension. The length of the system (1) remains fairly constant and therefore with the other constants (8/p) can be removed from consideration. The lung comprises many parallel tubes so that with this additional modification it is clear that pulmonary vascular resistance is related to blood viscosity, the number of resistance vessels and their radii. The latter two variables reflect the total cross sectional area of the pulmonary vascular bed. It is apparent that pulmonary vascular resistance is directly related to the viscosity of blood perfusing the lungs, and inversely related to the cross sectional area of the pulmonary vascular bed. Increasing viscosity or decreasing vessel radius or number therefore leads to an elevation of pulmonary vascular resistance .

By further rearrangement of the equations, pulmonary arterial pressure has the same relationships to viscosity and cross sectional area (or radius) and also has a direct relationship to pulmonary venous pressure. Consideration of these factors, particularly viscosity and cross sectional area of the vascular bed, is important in evaluating the pathophysiology of persistent pulmonary hypertension syndrome in the newborn infant.

D.   Normal physiology of the perinatal pulmonary circulation
          (See Chapters by McMurty and by Cassin for details).

1.   Mechanical factors affecting pulmonary vascular resistance

The fetal lung is fluid filled and normally spontaneous fetal breathing movements do not affect pulmonary vascular resistance. However, rhythmic ventilation of fetal lungs with a gas, but not a liquid, without changing arterial blood PO_2, decreases pulmonary vascular resistance (13). This fall is related in small part to surface tension factors acting at the alveolar air-liquid interface tending to reduce perivascular tissue pressure (14) but more importantly is due to the release of vasoactive substances, particularly prostaglandin I_2 (PGI_2), by the movement or distention of the lung tissue (see below).

2.   Oxygen

Under normal resting conditions in the fetal lamb, femoral arterial blood PO_2 is about 22-24 torr and pulmonary araterial blood PO_2 17-20 torr. Because reduction of PO_2 to similar levels in newborn animals produces a marked increase in pulmonary vascular resistance (15-17), it is likely that the low PO_2 found normally in the fetus is involved in maintaining pulmonary vasoconstriction and thereby an increased pulmonary vascular resistance. Further reducing fetal PO_2 below normal by inducing maternal hypoxemia (6) produces an additional significant increase in pulmonary vascular resistance. This response is marked close to term but at about 0.6 gestation very little pulmonary vasoconstriction occurs. The exact mechanisms responsible for hypoxic vasoconstriction are not clearly established (see chapter by McMurtry for details). Both reflex-mediated chemoreceptor stimulation and direct local effects have been considered.

Although gaseous expansion or ventilation of fetal lungs without increasing PO_2 leads to a significant fall in pulmonary vascular resistance, a further major fall occurs with the addition to the gas mixture of oxygen (13,18). This effect of oxygen has been further substantiated without expanding or ventilating the lungs by exposing fetal lambs to hyperbaric oxygenation (19,20). It is not known whether the effects of increased oxygen are directly on the pulmonary vascular smooth muscle or whether a rise in PO_2 results in the release of an intermediary substance which either actively dilates the pulmonary circulation or inhibits vasoconstriction.

3.   Vasoactive substances and hormones

Many vasoactive substances have been shown to affect the fetal pulmonary circulation. Whether or how they play a physiologic role in the maintenance of the high pulmonary vascular resistance in the fetus or in postnatal responses is not fully known. Those invoked include histamine, a pulmonary vasodilator in newborns (21); and angiotensin II, not as a pulmonary vasoconstrictor as in adults, but as a possible stimulator of PGI_2 production (22). The physiologic role of the various products of the prostaglandin (PG) cascade (cyclo-oxygenase products of arachidonic acid metabolism) is also not clear. In the fetus, PGE_1 and PGE_2 both are modest pulmonary vasodilators (23-25); PGI_2 (Prostacyclin) also is a pulmonary vasodilator and is somewhat more potent (26-27) than both PGE_1 and PGE_2. None of these PGs (23-26) are specific for the pulmonary circulation and they generally effect the systemic vascular resistance as well. It is possible that production of these substances may modulate the constrictor effects of, for example, the normally low PO_2, thromboxane A_2 or the leukotrienes. $PGF_{2\alpha}$ produces only pulmonary vasoconstriction in fetal goats (24) and therefore possibly could play some role in active pulmonary vasoconstriction.

Lung distension or mechanical stimulation of lungs leads to PG production (28-30), and ventilation of fetal lungs is associated with the net production and release of PGI_2 by the lungs (31-33). In the lungs of fetuses close to term, perfused *in situ*, inhibition of prostaglandin synthesis by indomethacin attenuated the progressive fall in pulmonary vascular resistance that normally occurred 30 seconds after ventilation was started; the initial rapid fall was unaltered (34). These studies strongly suggest a physiologic role for PGI_2.

More recently another prostaglandin, PGD_2, has been shown to be a pulmonary vasodilator in perfused fetal lungs (35). In intact, newly delivered term lambs with hypoxia induced pulmonary hypertension, PGD_2 produced a significant and specific fall in pulmonary arterial pressure and calculated pulmonary vascular resistance with an increase in both pulmonary and systemic blood flows and no change in systemic arterial blood pressure (17). This response disappears by about 1 week of age (36) and therefore these specific effects in the immediate newborn suggest a physiologic role for PGD_2 in the immediate perinatal period.

Bradykinin, a potent vasoactive peptide, also produces marked pulmonary vasodilatation when infused into fetal lambs (37). Because bradykinin is released transiently from fetal lungs either following ventilation of the lungs with air or during hyperbaric oxygenation (20) it is possible that bradykinin also has some direct physiologic role in the immediate postnatal pulmonary circulatory changes. A further possible role for bradykinin, as with angiotensin II, relates to its ability to stimulate local production of PGI_2 (30,32).

Another class of substances, the leukotrienes (LTs), also derived from arachidonic acid but via the lipoxygenase pathway, have generated considerable interest in view of their constricting effect on smooth muscle. The leukotrienes may be responsible, at least in part, for mediating hypoxic pulmonary vasoconstriction in adults (38,39) and in newborn lambs (40). We therefore considered that leukotrienes could be involved in regulating the normal pulmonary vasoconstriction in the fetus. End organ antagonism (receptor blockade) of leukotriene effect in fetal lambs increased pulmonary blood flow to the level expected with normal ventilation after birth (41). These studies strongly suggest a physiologic role for LTs in maintaining pulmonary vasoconstriction and thereby a low pulmonary blood flow in the fetus.

It is probable therefore that control of the perinatal pulmonary circulation reflects a balance between factors producing active pulmonary vasoconstriction and those leading to pulmonary vasodilatation. The dramatic increase in pulmonary blood flow after birth most likely reflects a shift from active pulmonary vasoconstriction to active pulmonary vasodilatation. It is possible that arachidonic acid metabolism shifts from lipoxygenase products (LTs) in the fetus towards cyclo-oxygenase products (PGs) due to either mechanical stimulation with lung expansion or the higher oxygen environment after birth.

III. PATHOPHYSIOLOGY OF PERSISTENT PULMONARY HYPERTENSION SYNDROME IN THE NEWBORN

A. General Features

The feature common to all infants with this syndrome is failure of the pulmonary vascular resistance to fall normally with initiation of ventilation. As a result, pulmonary blood flow is compromised and pulmonary arterial pressure remains elevated at or near fetal levels. Associated with the pulmonary hypertension, right-to-left shunting may occur across the ductus arteriosus (which remains persistently patent for several days in most of these infants). Right ventricular end-diastolic pressure is usually elevated and consequently right atrial pressure also is increased; as a result right-to-left shunting often occurs across the foramen ovale. Tricuspid valve insufficiency is often associated with the pulmonary hypertension and right ventricular dilatation will accentuate this. As described above, the elevation of pulmonary vascular resistance is related to several factors, the most important for this clinical syndrome being either pulmonary venous pressure, viscosity or the cross sectional area of the pulmonary vascular bed. Conditions which alter these can lead to persistent pulmonary hypertension in the newborn infant.

B. Increased Pulmonary Venous Pressure

1. General pathophysiology

Associated with pulmonary venous hypertension of any etiology is an increase in mean capillary and pulmonary arterial blood pressure. Secondary to this, there may be increased fluid transudation from the vascular compartment into interstitial spaces with the development of alveolar hypoxia and then pulmonary vasoconstriction leading to further pulmonary hypertension (42). In addition, the increased interstitial fluid may also physically compress the small pulmonary arteries. In the immediate newborn period much of the fetal alveolar lung liquid has passed into the interstitial spaces and has to be cleared from the lungs over a period of several hours (43). Pulmonary venous hypertension interfering with this normal process may lead to the development in some instances of significant pulmonary hypertension.

2.   Structural cardiac anomalies

Congenital malformations that produce left ventricular failure are the commonest cause of pulmonary venous hypertension in infants. Juxtaductal coarctation or aortic stenosis, although relatively uncommon, are most often seen in this group. Lesions such as pulmonary venous stenosis, anomalous pulmonary venous return, cor-triatriatum, congenital mitral stenosis or variants thereof which obstruct blood flow into the left ventricle also may lead to pulmonary venous hypertension. These lesions may cause pulmonary edema, tachypnea, rales, pulmonary hypertension and its consequences, and often cannot be distinguished clinically, electrocardiographically or radiologically from severe lung disease. Any infant in whom this picture persists without improvement should have careful echocardiography and, if necessary, cardiac catheterization, so that a treatable cause of pulmonary venous hypertension is not missed.

3.   Myocardial dysfunction

Left ventricular myocardial dysfunction may lead to an elevation of left ventricular end-diastolic pressure with secondary left atrial and pulmonary venous hypertension. Myocardial dysfunction may be associated with transient cardiomyopathy as seen in infants of diabetic mothers or after asphyxia. Less common are primary cardiomyopathies of unknown etiology and myocardial tumors such as rhabdomyomas. Infectious viral myocarditis also may lead to severe alterations in myocardial performance. Electrolyte imbalances, particularly hypocalcemia and hypoglycemia, too may adversely effect myocardial performance. Although rare, coronary occlusion or anomalous origin of the left coronary artery may produce global left ventricular ischemia and dysfunction. Most of these situations are clinically recognizable and generally are not confused with persistent pulmonary hypertension syndrome. However, secondary left ventricular dysfunction such as occurs with hypocalcemia, for example, certainly may aggravate the pulmonary hypertension in an infant with the syndrome of persistent pulmonary hypertension.

4.   Increased pulmonary vascular resistance.

a. Increased Viscosity. Viscosity of blood is related to red cell number, fibrinogen concentration and red cell deformability. An increased hematocrit will raise viscosity, and may be found following twin to twin or maternal to fetal transfusion or delayed cord clamping or in infants of diabetic mothers. Pulmonary vascular resistance rises approximately logarithmically with the increase in hematocrit (44). Chronic intrauterine hypoxemia (intrauterine growth retardation) also is associated with an increased hematocrit, as well as increased fibrinogen (45). Reduced red cell deformability, and therefore a potential increase in pulmonary vascular resistance, is a feature of newborn red cells, relative to adult cells, and this is accentuated by acidemia.

b. Reduced Cross-sectional Area. If increased blood viscosity does not explain the high pulmonary vascular resistance, then the number of vessels or their radii must be considered. During fetal development, there is a steady growth of acini and pulmonary arteries, most of which accompany the airways (8) with a rapid increase of arterial number in the last trimester (8,9). Disorders associated with failure of normal lung growth (oligohydramnios, diaphragmatic hernia, thoracodystrophy, lung cysts, etc.) may be associated with a proportional reduction in the number of pulmonary vessels.

The most common cause for reduction in total pulmonary vascular cross sectional area is failure of the pulmonary circulation to undergo normal postnatal vasodilatation. The exact mechanisms responsible for failure of the pulmonary vasculature to dilate normally are unknown. A likely, but not proven, common denominator is hypoxemia, which produces pulmonary vasoconstriction (15,16). Why some infants exposed to perinatal hypoxemia or asphyxia develop pulmonary hypertension whereas many others, equally stressed in the immediate perinatal period, do not, is unclear. Recent pathologic studies may shed some light on this. Morphologic evaluation of the pulmonary vasculature of infants dying with the pulmonary hypertension syndrome has shown clearly that there is an increased amount of medial smooth muscle in the walls of the small pulmonary arteries as well as an ontogenetically accelerated distribution of the smooth muscle along the length of the resistance vessels (46-49). Perhaps these abnormally developed vessels also have an increased constrictor response to low oxygen, either because of the increased muscle mass or because the developmental acceleration is functional as well as structural. In fetal animals, chronic intrauterine stress, such as chronic hypoxemia (50) or pulmonary hypertension, (51) increases medial muscle mass in the small pulmonary arteries. Infants exposed to similar intrauterine stresses are perhaps those at high risk for developing morphologic changes of the pulmonary vasculature and then pulmonary hypertension syndrome.

It is now clearly established that the administration to pregnant animals of inhibitors of prostaglandin synthesis such as aspirin or indomethacin produces constriction of the ductus arteriosus in utero (7,12). This produces pulmonary hypertension and the development of increased pulmonary vascular medial smooth muscle (52). Use of these pharmacologic agents during pregnancy has been linked to the development of pulmonary hypertension syndrome (47,53-55) but the association is not clear cut.

Another possible cause of a reduced cross sectional area of the pulmonary vascular bed is occlusion of the small pulmonary arteries by platelet emboli or thrombus formation. Recent evidence has been presented to suggest that microthromboembolism (56) may in fact play a significant part in the pathophysiology of the syndrome of pulmonary hypertension in the newborn and that this feature may be associated with the severest form of the disease and therefore therapeutically the least responsive group of infants. Not only will the thrombi block the vessel lumen but thromboxane A_2 may be released and produce secondary pulmonary vasoconstriction.

REFERENCES

1. Levin DL, Heymann MA, Kitterman JA, Gregory GA, Phibbs RH and Rudolph AM. (1976) *J Pediatr* **89**:626.
2. Goetzman BW and Riemenschneider TA. (1980) *Pediatr Rev* **2**:37.
3. Emmanouilides GC and Baylen BG. (1979) *Curr Probl Pediatr IX*. **7**:1.
4. Rudolph AM and Heymann MA. (1970) *Circ Res* **26**:289.
5. Heymann MA, Creasy RK and Rudolph AM. (1973) *In:* **Proceedings of the Sir Joseph Barcroft Centenary Symposium. Foetal and Neonatal Physiology.** Cambridge University Press:Cambridge.
6. Lewis AB, Heymann MA and Rudolph AM. (1976) *Circ Res* **39**:536.
7. Heymann MA and Rudolph AM. (1976) *Circ Res* **38**:418.
8. Hislop A and Reid LM. (1972) *J Anat* **113**:35.
9. Levin DL, Rudolph AM, Heymann MA and Phibbs RH. (1976) *Circulation* **53**:144.
10. Moss AJ, Emmanouilides G and Duffie ER Jr. (1963) *Pediatrics* **32**:25.
11. Rudolph AM, Auld PAM, Golinko RJ and Paul MH. (1961) *Pediatrics* **28**:28.
12. Clyman RI and Heymann MA. (1981) *Pediatr Clin N Am* **28**:77.
13. Cassin S, Dawes GS, Mott JC, Ross BB and Strang LB. (1964) *J Physiol (Lond)* **171**:61.
14. Enhorning G, Adams FH and Norman A. (1966)*Acta Paediatr Scand* **55**:441.
15. Stahlman M, Shepard F, Gray JR and Young W. (1964) *J Pediatr* **65**:1091.

16. Rudolph AM and Yuan S. (1966) *J Clin Invest* **45**:399.
17. Soifer SJ, Morin FC III and Heymann MA. (1982) *J Pediatr* **100**:458.
18. Cook CD, Drinker PA, Jacobson NH, Levison H and Strang LB. (1963) *J Physiol (Lond)* **169**:10.
19. Assali NS, Kirschbaum TM and Dilts PV Jr. (1968) *Circ Res* **22**:573.
20. Heymann MA, Rudolph AM, Nies AS and Melmon KL. (1969) *Circ Res* **25**:521.
21. Goetzman BW and Milstein JM. (1980) *J Appl Physiol* **49**:380.
22. Dusting AJ. (1981) *J Cardiovasc Pharm* **3**:197.
23. Cassin S, Tyler TL and Wallis R. (1975) *Proc Soc Exp Biol Med* **148**:584.
24. Tyler TL, Leffler CW and Cassin S. (1977) *Chest* **71S**:271S.
25. Tripp ME, Heymann MA and Rudolph AM. (1978) *In:* **Advances in Prostaglandin and Thromboxane Research.** Volume 4. (F Coceani and PM Olley, eds.) Raven Press:New York.
26. Leffler CW and Hessler JR. (1979) *Eur J Pharmacol* **54**:37.
27. Cassin S, Winikor I, Tod M, Philips J, Frisinger S, Jordan J and Gibbs C. (1981) *Pediatr Pharmacol* **1**:197.
28. Edmonds JF, Berry E and Wyllie JH. (1969) *Brit J Surg* **56**:622.
29. Gryglewski RJ, Korbut R and Ocetkiewics A. (1978) *Nature* **273**:765.
30. Gryglewski RJ. (1980) *Ciba Found Symp* **78**:147.
31. Leffler CW, Hessler JR and Terragno NA. (1980) *Am J Physiol* **238**:H282.
32. Leffler CW, Hessler JR and Green RS. (1984) *Prostaglandins* **28**:877.
33. Leffler CW, Hessler JR and Green RS. (1984) *Pediatr Res* **18**:938.
34. Leffler CW, Tyler TL and Cassin S. (1978) *Am J Physiol* **234**:H346.
35. Cassin S, Tod M, Philips J, Frisinger J, Jordan J and Gibbs C. (1981) *Am J Physiol* **240**:H755.
36. Soifer SJ, Morin FC III, Kaslow DC and Heymann MA. (1983) *J Dev Physiol* **5**:237-250.
37. Campbell AGM, Dawes GS, Fishman AP, Hyman AI and Perks AM. (1968) *J Physiol (Lond)* **195**:83.
38. Ahmed T and Oliver W Jr. (1983) *Amer Rev Respir Dis* **127**:566.
39. Morganroth ML, Reeves JT, Murphy RC and Voelkel NF. (1984) *J Appl Physiol* **56**:1340.
40. Schreiber MD, Heymann MA and Soifer SJ. (1985) *Pediatr Res* **19**:437.
41. Soifer SJ, Loitz RD, Roman C and Heymann MA. (1985) *Am J Physiol* **249**:H570.
42. Iliff LD, Greene RE and Hughes JMB. (1972) *J Appl Physiol* **33**:462.
43. Bland RD, McMillan PD and Bressack MA. (1977) *Ann Rech Vet* **8**:418.
44. Agarwal JB, Paltoo R and Palmer WH. (1970) *J Appl Physiol* **29**:866.

45. Pickart LR, Creasy RK and Thaler MM. (1976) *Am J Obstet Gynecol* **124**:268.

46. Haworth SG and Reid L. (1976) *J Pediatr* **88**:614.

47. Levin DL, Fixler DE, Morriss FC and Tyson J. (1978) *J Pediatr* **92**:478.

48. McKenzie S and Haworth SG. (1981) *Br Heart J* **46**:675.

49. Murphy JD, Rabinovitch M, Goldstein JD and Reid LM. (1981) *J Pediatr* **98**:962.

50. Goldberg SJ, Levy RA, Siassi B and Betten J. (1971) *Pediatarics* **48**:528.

51. Levin DL, Hyman AI, Heymann MA and Rudolph AM. (1978) *J Pediatr* **92**:265.

52. Levin DL, Mills LJ and Weinberg AG. (1979) *Circulation* **60**:360.

53. Manchester D, Margolis HS and Sheldon RE. (1976) *Am J Obstet Gynecol* **126**:467.

54. Csaba IF, Sulyok E and Ertl T. (1978) *J Pediatr* **92**:484.

55. Wilkinson AR, Aynsley-Green A and Mitchell MD. (1979) *Arch Dis Child* **54**:942.

56. Levin DL, Weinberg AG and Perkin RM. (1983) *J Pediatr* **102**: 299.

Potential Mechanisms of Hypoxic Pulmonary Vasoconstriction

IVAN F. MCMURTRY
University of Colorado
Health Sciences Center, Denver, CO

BERNADETTE RAFFESTIN
Universite Paris-Sud,
UER, Kremlin-Bicetre,
France

I. INTRODUCTION

The mechanism of hypoxic pulmonary vasoconstriction (HPV) has been the subject of numerous studies in man and other mammals (1-9) since 1946 when von Euler and Liljestrand (10) first described the pulmonary pressor response to acute airway hypoxia. Continued biomedical interest in HPV stems from its role in the shunting of blood flow from the unventilated fetal lung and the critical reversal of this process in the neonate, the local matching of pulmonary capillary blood flow to alveolar ventilation in the adult, and the development of pulmonary hypertension in patients with chronic ventilatory insufficiency. The mechanism of HPV also presents an interesting challenge to investigators concerned with the basic physiology of vascular control and the biochemistry of cellular O_2 sensing.

II.   INTRAPULMONARY MECHANISM

Although much has been learned of HPV in the past 40 years, the basic mechanism remains unknown (1-9). HPV is significantly influenced by systemic hemodynamic, neural, and humoral signals, but the essential mechanism comprising O_2 sensor, transduction process, and effector is intrapulmonary because hypoxic vasoconstriction occurs in isolated, artificially-perfused lungs. Blood cells and platelets may affect hypoxic pressor reactivity through effects on perfusate viscosity and the release of vasoactive substances, but they are not a necessary component of the hypoxic mechanism, as isolated lungs perfused with platelet-poor plasma or physiological salt solution show hypoxic pressor responses (11,12). The relatively poor hypoxic pressor reactivity of salt solution as compared to plasma-perfused lungs is probably due to a generalized decrease of vascular reactivity, rather than the absence or scarcity of a unique component of the hypoxic mechanism normally supplied by plasma.

We have recently observed that the composition of salt solution is an important determinant of hypoxic pressor reactivity in isolated rat lungs. In earlier experiments McMurtry *et al.* (12,13) found that lungs perfused with salt solution containing 50 mM sucrose showed little or no hypoxic vasoconstriction unless they were also exposed to vasoactive agents such as angiotensin II, vanadate, 4-aminopyridine, high levels of K^+, and dexamethasone. Within the past year we have observed that lungs perfused with the same salt solution (Earle's balanced salts, Sigma) not containing the sucrose will often, but not always, develop significant hypoxic pressor responses without exposure to any other agent (Figure 1). It is also our experience that lungs perfused with HEPES-buffered salt solution have greater hypoxic pressor reactivity than those perfused with HCO_3/CO_2-buffered solution. Hypoxic vasoconstriction in salt solution-perfused rat lungs is generally enhanced by the inhibitor of cyclooxygenase, meclofenamate (12,13). We do not fully understand what is happening in these experiments, but we believe the bottom line is that the basic mechanism of HPV resides in pulmonary parenchymal and/or vascular tissue and that its full expression requires an optimal degree of vascular smooth muscle excitability, *i.e.*, HPV is particularly dependent on "initial vascular tone" (3,12). It is also possible that some of the numerous physiological and methodological factors found to influence hypoxic pressor reactivity (1-9,12,13) affect more directly the specific process of O_2 sensing than the degree of vascular excitability *per se*.

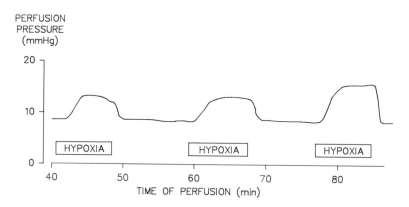

Figure 1. Tracing of normoxic ($F_IO_2=21\%$) and hypoxic ($F_IO_2=0\%$) perfusion pressure in rat lungs perfused with Earle's balanced salt solution buffered with HEPES (10mM) and containing F_ICO_2 (4g/100 ml) and meclofenamate (3.1 μM). Significant hypoxic pressor responses occurred without addition of other vasoactive agents to perfusate. In similar experiments the first three hypoxic pressor responses after 20 min of equilibration were 4.9 ±1.0, 6.4 ±0.9, and 7.5 ±0.9 mmHg in 10 HEPES-buffered lungs and 3.5 ±0.7, 4.1 ±1.0, and 3.7 ±0.9 mmHg in 10 HCO_3/CO_2-buffered lungs (p<0.05).

III. MEDIATOR VERSUS DIRECT EFFECT

It is generally believed that smooth muscle of small, peripheral pulmonary arteries is the effector of HPV (1-9), but the cellular site and biochemical nature of the O_2 sensor and the sequence of events which converts sensing of hypoxia to contraction of vascular smooth muscle, *i.e.*, the transduction process, are unknown. Historically, the two main proposals for the mechanism of HPV have been that hypoxia either elicits release of a vasoconstrictor (a mediator) from some lung cell other than the arterial smooth muscle or acts directly to excite the smooth muscle cell. Numerous substances have been examined as the hypothetical intercellular mediator of HPV. However, when the criteria shown in Table I are applied, neither catecholamines, histamine, serotonin, prostaglandins, thromboxane, angiotensin II, bradykinin, vasopressin, acetylcholine, VIP, substance P, ATP, nor lactic acid fill the bill (1-9). It is also unlikely that platelet activating factor, a pulmonary pressor substance in many species, is the mediator because we have found it to be a potent inhibitor of HPV in intact rats and isolated rat lungs (14).

TABLE I. Criteria for a unique intercellular mediator of HPV (3).

The potential mediator should be:
- A potent pulmonary vasoconstrictor
- Synthesized and/or stored in or near small pulmonary arteries
- Released or activated by hypoxia
- Rapidly sequestered or inactivated upon re-exposure to normoxia

HPV should be specifically blocked by:
- Mediator antagonists
- Inhibitors of mediator synthesis and/or storage

A recent, serious candidate for mediator of HPV is leukotriene C_4 (LTC_4) or some other metabolite of the lipoxygenase pathway of arachidonic acid metabolism (8,9). LTC_4 is a pulmonary vasoconstrictor synthesized by lung tissue and, at least in the rat lung (15), released during HPV and metabolized upon return to normoxia. In addition, HPV has been inhibited in some studies by the blockers of leukotriene synthesis, diethylcarbamazine, U-60257, and nordihydroquaiaretic acid (15-18), the putative blocker of mast cell leukotriene release, cromolyn sodium (19), and the LTC_4 end-organ antagonists, FPL-55712 and -57231 (16,19-21). Although these findings seemingly indicate that LTC_4 fulfills the criteria for mediator of HPV (Table 1), there are numerous discordant observations (Table II). These negative reports are not conclusive, but they render the evidence for LTC_4 or some other lipoxygenase metabolite as the hypoxic mediator qualitatively similar to that used more than a decade ago to argue the same role for catecholamines and histamine (2,3,6). Further work is clearly required to establish whether or not a lipoxygenase metabolite mediates HPV. Even though there is currently no other viable candidate, a decision against a lipoxygenase product would not eliminate the mediator hypothesis — in other words, "absence of evidence is not evidence of absence."

Various attempts have been made with isolated pulmonary arteries to test if HPV is due to a direct hypoxic excitation of the smooth muscle. Although it is now clear that isolated pulmonary (and systemic) arteries can be made to contract in response to hypoxia (5,34-40), an important question is whether these *in vitro* hypoxic responses involve the same mechanism as HPV in intact animals and isolated lungs. Based on the characteristics of the hypoxic response in the latter two preparations (1-9), we believe a valid *in vitro* model of HPV should show the following behavior. The hypoxic contraction should show a stimulus-response curve over a certain range of O_2 tension, *i.e.*, the contraction should be elicited by

TABLE II. List of observations which tend not to support role for leukotrienes as mediator of HPV.

Preparation	Observation	Reference
Dog, Cat lung	Inhibition of mast cell release by cromolyn did not block HPV	22,23
Piglet	DEC, NDGA, and FPL 55712 did not inhibit HPV	24
Dog, Cat	DEC did not inhibit HPV	25,26
Dog	LY-83583 did not inhibit HPV	26
Dog	BW755C did not inhibit HPV	27,28
Dog	Phenidone did not inhibit HPV	29
Rat lung	Dexamethasone and caffeic acid did not inhibit HPV	13[a]
Rat lung	HPV inhibited only by high concentration of phenidone	30
Dog, Rat lung	HPV inhibited only by high concentration of FPL-57231	29,30
Lamb	Inhibitory effect of FPL-57231 not specific for HPV	31
Sheep lung	HPV not associated with release of leukotrienes	32
Human lung fragments	Hypoxia did not release leukotrienes	33

[a] Unpublished observation by IFMc that in salt solution plus meclofenamate-perfused rat lungs (n=6) the pressor response to hypoxia (F_IO_2 = 0% O_2) was 10.7 ± 3.1 mmHg before and 13.0 ± 2.8 mmHg after addition of 10^{-3} M caffeic acid to perfusate.

hypoxia rather than only by anoxia. In fact, it could be expected that the contraction might be depressed by severe hypoxia (8). The contraction should develop within five minutes or less of the hypoxic exposure and be rapidly reversed by reexposure to normoxia. It should be potentiated by BAY K8644 (41,42) and readily inhibited by verapamil, nifedipine, Ca^{++}-free incubation, or a sudden, moderate decrease in temperature (43). The hypoxic contraction should not be mediated by catecholamines, histamine, cyclooxygenase metabolites, serotonin, angiotensin II, or any other substance shown not to be the mediator of HPV. Whether it should involve the action of a lipoxygenase metabolite remains to be determined. It might be potentiated by inhibition of cyclooxygenase activity.

When the above criteria are applied to various isolated artery preparations reported to develop "hypoxic contractions" (5,34-40), the one recently described by Madden *et al.* (37,38) is the most convincing as an *in vitro* model of HPV. J. Madden and D. Harder, systemic vascular smooth muscle electrophysiologists, were apparently prompted by J. Linehan and C. Dawson, pulmonary physiologists, to use their skills in isolating and studying small systemic arteries to test if hypoxia would constrict isolated small pulmonary arteries. In their subsequent studies with cat isolated pulmonary arteries they found whereas hypoxia elicited significant constriction of arteries < 300 μm in diameter, it caused only small inconsistent responses in those > 500 μm. The cause of this difference between the small and large vessels is unknown. The hypoxic contraction was rapid in onset, relatively well sustained, and rapidly reversed by normoxia. The contraction was inversely related to O_2 tension until the response began to decline with severe hypoxia. Verapamil, but not phentolamine, blocked the response and indomethacin potentiated it. Thus, this hypoxic response shows many similarities to HPV and can probably be considered a valid *in vitro* model. It is apparent that two to three other groups of investigators have not been able to duplicate these results with similar preparations within the past year. Although this is a bit disconcerting, it should be noted that it often takes considerable practice to establish the techniques and conditions necessary for obtaining consistent hypoxic pressor reactivity in isolated lungs.

If the above hypoxic constriction is due to the same mechanism responsible for HPV, then what more do we know about whether HPV is due to release of a mediator or to direct hypoxic excitation of the vascular smooth muscle? We are hopefully closer to the answer — but because the arteries studied presumably contained endothelial cells and perhaps some adventitial fibroblasts and mast cells, the possible involvement of a mediator has not been ruled out. We are unaware of any direct evidence for mediator release by fibroblasts, and a necessary role for mast cells in HPV is doubtful (3,8,44). In contrast, there is currently much interest in the control of vascular tone by endothelium-derived substances (45-47). The predominant effect of endothelial "stimulation" on vascular tone is dilation caused by release of agents such as prostaglandin I_2 and endothelium-derived relaxing factor (EDRF), but there is also evidence for endothelial production of vasoconstrictors (39,48,49). For example, dog isolated coronary and femoral arteries incubated with indomethacin and exhibiting some degree of either spontaneous or agonist-induced active tone were found by Rubanyi and Vanhoutte (39) to develop endothelial-dependent hypoxic and anoxic contractions. Arteries denuded of endothelium did not contract to stepwise decreases in O_2 tension unless they were apposed to an endothelial-intact vascular strip. The hypoxic contraction was not blocked by inhibitors of either phospholipase A_2 or lipoxygenase. Thus, this hypoxic contraction was apparently mediated by release of a vasoconstrictor from endothelial cells. A somewhat similar finding with the main pulmonary artery of the pig has been reported by Holden and McCall (36). Whether the same or a similar mechanism was operating in the hypoxic response observed by Madden *et al.* (37,38) is unclear. The latter investigators have found in preliminary experiments (50) that removal of endothelium from the small pulmonary arteries depresses contractile responses to hypoxia, KCl, and serotonin. This generalized depression of vasoreactivity precludes any decision about an endothelium-derived mediator of HPV. The possible effects of increased production of vasodilator prostaglandins should be considered in experiments involving removal of the endothelium (51,52).

IV. MEMBRANE DEPOLARIZATION AND CA⁺⁺ INFLUX

Regardless of whether HPV is due to release of an intercellular mediator or a direct action on the arterial smooth muscle, there is strong support for the idea that membrane depolarization and Ca^{++} influx through voltage-dependent channels are key components of the transduction process. Early studies showed in isolated rat lungs that the Ca^{++} channel blocker verapamil inhibited hypoxic vasoconstriction more readily than that elicited by angiotensin II or prostaglandin $F_{2\alpha}$ (53). This finding suggested that whereas the pulmonary vasoconstriction elicited by some agonists could be transduced partly by release of intracellular Ca^{++} and/or Ca^{++} influx through receptor-operated channels, HPV was critically dependent on Ca^{++} influx through voltage-dependent channels. Recent experiments show that HPV is potentiated in isolated lungs (41,42) and anesthetized dogs (42) by BAY K 8644, a structural analog of nifedipine which binds to the "dihydropyridine receptor" and facilitates Ca^{++} influx through partially activated, voltage-dependent Ca^{++} channels. Further support for the role of membrane depolarization and Ca^{++} influx in the mechanism of HPV is provided by the electrophysiological studies of Harder *et al.* (38). These investigators observed that the hypoxic contraction of isolated small pulmonary arteries was associated with smooth muscle membrane depolarization and generation of action potentials. The hypoxic contraction, membrane depolarization, and action potentials were inhibited by verapamil and depletion of extracellular Ca^{++}. Similar findings have been reported in preliminary form by Hottenstein *et al.* (40). Collectively, these observations indicate that hypoxia can lead to the membrane depolarization, Ca^{++} influx, and contraction of some pulmonary arterial smooth muscle, but they do not differentiate between a mediated or a direct action of hypoxia.

V. O_2 SENSOR

Sylvester *et al.* (8) recently discussed the airway hypoxia stimulus-pressor response relationships observed in isolated lungs of various species. In general, the stimulus-response curve shows a typical sigmoid relationship until the response begins to fail with severe hypoxia. It is apparent that in some cases the unidentified O_2 sensor can detect very mild degrees of airway hypoxia and track closely a progressive fall in airway O_2 tension. Whether this distinctive sensitivity to O_2 tension is due to a particularly high affinity of the sensing molecule for O_2 or to a large O_2 diffusion gradient (64) is unknown. Although O_2 tension of the sensor is determined primarily by airway O_2 tension, perfusate O_2 tension has an effect (55, 56). The exact cellular site of the O_2 sensor has not been determined, but it is presumably located in or near the wall of small pulmonary arteries (1,3,8,56).

The primary O_2 sensing process in the mechanism of HPV could theoretically involve either allosteric changes in an O_2 binding protein that controls transmembrane ion flux or alterations in activity of an O_2 dependent enzyme. There is no direct evidence for the former in HPV, but such a mechanism has been proposed for the hypoxic excitation of Aplysia neurons (57). As was noted by Sylvester *et al.* (8), this possibility is attractive in its economy and should probably be given more consideration than it has received.

Although there are numerous O_2-dependent enzymes, oxygenases and oxidases, whose activity can be altered by various degrees of hypoxia (8,54), the only two that have received much attention as the possible O_2 sensor of HPV are the microsomal cytochrome P-450 and the mitochondrial cytochrome oxidase. Sylvester and McGowan (58) tested whether HPV was initiated by desaturation of the heme iron of cytochrome P-450 and observed blunting of HPV in pig lungs by the inhibitors of P-450, metyrapone and CO. Similar results have been obtained in rat lungs (59), dogs (60), and sheep (61), but not in lambs (61). A major question raised in these experiments is whether the high concentrations of inhibitors used had nonspecific effects. In this regard it is interesting that glucose-free perfusion, which may inhibit cytochrome P-450 by depletion of NADPH (62), potentiated HPV in rat lungs (63). Thus, the exact role of cytochrome P-450 activity in the mechanism of HPV remains to be determined.

Recent evidence that the O_2 dependence of cytochrome c oxidase is greater in intact cells than in isolated mitochrondria (54,64), and that hypoxic depression of mitochondrial oxidative phosphorylation does not necessarily lead to a decrease in respiration or in total cellular [ATP], [ATP]/[ADP], or the adenylate energy charge (64), have alleviated some of the doubt about whether mitochondrial cytochrome oxidase can act as an O_2 sensor for physiological responses to hypoxia. It is uncertain how mild to moderate decreases in cytochrome c oxidation and oxidative phosphorylation might signal changes in cell function, but shifts in the intracellular levels of [ATP]/[ADP][Pi], phosphocreatine, Pi, pyridine nucleotides, and H^+ are possibilities (54,64).

The idea that HPV involves a decrease in mitochondrial cytochrome oxidase activity and oxidative phosphorylation stems largely from the above evidence that the latter are sensitive to physiological levels of hypoxia, and from Lloyd's (65) and Rounds' and McMurtry's (66) observations that numerous chemically-different inhibitors of oxidative phosphorylation, e.g., antimycin, azide, cyanide, dinitrophenol, and rotenone, can mimic airway hypoxia and elicit pulmonary vasoconstriction in normoxic lungs. The pressor responses to hypoxia and the chemical inhibitors show many physiological and pharmacological similarities (65) including sensitivity to inhibition by verapamil (68). Chemical inhibitors of oxidative phosphorylation can also cause Ca^{++}-dependent contraction of isolated arteries (5). However, it is unknown if the vasoconstrictions elicited by the two forms of stimulus are preceded or accompanied by similar, if any, changes in either lung or vascular tissue bioenergetics.

Because increased glycolysis buffers the metabolic and functional effects of decreased mitochondrial oxidative phosphorylation in many tissues, Stanbrook and McMurtry (63) reasoned that if HPV were signaled by depression of oxidative phosphorylation, then hypoxic pressor sensitivity might be increased by inhibition of glycolysis. They observed in rat lungs that inhibition of glycolysis by iodoacetate, 2-deoxyglucose, or glucose-free perfusion potentiated hypoxic pressor sensitivity. The potentiation by glucose-free perfusion was prevented by addition of lactate and pyruvate to the perfusate, and this inhibitory effect of lactate plus pyruvate was partly reversed by the citric acid cycle blocker, malonate. These results show that inhibition of glucose metabolism potentiates HPV in rat lungs, but the biochemical link between the two events is not clear. The results are consistent with the idea that the potentiation is due to limitation of mitochondrial oxidative phosphorylation and some change in bioenergetics, but it is also possible that it is related to a change in level of an unidentified intra- or intercellular modulating peptide, fatty acid, or lipid. The results clearly eliminate the possibility that HPV is due to increased production of lactate.

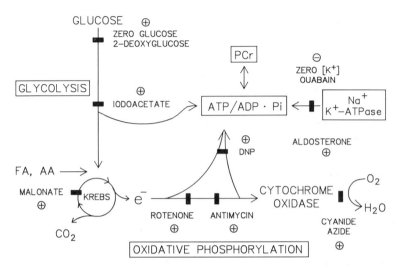

Figure 2. Diagram of sites of action of various "metabolic agents" which alter hypoxic pressor reactivity of isolated rat lungs. Agents labelled with plus sign have been found to potentiate and/or mimic HPV and have in common the potential to cause a decrease in cellular energy state. Agents labelled with minus sign have been found to blunt HPV and could theoretically lead to an increase in energy state.

Because the sensitivity of mitochondrial oxidative phosphorylation and cellular energy state to hypoxic depression is related to the underlying rate of energy utilization and respiration (64), Herget and McMurtry (67) tested if agents or conditions which could be expected to increase or decrease lung tissue energy metabolism and respiration would, respectively, increase and decrease hypoxic pressor sensitivity. They observed in rat lungs that hypoxic pressor sensitivity was blunted by two inhibitors of Na^+, K^+-ATPase, ouabain and low perfusate $[K^+]$, and potentiated by aldosterone, an agent that may increase membrane permeability to Na^+ and lead to increased Na^+, K^+-pumping. These findings provide no support for the suggestion that membrane depolarization due to inhibition of electrogenic Na^+, K^+-pumping is a necessary component of HPV (68). They do suggest a positive relationship between Na^+,K^+-ATPase activity and hypoxic pressor sensitivity, and are consistent with the idea that the former may influence the latter indirectly by altering cellular energy metabolism. However, it is also possible that the results were in some way due to changes in intracellular $[Na^+]$ or transmembrane Na^+ gradient, rather than to changes in energy metabolism.

In summary, these experiments provide consistent pharmacological evidence that depression of mitochondrial oxidative phosphorylation and a decrease in cellular energy state are involved in the mechanism of HPV (Figure 2). Because the effect of hypoxia (and of chemical inhibitors of oxidative phosphorylation) on pulmonary vascular tone is biphasic, *i.e.*, constriction with mild and moderate hypoxia and dilation with severe hypoxia or anoxia (8,65,66), we believe it possible that whereas a decrease in either lung or vascular tissue [PCr]/[Cr] or [ATP]/[ADP][Pi] with moderate hypoxia (84) somehow leads to membrane depolarization, Ca^{++} influx, and vasoconstriction, further inhibition of energy metabolism and a fall in [ATP] cause vasodilation. The major problem with the available evidence for this idea is that it is all indirect. Perhaps the *in vitro* model described by Madden *et al.* (37,38) will allow more rigorous testing of the working hypothesis shown in Figure 3 and the alternatives proposed by other investigators of the mechanism of HPV (7,8,9).

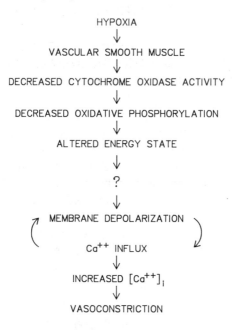

HYPOXIA
↓
VASCULAR SMOOTH MUSCLE
↓
DECREASED CYTOCHROME OXIDASE ACTIVITY
↓
DECREASED OXIDATIVE PHOSPHORYLATION
↓
ALTERED ENERGY STATE
↓
?
↓
MEMBRANE DEPOLARIZATION
Ca^{++} INFLUX
↓
INCREASED $[Ca^{++}]_i$
↓
VASOCONSTRICTION

Figure 3. Working hypothesis for direct mechanism of HPV. Evidence relating to this hypothesis is reviewed in text.

REFERENCES

1.   Bergofsky EH. (1974) *Am J Med* **57**:378.
2.   Barer GR. (1976) *Pharmacol Ther B* **2**:247.
3.   Fishman AP. (1976) *Circ Res* **38**:221.
4.   Harris P and Heath D. (1977) **The Human Pulmonary Circulation.** Churchill Livingstone:New York.
5.   McMurtry IF, Rounds S and Stanbrook HS. (1982)*Adv Shock Res* **8**:21.
6.   Grover RF, Wagner WW Jr, McMurtry IF and Reeves JT. (1983) *In* **Handbook of Physiology -The Cardiovascular System III** (JT Shepherd, FM Abboud, and SR Geiger, eds) American Physiol Soc: Bethesda, MD.
7.   Weir EK. (1984) *In* **Pulmonary Hypertension.** (EK Weir and JT Reeves, eds) Futura:New York.
8.   Sylvester JT, Gottlieb JE, Rock P and Wetzel RC. (1986) *In* **Abnormal Pulmonary Circulation.** (EH Bergofsky ed), Churchill Livingstone: New York.
9.   Voelkel NF. (1986) *Am Rev Respir Dis* **133**:1186.
10. Euler US v and Liljestrand G. (1946) *Acta Physiol Scand* **12**:301.
11. McMurtry IF, Hookway BW and Roos SD. (1978) *Am J Physiol* **234**:H186.
12. McMurtry IF. (1984) *J Appl Physiol* **56**:375.
13. McMurtry IF and Herget J. (1986) *Fed Proc* **45**:552.
14. McMurtry IF and Morris KG. (1986) *Am Rev Respir Dis* **133**:A227.
15. Morganroth ML, Stenmark KR, Zirrolli JA, Mauldin R, Mathias M, Reeves JT, Murphy RC and Voelkel NF. (1984) *Prostaglandins* **28**:867.
16. Morganroth ML, Reeves JT, Murphy RC and Voelkel NF. (1984) *J Appl Physiol* **56**:1340.
17. Morganroth ML, Stenmark KR, Morris KG, Murphy RC, Mathias M, Reeves JT and Voelkel NF. (1985) *Amer Rev Respir Dis* **131**:488.
18. Gottlieb J, McGeady M, Adkinson NF, Hayes E and Sylvester JT. (1984) *Am Rev Resp Dis* **129**:A343.
19. Ahmed T and Oliver W Jr. (1983) *Amer Rev Respir Dis* **127**:566.
20. Soifer SJ, Loitz RD, Roman C and Heymann MA. (1985) *Am J Physiol* **249**:H570.
21. Goldberg RN, Suguihara C, Ahmed T, Deseda de Cudemus B, Barrios P, Setzer ES and Bancalari E. (1985) *Pediatr Res* **19**:1201.
22. Rengo F, Trimarco B, Ricciardelli B, Volpe M, Violini R, Sacca L and Chiariello M. (1979) *J Pharmacol Exp Ther* **211**:686.
23. Porcelli RJ, Ventura DF, Mahoney WA and Bergofsky EH. (1981) *J Appl Physiol* **51**:1320.

24. Leffler CW, Mitchell JA and Green RS. (1984) *Circ Res* **55**:780.
25. Dennis DR and Schuster DP. (1986) *Amer Rev Respir Dis* **13**:A398.
26. Mammel MC, Edgren BE, Gordon MJ and Boros SJ. (1986) *Clin Res* **234**:153A.
27. Rubin LJ, Hughes JD and Lazar JD. (1985) *Am Rev Respir Dis* **132**:93.
28. Foster S, Garrett RC and Thomas HM. (1986) *Amer Rev Respir Dis* **133**:A226.
29. Holroyde MC. (1986) *Br J Pharmacol* **88**:395P.
30. Holroyde MC and Murphy IJ. (1986) *Br J Pharmacol* **88**:396P.
31. Kulik TJ, Schutjer RK, Howland DF and Lock JE. (1985) *Am J Physiol* **249**:H986.
32. Schnader J, Undem B, Adams K, Peters S and Sylvester J. (1986) *Amer Rev Respir Dis* **133**:A226.
33. Peter SP, Lichtenstein LM and Adkinson NF Jr. (1986) *J Pharmacol Exp Ther* **238**:8.
34. Lloyd TC Jr. (1970) *J Appl Physiol* **28**:566.
35. DeMey JG and Vanhoutte PM. (1982)*Circ Res* **51**:439.
36. Holden WE and McCall E. (1984) *Exp Lung Res* **7**:101.
37. Madden JA, Dawson CA and Harder DR. (1985) *J Appl Physiol* **49**:113.
38. Harder DR, Madden JA and Dawson C. (1985) *J Appl Physiol* **59**:1389.
39. Rubanyi GM and Vanhoutte PM. (1985) *J Physiol* **364**:45.
40. Hottenstein OO, Mitzner WA and Sylvester JT. (1984) *Fed Proc* **43**:923.
41. McMurtry IF. (1985) *Am J Physiol* **249**:H741.
42. Tolins M, Weir EK, Chesler E, Nelson CP and From AHL. (1986) *J Appl Physiol* **60**:942.
43. Haavik Nilsen K, Hauge A. (1968) *Acta Physiol Scand* **73**:111.
44. Zhu YJ, Kradin R, Brandstetter D, Staton G, Moss J and Hales CA. (1983) *J Appl Physiol* **54**:680.
45. Furchgott RF. (1983) *Circ Res* **553**:557.
46. Peach MJ, Singer HA and Loeb A. (1985) *Biochem Pharmacol* **34**:1867.
47. Vanhoutte PM, Rubanyi GM, Miller VM and Houston DS. (1986) *Ann Rev Physiol* **48**:307.
48. Hickey KA, Rubanyi G, Paul RJ and Highsmith RF. (1985) *Am J Physiol* **248**:C550.
49. O'Brien RF and McMurtry IF. (1984) *Amer Rev Respir Dis* **129**:A337.
50. Madden J, Dawson C, Gradall K and Harder D. (1986) *Fed Proc* **45**:277.
51. Boeynaems JM, Galand N and Ketelbant P. (1985) *J Clin Invest* **76**:7.
52. Forstermann U, Hertting G and Neufang B. (1986) *Br J Pharmacol* **87**:521.

53. McMurtry IF, Davidson AB, Reeves JT and Grover RF. (1976) *Circ Res* **38**:99.

54. Jones DP. (1986) *Ann Rev Physiol* **48**:33.

55. Hauge A. (1969) *Acta Physiol Scand* **76**:121.

56. Marshall C and Marshall B. (1983) *J Appl Physiol* **55**:711.

57. Chalazonitis N and Arvanitaki A. (1970) *Adv Biochem Psychopharmacol* **2**:245.

58. Sylvester JT and McGowan C. (1978) *Circ Res* **43**:429.

59. Chang S, Stearns R, Ortiz de Montellano PR and Voelkel NF. (1986) *Fed Proc* **45**:278.

60. Miller MA and Hales CA. (1979) *J Clin Invest* **64**:666.

61. Custer J, Zhu Y and Hales C. (1985) *Amer Rev Respir Dis* **131**:A399.

62. Aldrich TK, Fisher AB and Forman HJ. (1983) *J Appl Physiol* **54**:1089.

63. Stanbrook HS and McMurtry, IF. (1983) *J Appl Physiol* **55**:1467.

64. Erecinska M and Wilson DF. (1982) *J Membrane Biol* **70**:1.

65. Lloyd TC Jr. (1965) *J Appl Physiol* **20**:488.

66. Rounds S and McMurtry IF. (1981) *Circ Res* **48**:393.

67. Herget J and McMurtry IF. (1985) *Am J Physiol* **248**:H55.

68. Haas F, Foster WM and Bergofsky EH. (1975) *Prog Respir Res* **9**:273.

Mechanisms of Control of the Perinatal Pulmonary Circulation

SIDNEY CASSIN

Department of Physiology
College of Medicine
University of Florida
Gainesville, FL 32610

I.   INTRODUCTION

Successful adaptation to extrauterine life depends on necessary
maturational changes which occur during fetal life. Without these changes,
survival of healthy individuals during the newborn period would not be possible.
The two most important extrauterine adaptations that occur are: (a) interruption of
circulation through the placenta; and (b) expansion of the lungs with air. With
these events, the function of gas exchange is rerouted from the placenta to the
lungs, and there is a unique rearrangement of the circulation. Of prime importance
to the sequence of adaptive alterations that occur in the circulation at birth is the
nature of the pulmonary vasculature at this time and the changes that occur in
function when the lungs are ventilated.

In the transition from a liquid-breathing fetus to an air-breathing newborn,
pulmonary vascular resistance is decreased about 5-fold. Factors which may be
involved in this change in blood flow have been studied extensively (1-3);
however, the specific basic mechanisms by which these changes occur in the fetal
pulmonary circulation are not known.

It is now clear that the pulmonary vasculature of fetal animals is
exquisitely sensitive, not only to alterations in blood gases and pH, but to a
variety of vasoactive materials. Thus, over the last few years, we have

concentrated our efforts on evaluating the effects of vasoactive eicosanoids, precursors of prostaglandins and leukotrienes, metabolites of these compounds, and inhibitors of the cyclooxygenase and lipoxygenase pathways on the perinatal pulmonary circulation.

Table I lists the eicosanoids we have examined, as well as their relative vasoactive potencies in the fetal pulmonary circulation. Details of our studies for most of these substances have been presented elsewhere and are summarized to a large extent in prior reviews (4,5). This review will focus on our more recent work dealing with prostaglandin precursors, PGD_2, PGD_3, PGI_2, LTD_4, and the end organ antagonist FPL 57231.

TABLE 1. Responses of fetal pulmonary circulation to prostaglandins, precursors, metabolites and leukotrienes.

Agent	Effect	Relative activity	Species
D_2	Dilation	+++	Goats, Sheep
D_3	Dilation	++++	Sheep
E_I	Dilation	+++	Goats, Sheep
E_2	Dilation	++	Goats, Sheep
$F_{1\alpha}$	Constriction	++	Goats
$F_{2\alpha}$	Constriction	+++	Goats
I_2	Dilation	++++	Goats, Sheep
AA	Constriction	++	Goats, Sheep
DGLA	Constriction	++	Goats
ENDO I*	Constriction	+++	Goats
ENDO II**	Constriction	++	Goats
PGH_2	Dilation	++	Sheep
15-keto-PGE metabolite	No Effect		Goats
6-keto-$PGF_{1\alpha}$	Dilation	+	Goats
6-keto-PGE_1	Dilation	++	Goats
LTD_4	Constriction	++	Sheep

++++ = greatest activity; + = least activity
*   ENDO I = 9,11-dideoxy-11α,9α-epoxymethano-$PGF_{2\alpha}$
** ENDO II = 9,11-dideoxy-9α,11α,epoxymethano-$PGF_{2\alpha}$

II.   PRECURSORS OF PROSTAGLANDINS

A wide variety of body tissues (6) are capable of synthesizing, releasing, and metabolizing prostaglandins. A rather large tissue source of prostaglandins is found in the lungs (7). To evaluate the effects of infusions into the pulmonary circulation of several prostaglandin precursors and synthetic analogs of endoperoxide intermediates, studies have been carried out in adult and perinatal animals (8-13). Arachidonic acid and di-homo-gamma-linolenic acid were used as precursors of monoenoic and bisenoic prostaglandins. Infusions of either arachidonic acid or dihomo-gamma-linolenic acid directly into the perinatal pulmonary circulation always produced an increase in pulmonary vascular resistance, which was associated with systemic hypotension (13). Dose dependent increases in pulmonary vascular resistance were seen over a range of 2 - 1000 μg/kg/min with either of these compounds. These results, however, are not totally in accord with other data published on the effects of arachidonic acid on the pulmonary circulation of adult animals. Thus, it has been reported that intrapulmonary arterial bolus injections of arachidonate in dogs (8,10), cats (14), and monkeys (15) produced an increase in pulmonary vascular resistance. In contrast to these studies, Mullane et $al.$ (15) showed that intravenous infusions of arachidonic acid resulted in reduced pulmonary arterial pressures in dogs. To further complicate matters, Hyman et $al.$ (11) showed that infusions of arachidonate may cause either increases or decreases in the adult feline pulmonary vascular resistance. It is interesting that investigators reporting an increase in pulmonary vascular resistance following arachidonate infusion into the pulmonary circulation have suggested that there are increases in the concentration of PGE_2 and $PGF_{2\alpha}$ in pulmonary venous blood. Both of these substances are constrictors of the adult pulmonary circulation (10). In contrast, the investigators reporting a decrease in pulmonary vascular resistance have suggested that there is an increased production of prostacyclin-like material (15).

Gerber et $al.$ (12) reported that infusion of arachidonic acid into the pulmonary circulation resulted in a release of PGI_2, which reversed the pulmonary pressor response to hypoxia. In fetal and newborn goats and sheep, infusion of arachidonic acid results in pulmonary hypertension and systemic hypotension. Although all of the products of exogenous arachidonic acid metabolism have not been identified in the sheep or goat perinatal pulmonary vasculature, it is conceivable that similar substances to those seen in adults are produced. In perfused fetal rabbit lungs close to term (31 days gestation), archidonic acid is converted primarily to PGE_2 and its metabolites (mainly, 15-keto metabolites); however, fairly high levels of $PGF_{2\alpha}$ and TXB_2 are present (16). Friedman et $al.$ (17) have shown that fetal lamb lung microsomes are capable of producing PGE_2,

PGI_2, and TXA_2 enzymatically from PGH_2. Prostacyclin synthetase exhibited enzyme saturation at low levels of PGH_2, and resulted in low output of PGI_2 throughout gestation. Thromboxane synthetase showed low activity when PGH_2 was in low concentration; but at high concentration (400 mg PGH_2/250 µg lung homogenate protein), thromboxanes were a major product of prostaglandin synthesis in late term fetal lung. The product formed in greatest quantities from PGH_2 by fetal lamb lung homogenates was PGE_2. McNamara et al. (18) reported that PGE_2 formation by fetal goat lung homogenates was enhanced by GSH. Thus, it appears that endogenous levels of GSH in fetal lung may exert an importantcontrol over products of PGH_2 metabolism, with greater amounts of thromboxanes formed in the absence of GSH and more PGE_2 formed in its presence (18). Factors involved in the regulation of GSH in fetal lung are presently unknown.

It is clear at this time that pulmonary vascular responses of the fetal and neonatal animal to metabolites of arachidonic acid may, in fact, be different in many instances from those responses reported for adult animals of the same and other species. Thus, PGE_2 is a dilator of the fetal pulmonary circulation and a constrictor of the adult pulmonary circulation (19). Since $PGF_{1\alpha}$ and $PGF_{2\alpha}$ are reported as constrictors of the perinatal pulmonary circulation, one might be tempted to explain the effects of arachidonic acid and di-homo-gamma-linolenic acid as being due to a release of the F-series prostaglandins. However, $PGF_{1\alpha}$ and $PGF_{2\alpha}$ are constrictors of the systemic circulation, while the precursors produce systemic hypotension. Thus, it becomes obvious that one cannot explain the divergent effects of precursors on the pulmonary and systemic circulations by means of a single prostaglandin. One might, however, consider the possibility that pivotal endoperoxides per se (20,21) might produce vasoconstriction in the lungs and subsequently be converted to dilator prostaglandins, which in turn could have a systemic hypotensive effect. In order to test these possibilities, Tyler et al. (13) used synthetic analogs of the cyclic endoperoxides (Table I). These analogs are pressors in the pulmonary circulation, but are not metabolized by the lung (as is authentic PGH_2) and are, therefore, pressors in the systemic circulation also. More recent studies have provided evidence that these PGH_2 analogs are, in fact, selective TXA_2 mimetics (22).

To further evaluate the possibility that endoperoxides could cause vasoconstriction in the lung and be converted to dilator agents, we (23) infused authentic PGH_2 (0.24 - 0.61 µg/kg) directly into the pulmonary arteries of six unventilated fetal lambs. PGH_2 was prepared from arachidonic acid, isolated, and purified as described by Egan et al. (24) and She et al. (25). The infusions produced decreases in pulmonary vascular resistance of 10% - 21%. The fall was rapid in onset, reaching a peak 10 seconds after injection and returning to baseline within 35 seconds. Similar infusions in ventilated mature fetal lambs result in increases in pulmonary vascular resistance. The pulmonary pressor response to PGH_2 in the ventilated fetus was reduced by about 50% when the thromboxane synthetase inhibitor OKY 1581 (Ono Company, Japan) was used. These data suggest a metabolism of PGH_2 to dilator PG's before ventilation and to constrictor PG's as well as thromboxanes after ventilation, and/or direct effects of PGH_2 on vascular smooth muscle that is dependent on existing vascular smooth muscle tone. To eliminate the possibility of platelet involvement (aggregation or thromboxane release) in the pressor response to arachidonic acid, we (26) perfused isolated lamb lungs with Krebs solution and obtained a pressor response when arachidonate was added. Resolution of the divergent responses to arachidonic acid and PGH_2 on the pulmonary circulation of the fetal lamb is still incomplete. Thus, analyses of pulmonary venous concentrations of 6-keto-$PGF_{1\alpha}$ and TXB_2 were made (27) before and after infusions of arachidonic acid directly into the pulmonary artery (200 $\mu g/kg/min$). The data indicated a significant increase in thromboxane B_2 (64% above control levels) after injection. Although there was a small increase in the pulmonary venous plasma concentration of 6-keto-$PGF_{1\alpha}$ following arachidonic acid infusion, the increment was not statistically significant.

Recently, we investigated the effects of hypoxia on the arachidonic acid-induced increment in pulmonary vascular resistance in ventilated fetal and neonatal lambs (28). Infusion of arachidonic acid in the fetus resulted in a greater pressor response during hypoxia than during normoxia. In contrast, the pulmonary vascular effects of arachidonic acid in the newborn are unaltered by hypoxia.

The pressor response to arachidonic acid alone in the fetus or newborn is blocked by indomethacin or meclofenamate and is diminished by a thromboxane synthetase inhibitor (OKY 1581). In contrast, there are no significant differences in the hypoxic pulmonary pressor response of lambs with and without thromboxane synthetase inhibition (29). Thus, the pulmonary response to arachidonic acid involves, at least to some extent, the cyclooxygenase metabolite thromboxane. However, the pressor response to hypoxia does not involve cyclooxygenase metabolites directly. The vasoconstriction of hypoxia may, in turn, cause release of dilator agents such as PGI_2. This would account for the increased pressor response to hypoxia following indomethacin. With infusion of arachidonic acid in either unventilated or ventilated fetal and newborn lambs, there is an associated systemic hypotension. It is unlikely that the products of the lipoxygenase pathway are involved in this response, since leukotrienes A_4, B_4, C_4, D_4, and E_4 appear to be constrictors in adult lungs of guinea pigs and monkeys (30), and leukotriene D_4 is a potent constrictor of the neonatal lamb circulation (31). If, in fact, the leukotrienes were involved, one might anticipate a marked pressor response to pulmonary arterial infusion of arachidonate following administration of indomethacin or meclofenamate.

III.   PROSTAGLANDINS OF THE D-SERIES

Prostaglandin D_2 was originally described as being biologically inactive (32). In 1975, Hamberg *et al.* (33) described vasopressor responses to PGD_2 as well as bronchoconstrictor activity in guinea pigs. Since then, several studies have demonstrated that PGD_2 acts to constrict the adult canine pulmonary circulation (34-36) and causes contraction of isolated bovine and canine pulmonary vessels (37). As a result of the above data, we attempted to use PGD_2 to elevate the pulmonary vascular resistance in an experimentally dilated fetal pulmonary circulation. Much to our surprise, we managed only to produce a further dilatation. Thus, we investigated the action of this primary prostaglandin in the perinatal pulmonary circulation (38). With infusions of PGD_2 directly into the pulmonary artery of the isolated perfused lower left lobe of fetal (0.9 - 1.0 gestation) animals, we obtained a dose related decrease in pulmonary vascular resistance. Over the range of infusions used (0.05 µg/kg/min - 70 µg/kg/min) we always noted pulmonary vasodilation with approximately a 45% decrease at 70 µg/kg/min. In those aminals receiving indomethacin prior to PGD_2, the response to similar doses was even greater. Thus, the following are dose response regression curves for the fetal animals:

control: % ΔPVR = - 8.73 (log dose) – 28.37
                      r = 0.70; P < 0.0001

indomethacin: % ΔPVR = -19.49 (log dose) – 46.76
                      r = 0.83; P < 0.01

In newborn animals (1 - 12 days old), we noted a biphasic response, with dilation occuring at infusions of 2.5 µg/kg/min or less. However, at infusion rates of greater than 8 µg/kg/min, we noted only a pulmonary pressor response. With infusions of 0.03 - 4.29 µg/kg/min in three adult animals, we always saw a pulmonary pressor response (4% - 64% increment in pulmonary vascular resistance). Of additional interest is the fact that we did not observe any significant systemic hypotension in any of the three groups studied. This is very important, in view of the systemic hypotensive effect seen with other pulmonary vasodilators in the perinatal period (39,40,41).

Mechanisms for the age-related divergent responses of the pulmonary circulation to prostaglandin D_2 are not known. It is possible that these differences are due to: (a) an increase in smooth muscle and tone in the fetal pulmonary circulation; (b) differences in the number and type of prostaglandin D_2 receptors in the perinatal and adult lung; and (c) differences in the enzymatic conversion of PGD_2 to $PGF_{2\alpha}$ in the perinatal and adult pulmonary and systemic circulations. It is conceivable that "dilator receptors" in the newborn have a greater affinity for PGD_2 than "constrictor receptors." Thus, one would anticipate that at low concentrations of PGD_2, the "dilator receptors" would bind to the drug to a greater extent than "constrictor receptors." As the concentration of PGD_2 increased, "dilator receptors" would become saturated, and more drug would be bound to the "constrictor receptors." As of this time, studies concerned with receptor mechanisms for PGD_2 in the perinatal pulmonary circulation have not been carried out.

PGD_2 is apparently released in very small amounts by homogenates of fetal pulmonary arteries (42), and also from Krebs-perfused perinatal lungs of sheep and goats (43). However, this material appears to selectively dilate the pulmonary circulation of fetal lambs and goats. For this reason, it was recommended as a potentially useful agent in the treatment of persistent pulmonary hypertension in the newborn (38). However, since we had infused PGD_2 directly into the left pulmonary artery below the ductus, we were concerned that this would provide an obstacle to its clinical use. As a result, we carried out a series of experiments designed to evaluate the hemodynamic effects of postpulmonary infusion of the drug in fetal animals. Thus, 18 one-minute infusions of PGD_2 at various doses into the left atrium of five fetal lambs produced a dose-dependent decrease in pulmonary vascular resistance. Again, there was no systemic hypotension. If any change occurred, it was an increase in systemic arterial pressure and heart rate with the left atrial infusion (44). These data showed that exposure of the systemic circulation to PGD_2 prior to its entering the pulmonary vasculature does not modify the preferential pulmonary dilator action, nor does it produce significant hypotension. Drummond et al. confirmed that PGD_2 in newborn lambs is a moderate systemic pressor agent. However, these authors also suggested that PGD_2 is a cardiac depressant (45). In contrast, Uemura et al. suggested that PGD_2 has a positive inotropic effect on the newborn (4 - 7 days) rabbit heart (46).

In contrast to the biphasic response to PGD_2, which we reported, Lock et al. (47) found only a pulmonary pressor response to PGD_2 in newborn sheep (6 - 26 days of age), whether they were normoxic or hypoxic. Other studies (48-50) have corroborated our data, demonstrating that PGD_2 is a dilator in ventilated, near term fetal and newly born lambs. A recent paper by Soifer et al. (51) on newborn lambs (1 - 30 days of age), chronically instrumented, made hypoxic, and treated with PGD_2, has provided further evidence of an age-related effect of this drug.

Recently, some interest has been shown in the prostaglandin D metabolite of eicosapentanoic acid, prostaglandin D_3. Thus, studies have demonstrated that prostaglandin D is an inhibitor of platelet aggregation and a pulmonary pressor agent (52,36). Since similar properties were attributed to PGD_2, we decided to evaluate PGD_3 on the fetal pulmonary circulation. Although PGD_3 behaves qualitatively like PGD_2 as a dilator of the fetal pulmonary circulation, it is quantitatively more powerful than PGD_2. Also, PGD_3, like PGD_2, has the property in fetal animals of not decreasing systemic pressure when injected into the pulmonary circulation. We demonstrated a dose-dependent decrease in pulmonary vascular resistance over the range of 0.1 - 5 $\mu g/kg/min$, with one-minute infusions of PGD_3. In contrast to PGD_2, which produced a decrease in pulmonary vascular resistance of 36% with an infusion of 5 $\mu g/kg/min$, PGD_3 produced close to a 60% reduction in pulmonary vascular resistance at this dose. Thus, we suggest further animal and clinical evaluation of this compound for its potential use in persistent pulmonary hypertension.

IV.   LEUKOTRIENES

Leukotrienes are a family of local hormones derived from arachidonic acid via the 5-lipoxygenase pathway, rather than through the cyclooxygenase system. Leukotrienes have a conjugated triene structure, and a peptide chain containing 1-3 amino acid residues, attached by way of a sulphur atom to carbon atom 5. The "slow reacting substance" of anaphylaxis (53,54) has now been identified as a mixture of several leukotrienes.

Kadowitz and Hyman (55) have analyzed the responses of leukotriene D_4 in the adult sheep and cat. While LTD_4 is a powerful constrictor of the ovine pulmonary circulation, it is a relatively modest constrictor of the pulmonary vascular bed of the cat. These investigators concluded that the vasoconstrictor effect of leukotriene D_4 is partly due to direct effect, but also was dependent on formation of cyclooxygenase products, including thromboxane. They also suggested that the increase in pulmonary vascular resistance was a result of an intrapulmonary venous constriction. In contrast to its moderate feline pulmonary vasoconstrictor activity, LTD_4 was found to be a vasodilator or relaxant of canine renal and superior mesenteric arteries (56). Morganroth et al. (57) hypothesized that the leukotrienes were involved in the hypoxic pulmonary vasoconstrictor response. As a result, these investigators evaluated, in isolated perfused rat lungs, the effects of structurally unrelated antagonists of leukotriene synthesis or receptors (diethylcarbamazine citrate, U-60257, and FPL 55712). All three of the these compounds blocked the pressor response to hypoxia in this particular preparation.

Recently, interest has turned towards the role of leukotrienes in the fetal and neonatal period. Saeed and Mitchell (58) provided suggestive evidence that lipoxygenase activity is present in human fetal lungs of 12 - 18 weeks gestational age. More recently, Stenmark et al. (59) demonstrated the presence of leukotrienes (LTC_4 and LTD_4) in lung lavage fluid of human neonates with persistent pulmonary hypertension. Lavage fluid obtained from ventilated infants without neonatal pulmonary hypertension did not have these substances present. Yokochi et al. (31) demonstrated that LTD_4 is a powerful vasoconstrictor of the pulmonary and systemic circulation of newborn lambs.

These studies were followed by an interesting series of investigations by Leffler et al. (60), in which experiments were carried out on mechanically ventilated neonatal piglets (with a constant left pulmonary arterial blood flow) on the effects of LTD_4, leukotriene synthesis inhibitors, and leukotriene receptor antagonists. LTD_4 (100 - 10,000 ng IV) caused a dose-dependent increase in pulmonary and systemic vascular resistance. These investigators were unable to show any alteration in baseline cardiovascular parameters following treatment with diethylcarbamazine, nordihydroguaiaretic acid, or FPL 55712. Similarly, they were unable to show any effect of treatment with these compounds on the hypoxic pulmonary pressor response. Although, in this particular study, all of the cardiovascular responses to LTD_4 were blocked by continuous infusions of 100 μg/kg/min of FPL 55712, this concentration of the putative receptor antagonist may not have been large enough to block the pressor response to hypoxia.

More recently, Shreiber et al. (61) evaluated the effects of FPL 57231, another putative leukotriene receptor antagonist, in newborn lambs subjected to hypoxic pulmonary vasoconstriction. Studies were carried out on spontaneously breathing unanesthetized newborn lambs, varying from 3 to 7 days of age. When FPL 57231 was infused intravenously (1 mg/kg/min) during the hypoxic pressor response, the response was diminished to control or normoxic levels. These authors have, therefore, suggested that leukotrienes play a significant role in the mediation of the hypoxic pressor response.

Subsequent studies by Soifer et al. (62), in six fetal lambs with catheters chronically implanted (130 - 134 days gestation), showed that FPL 55712 reduced pulmonary vascular resistance by some 45%. In six other fetal lambs studied at 130 - 140 days, FPL 57231 decreased pulmonary vascular resistance by 87%. As a result of these studies, it was suggested that the leukotrienes may play a role in the normal physiological control of the fetal pulmonary circulation.

Recently, we also investigated the effects of LTD_4 and the putative leukotriene end-organ antagonist FPL 57231 on the fetal pulmonary circulation.

The studies were carried out in 24 fetal lambs which were delivered by cæsarian section from chloralose-anesthetized ewes; the fetuses were prevented from breathing. Measurements were made of pulmonary arterial pressure, left atrial pressure, pulmonary blood flow, systemic arterial pressure, and heart rate. Bolus injections of LTD_4 in this preparation (0.1 to 10 µg) into the left pulmonary artery produced dose-dependent increases in pulmonary vascular resistance. On the other hand, administration of the FPL 57231 produced dose-dependent decreases in pulmonary vascular resistance in the fetal state (% ΔPVR = -29.4 – 31.27 log dose [mg/kg]). We appraised the effectiveness of FPL 57231 as a blocker of the LTD_4 vasoconstriction by evaluating the doses of FPL 57231 necessary to inhibit the pressor response to LTD_4, which was given over a range of 0.3 to 10 µg. With bolus injections of 4.35 to 9.80 mg/kg of FPL 57231, we were able to achieve an 82%-100% reduction in the PVR increase produced by LTD_4. However, on further investigation, it became apparent that FPL 57231 may not be a specific blocker of the leukotriene pressor response. The endoperoxide (PGH_2) analog (9,11-dideoxy-11α,9α-epoxymethano-prostaglandin $F_{2\alpha}$) is a powerful pressor agent and thought to be a mimic of thromboxane [22]) in the perinatal pulmonary circulation. Response to infusion of this agent is also blocked by FPL 57231. Doses of FPL 57231 used to produce inhibition of the LTD_4 pressor response were also seen to produce a 67% - 79% reduction in the pressor response to the endoperoxide. Similarly, we were able to demonstrate that the pressor response to phenylephrine could be reduced by some 72% with doses generally used to reduce responses to LTD_4. Thus, it was concluded that, although FPL 57231 may block endogenous leukotrienes in the fetal pulmonary circulation, this compound may not be entirely specific for leukotrienes.

Recently, it has been suggested that FPL 55712 and its analog 57231 have other pharmacologic actions and are thus not specific leukotriene antagonists (63). Also, evidence is presented by Foster et al. (64) that the pulmonary pressor response to hypoxia in dogs is not reduced by complete blockade of both cyclooxygenase and lipoxygenase systems with BW 755C, an analog of phenidone, which has been studied extensively (65).

Other related experiments lead one to believe that leukotrienes per se are not responsible for the pulmonary pressor response to hypoxia and/or the high pulmonary vascular resistance of the fetus. Thus, Naeije et al. (66) were unable to confirm the finding of Morganroth et al. (57) in the dog, namely, that diethylcarbamazine inhibits hypoxic pulmonary vasoconstriction. Furthermore, interpretations of these data are complicated by side effects of the agents used, which may also influence vasoconstriction. Thus, diethylcarbamazine has calcium-dependent depressant effects on the myocardium (67) and nicotine-like effects on the pulmonary and systemic circulations (68).

Investigations in the area of leukotrienes and leukotriene antagonists are currently the most exciting information to have surfaced in the last few years, with regard to control of the pulmonary circulation in the fetal state in health and disease. Clearly, they deserve further investigation.

V. EFFECTS OF PROSTACYCLIN

The discovery of thromboxanes (72,73) and prostacyclin (PGI_2) (74-76) are recent landmarks in eicosanoid research. Thromboxane A_2 causes platelet aggregation and vasoconstriction, whereas prostacyclin is a powerful vasodilator and inhibitor of platelet aggregation. These two substances are probably responsible for maintenance of normal vascular integrity, as well as production of atheromatous plaques (77).

Actions of PGI_2 as a vasodilator have been described for the pulmonary circulation of adult dogs (78) and cats (79). Dilator material(s) appear to be released from the lungs following tissue distortion or distension (69). Also, PGI_2 has been shown to be released from lungs following hyperventilation (70). In addition, Terragno and coworkers (80,81) and Remuzzi et al. (82) have shown that prostacyclin is a major prostaglandin produced in vitro by fetal blood vessels, including the pulmonary artery. These data and our own research — which established that following cyclooxygenase inhibition there was: (a) an augmentation of the pressor response to $PGF_{2\alpha}$ and hypoxia; and (b) a depression of the pulmonary vasodilation that occurs normally with initiation of breathing (83) — suggested to us that at the time of ventilation of fetal lungs, endogenous dilator prostaglandins (probably of the E- and I-series) were released. Since our studies, Leffler et al. (71) demonstrated that there was indeed production of PGI_2 by the newly ventilated lungs. In 1981, Leffler and Hessler (43) demonstrated that Krebs-perfused lungs of fetal lambs and goats after ventilation increased production of 6-keto-$PGF_{1\alpha}$ and 6,15-diketo[13,14-dihydro]$PGF_{1\alpha}$ (hydrolyzed metabolite of PGI_2 by 50% and 230%, respectively. Although the relative values obtained for PGI_2 concentrations in these studies before and after ventilation clearly substantiate that PGI_2 is released from fetal lungs which are ventilated, the values were apparently abnormally high. Thus, Leffler et al. (84) investigated the effects of the stress of anesthesia, surgery and exteriorization on fetal pulmonary arterial levels of PGI_2. They found that, in animals with indwelling cathers, in situ and without anesthesia: (a) pulmonary arterial plasma levels of 6-keto-$PGF_{1\alpha}$ were approximately 1 mg/ml at the conclusion of surgery, in contrast to 43 mg/ml in exteriorized anesthetized fetal goats subjected to extensive surgery; and (b) three days after surgery, 6-keto-PGF$_{1\alpha}$ had decreased to about 1/2 the value at the conclusion of surgery.

Additional supportive evidence for the importance of PGI$_2$ as a regulatory agent of pulmonary blood flow has been provided recently (85). In unanesthetized, *in utero* fetal lambs and goats with cannulæ implanted (in the pulmonary artery and vein) and flow cuffs on the pulmonary artery, prostacyclin production increased from an undetectable level to 30 ± 12.3 µg/kg/min when fetuses were delivered (0.95 term) and began spontaneous ventilation. The mechanism of PGI$_2$ production in response to ventilation seems to be related to distortion or stress of pulmonary tissue with alveolar distension, rather than to the composition of the inspired gas (86).

Furthermore, PGI$_2$ appears to be the major metabolite of arachidonic acid in fetal lamb pulmonary artery homogenate (87-89). Because of its endogenous release by the lungs and its potential significance in regulating pulmonary vascular tone, we studied the effects of infusions of PGI$_2$, as well as its metabolites 6-keto-PGF$_{1\alpha}$ and 6-keto-PGE$_1$, on pulmonary and systemic circulation of perinatal goats and sheep (89-91). PGI$_2$ infusions directly into the left pulmonary arterial circulation resulted in dose-dependent decreases in pulmonary vascular resistance and mean systemic arterial pressure. Two-minute infusions produced more pronounced decreases in pulmonary vascular resistance than did 1-minute infusions. Species variability was also noted with pulmonary depressor response in fetal goats, greater than that in fetal lambs. Since PGI$_2$ is not well metabolized by fetal or adult lungs (89,92), and its metabolites are vasoactive, systemic hypotensive responses and increases in heart rate were noted in both species. In our studies (90), PGI$_2$ was found to be the most powerful dilator of the fetal pulmonary circulation, followed by PGE$_1$ and PGE$_2$. Similar data have been described for the adult pulmonary circulation (79). However, these data are in contrast to those of Leffler and Hessler (93), who reported that PGE$_1$ was a more powerful dilator than either PGE$_2$ or PGI$_2$. Confirmatory data on the dilator properties of PGI$_2$ in the circulation system have been presented by Lock *et al.* (47) for newborn lambs, and Starling *et al.* for neonatal swine (94). A subsequent study by Starling *et al.* (95) in neonatal swine with elevated pulmonary vascular resistance suggests that PGI$_2$ is a better dilator than PGE$_1$ or tolazoline. In 1980, Lock *et al.* (96) evaluated effects of three prostaglandin I$_2$ analogs and found that each had pulmonary and systemic vasodilator effects. Although PGI$_2$ and its metabolites produce not only a pulmonary but systemic effect, it appeared that the pulmonary dilator effects exceed systemic effects. As a result, Lock *et al.* (97) used PGI$_2$ in the treatment of persistent pulmonary hypertension in a single human neonate. Although the results of his effort are variously described as "quite encouraging" (98) or "very successfully treated" (41), we were quite concerned with the approach because of potential systemic hypotension (99).

Clinical collaborative efforts were initiated (100) in which PGI$_2$ was to be evaluated (along with other agents) in children with persistent fetal circulation. Of 13 severely hypoxemic infants treated with PGI$_2$, 5 responded, 8 showed no significant response, and only 2 survived. In their review of pulmonary vasodilator agents, Drummond and Lock (41) conclude that PGI$_2$ can be very effective in some cases, but a large percentage of infants with pulmonary vasoconstriction will be unresponsive and at high risk for complications. It is reasonable to assume that because of its complex and multi-etiologic nature, one drug or therapy is not likely to be uniformly effective (101).

REFERENCES

1. Dawes GS, Mott JC and Widdicombe JG. (1954) *J Physiol* **126**:563.
2. Cassin S, Dawes GS, Mott JC *et al.* (1964) *J Physiol* **171**:61.
3. Gilbert RD, Hessler JR, Eitzman DV and Cassin S. (1972) *J Appl Physiol* **32**:47.
4. Cassin S. (1981) *In* **Platelets and Prostaglandins in Cardiovascular Disease.** (J Mehta and Mehta, eds) Futura:Mount Kisco, New York.
5. Cassin S. (1983) *In* **Developmental Pharmacology. Progress in Clinical and Biological Research.** (SM MacLeod, AB Okey and SP Spielberg, eds) Vol. 135. Alan R. Liss, Inc:New York.
6. Katz RL and Katz GJ. (1974) *Anesthesiology* **40**:471.
7. Pike J. (1971) *Sci Amer* **225**:84.
8. Wicks FC, Rose JC, Johnson M *et al.* (1976) *Circ Res* **38**:167.
9. Wicks, FC, Ramwell, PW, Rose, JC *et al.* (1977) *J Pharmacol Exp Ther* **201**:417.
10. Hyman AL, Mathe AA, Matthews CC *et al.* (1978) *J Pharmacol Exp Ther* **207**:388.
11. Hyman AL, Chapnick BM, and Kadowitz PJ. (1980) *Am J Physiol* **239**:H40.
12. Gerber JG, Voelkel N, Nies AS *et al.* (1980) *J Appl Physiol* **49**:107.
13. Tyler TL, Leffler CW and Cassin S. (1978) *Prostaglandins Med* **1**:213.
14. Hyman AL, Chapnick BM, Kadowitz PJ *et al.* (1977) *Proc Natl Acad Sci USA* **12**:5711.
15. Mullane KM, Dusting GJ, Solmon JA *et al.* (1979) *Eur J Pharmacol* **54**:217.
16. Simberg N and Uotila P. (1983) *Prostaglandins* **25**:629.

17.   Friedman WF, Printz MF, Skidgel RA *et al.* (1983) *In* **Prostaglandins and the Cardiovascular System.** (JA Oates, ed) Raven Press:New York.

18.   McNamara DB, Laird M, Hyman AL *et al.* (1982) *Fed Proc* **41**:1251.

19.   Cassin S, Tyler TL, Leffler CW *et al.* (1979) *Am J Physiol* **236**:H828.

20.   Kadowitz PJ, Gruetter CA, McNamara DB *et al.* (1977) *J Appl Physio.* **42**:953.

21.   Bowers RE, Ellis EF, Brigham KL *et al.* (1979) *Clin Invest* **63**:131.

22.   Coleman, RA, Humphrey, PPA, Kennedy, I *et al.* (1981) *Br J Pharmacol* **73**:773.

23.   Tod ML, Cassin S, McNamara DB *et al.* (1986) *Ped Res* **20**:565.

24.   Egan RW, Paxton J and Kuehl FA Jr. (1976) *J Biol Chem* **251**:7329.

25.   She HS, McNamara DB, Spannhake EW *et al.* (1981) *Prostaglandins* **21**:531.

26.   Leffler CW, Green RS, Jerkins RV *et al.* (1984) *Prost Leuko Med* **15**:115.

27.   Cassin S and Tod ML. (1985) *In* **The Physiological Development of the Fetus and Newborn.** (CP Jones and PW Nathanielsz, eds) Academic Press:London.

28.   Tod ML and Cassin S. (1984) *J Appl Physiol* **57**:977.

29.   Tod ML and Cassin S. (1985) *J Appl Physiol* **58**:710.

30.   Hedqvist P, Dahlen SE and Bjork J. (1982) *In* **Advances in Prostaglandin, Thromboxane, and Leukotriene Research.** (B Samuelsson and R Paoletti, eds) Raven Press:New York, Vol 9 [Leukotrienes and Other Lipoxygenase Products].

31.   Yokochi K, Olley PM, Sideris E *et al.* (1982) *In* **Advances in Prostaglandin, Thromboxane, and Leukotriene Research.** (B Samuelsson and R Paoletti eds) Raven Press:New York, Vol 9 [Leukotrienes and Other Lipoxygenase Products].

32.   Nugteren DH and Hazelhof E. (1973) *Biochim Biophys Acta* **326**:448.

33.   Hamberg MP, Hedqvist K, Strandberg P *et al.* (1975) *Life Sci* **16**:451.

34.   Kadowitz PJ, Spannhake EW, Greenberg S *et al.* (1977) *Can J Physiol Pharmacol* **55**:1369.

35.   Wasserman MA, Du Charme DW, Griffen RL *et al.* (1977) *Prostaglandins* **13**:255.

36.   Wendling MG and Du Charme DW. (1981) *Prostaglandins* **22**:235.

37.   Gruetter CA, McNamara DB, Hyman AL *et al.* (1978) *Am J Physiol* **234**:H139.

38.   Cassin S, Tod ML, Philips J *et al.* (1981) *Am J Physiol* **240**:H755.

39.   Cassin S, Tyler TL, Leffler CW *et al.* (1979) *Am J Physiol* **236**:H828.

40.   Cassin S, Winikor I, Tod ML *et al.* (1981) *Pediatr Pharmacol* **1**:197.

41. Drummond WH and Lock JE. (1984) *Dev Pharmacol Ther* **7**:1.
42. Printz MP, Friedman WF and Skidgel PA. (1983) *In* **Advances in Prostaglandin, Thromboxane, and Leukotriene Research** [B. Samuelsson, R Paoletti and PW Ramwell, eds) Vol 12. Raven Press:New York.
43. Leffler CW and Hessler JR. (1981) *Am J Physiol* **241**:H756.
44. Gause GE, Tod ML and Cassin S. (1985) *Proc Soc Exp Biol Med* **179**:373.
45. Drummond WH, Shrager HH, Dailey WA *et al.* (1984) *Ped Res* **18**:152A.
46. Uemura S, Nakanishi T, Matsuoka S *et al.* (1984) *Ped Res* **18**:1277.
47. Lock JE, Olley PM and Coceani F. (1980) *Am J Physiol* **238**:H631.
48. Soifer SJ, Morin FC III and Heymann MA. (1982) *Pediatrics* **100**:458.
49. Philips JB III, Lyrene RK, McDevitt M *et al.* (1983) *J Appl Physiol* **54**:1585
50. Sideris EB, Yokochi K, Van Helder T *et al.* (1983) *In* **Advances in Prostaglandin, Thromboxane, and Leukotriene Research.** (B Samuelsson, R Paoletti and PW Ramwell, eds) Vol 12. Raven Press:New York.
51. Soifer SJ, Morin FC III, Kaslow V *et al.* (1983) *J Dev Physiol* **5**:237.
52. Whitaker MO, Wyche A, Fitzpatrick F *et al.* (1979) *Proc Nat Acad Sci USA* **76**:5919.
53. Hedqvist P, Dahlen SE and Bjork J. (1982) *In* **Advances in Prostaglandin, Thromboxane, and Leukotriene Research.** (B Samuelsson and R Paoletti, eds), Vol 9 [Leukotrienes and Other Lipoxygenase Products]. Raven Press:New York.
54. Piper PJ. (1984) *Physiol Revs* **64**:744.
55. Kadowitz PJ and Hyman AL. (1984) *Circ Res* **55**:707.
56. Secrest RJ, Olson EJ and Chapnick BM. (1985) *Circ Res* **57**:323.
57. Morganroth ML, Reeves JT, Murphy RC *et al.* (1984) *J Appl Physiol:* **56**:1340.
58. Saeed SA and Mitchell MD. (1982) *Eur J Pharmacol* **78**:389.
59. Stenmark KR, James SL, Voelkel N *et al.* (1983) *N Engl J Med* **309**:77.
60. Leffler CW, Mitchell JA and Green RS. (1984) *Circ Res* **55**:780.
61. Schreiber MD, Heymann MA and Soifer SJ. (1985) *Ped Res* **19**:437.
62. Soifer SJ, Loitz RD, Roman C *et al.* (1985) *Am J Physiol* **249**:H570.
63. Weichman BM, Wasserman MA, Holden DA *et al.* (1983) *J Pharmacol Exp Ther* **227**:700.
64. Foster S, Garett RC and Thomas HM III. (1986) *Am Rev Respir Dis* **133**(4):A226.
65. Higgs GA and Vane JR. (1983) *Br Med Bull* **39**:265.

66. Naeije R, Leeman M, and Lejeune P. (1986) *Bull Eur Physiopathol Respir* **22**:75.

67. Ojewole JA and Onejeme IV. (1983) *Eur J Pharmacol* **87**:245.

68. Abartey AK and Parrat JR Jr. (1976) *Br J Pharmacol* **56**:219.

69. Edmonds JF, Berry E and Wyllie JH. (1969) *Br J Surg* **56**:622.

70. Gryglewski RJ, Korbut R and Ocetkiewiez A. (1978) *Nature* **273**:765.

71. Leffler CW, Hessler JR and Terragno NA. (1980) *Am J Physiol* **238**:H282.

72. Hambery M, Svensson J and Samuelsson B. (1974) *Proc Nat Acad Sci USA* **71**:3824.

73. Hambery M, Svensson J, and Samuelsson B. (1975) *Proc Nat Acad Sci USA* **72**:2994.

74. Gryglewski RJ, Bunting S, Moncada S *et al.* (1976) *Prostaglandins* **12**:685.

75. Moncada S, Gryglewsski R, Bunding S *et al.* (1976) *Nature* **263**:663.

76. Johnson RA, Morton DR, Kinner JH *et al.* (1976) *Prostaglandins* **12**:915.

77. Moncada, S. (1982) *Br J Pharmacol* **76**:3.

78. Kadowitz PJ, Chapnick BM, Feigen LP *et al.* (1978) *J Appl Physiol* **45**:408.

79. Hyman AL and Kadowitz PJ. (1979) *Circ Res* **45**:404.

80. Terragno NA and Terragno A. (1979) *ed Proc* **38**:75.

81. Terragno NA, Terragno A, McGiff JC *et al.* (1977) *Prostaglandins* **14**:721.

82. Remuzzi G, Misiani R, Muratore D *et al.* (1979) *Prostaglandins* **18**:341.

83. Leffler CW, Tyler TL and Cassin S. (1978) *Am J Physiol* **234**:H346.

84. Leffler CW, Hessler JR and Green RS. (1982) *Prostaglandins* **24**:387.

85. Leffler CW, Hessler JR and Green RS. (1984) *Ped Res* **18**:938.

86. Leffler CW, Hessler JR and Green RS. (1984) *Prostaglandins* **28**:877.

87. Printz MP, Friedman WF and Skidgel PA. (1983) *In* **Advances in Prostaglandin, Thromboxane, and Leukotriene Research** (B Samuelsson, R Paoletti and PW Ramwell, eds) Vol 12. Raven Press:New York.

88. Skidgel PA, Friedman WF and Printz MP. (1983) *Ped Res* **18**:12.

89. Cassin S, Winikor I and Tod ML. (1978) *Physiologist* **21**:17.

90. Cassin S, Winikor I, Tod ML *et al.* (1981) *Pediatr Pharmacol* **1**:197.

91. Tod ML and Cassin S. (1981) *Proc Soc Exp Biol Med* **166**:148.

92. Gerkins JF, Freisinger GC, Branch RA *et al.* (1978) *Life Sci* **22**:1837.

93. Leffler CW and Hessler JR. (1979) *Eur J Pharmacol* **54**:37.

94. Starling MB, Neutze JM, Elliott RL *et al.* (1979) *Prostaglandins Med* 3:105.

95. Starling MB, Neutze JM, Elliott RL *et al.* (1981] *Prostaglandins Med* 7:349.

96. Lock JE, Coceani FM, Hamilton F *et al.* (1980) *J Pharmacol Exp Ther* 215:156.

97. Lock JE, Olley PM, Coceani I *et al.* (1979) *Lancet* 1:1343.

98. Philips JB III. (1984) *Pediatr Pharmacol* 4:129.

99. Cassin S, Tod ML, Frisinger JE *et al.* (1979) *Lancet* 2:638.

100. Peckham GJ. (1982) *In* **Cardiovascular Sequelæ of Asphyxia in the Newborn. Report of the Eighty-Third Ross Conference on Pediatric Research.** (GJ Peckham and MA Heymann, eds) Ross Laboratories: Columbus, Ohio, p 110.

101. Philips JB III and Lyrene RK. (1984) *Clinics in Perinatology* 11:565.

Summary

A large number of poster presentations formed an important part of the session on mechanisms of pulmonary hypertension. R.L. Gibson and G.J. Redding from the University of Washington, Seattle reported that hypoxic pulmonary vasoconstriction persists after infusion of Group B streptococci in newborn piglets. The stimuli for this work were the observations (Reeves JT and Grover RF *JAP* **36**:328, 1974; Hutchinson A *et al. JAP* **58**:1463,1985) that endotoxin attenuates hypoxic vasoconstriction in adult dogs and sheep. There are several possible reasons for the failure to alter the hypoxic pressor response: the dose of streptococci (3 X 10^{-8} CFU/kg infused over 1 hour) may have been too low, the attenuation may not occur in neonates, there may be species differences; the streptococci may not initiate the alternate pathway of complement activation which appears to be involved in the adult model (Weir EK *et al., Resp Physiol* **53**:295,1983). All these questions could be resolved by further studies.

A series of very elegant experiments was presented by J.A. Madden, C.A. Dawson and D.R. Harder from the Medical College of Wisconsin and the Milwaukee VAMC. They have shown that isolated small pulmonary artery segments (less than 300 μm diameter) contract as the oxygen tension of the bath is reduced from 300 to 50 torr. The contraction is potentiated by indomethacin (10^{-9} M) or an increase in extracellular calcium (from 2.5 to 4.0 mM); it is unaltered by phentolamine and decreased by indomethacin (10^{-3} M) or a reduction in calcium (from 1.5 to 1.0 mM). In other small pulmonary arterial segments, membrane potential was measured by impalement of cells from the adventitial surface using glass microelectrodes. The membrane potential changes from -51 ±1.4 mV under control conditions to -37 ±2.0 mV during hypoxia. In some vessels, action potentials occur during hypoxia. These can be inhibited by verapamil, which partially repolarizes the membrane. It appears that increased conductance of calcium during hypoxia may account for the depolarization and generation of action potentials. Preliminary work suggests that the removal of pulmonary vascular endothelium may prevent hypoxic contraction, while the response to added 5-hydroxytryptamine or potassium is unchanged or modestly

The Pulmonary Circulation
in Health and Disease

reduced. Further studies in this series need to be performed before the endothelium can be considered essential for hypoxic pulmonary vasoconstriction.

A presentation by M. Murayama of the Laboratory of Cellular and Developmental Biology, NIH, Bethesda, indicated that platelets will spontaneously aggregate *in vitro* when decompressed from 768 to 380 torr, regardless of the oxygen tension (0 to 316 torr). This is thought to be due to an increased rate of fibrin polymerization. Platelets subjected to a high hydraulic pressure (680 atmospheres) do not show spontaneous aggregation. These observations may be helpful in elucidating the role of fibrin and platelets in the etiology of high altitude pulmonary hypertension.

L.J. Rubin *et al.* from the University of Maryland, Baltimore, described a model of emphysema, induced in dogs by the repeated intra-tracheal insufflation of 16% papain. After six months, mean pulmonary arterial pressure inceased from 11.8 ±1.5 to 18.2 ±7.4 mmHg, and pulmonary vascular resistance from 2.0 ±0.7 to 6.2 ±5.2 units. PaO_2 fell from 95±8 to 79±7.1 mmHg and there was an unexplained reduction in cardiac output from 5.2±1.4 to 3.0±0.9 L/min. Histopathology showed pan-lobular emphysema with medical hypertrophy in the smallest pulmonary arteries (<50 μ). This model will be useful in studying changes in pulmonary vascular reactivity related to chronic lung disease.

An interesting presentation by F.W. Cheney, M.J. Bishop and B.L. Eisenstein from the University of Washington, Seattle, suggested that hypoxic pulmonary vasoconstriction decreases edema formation in the presence of oleic acid induced permeability edema. Lobar weight, bloodless lobar weight, absolute bloodflow and percent of cardiac output to the lower left lobe were significantly less in animals ventilated with a hypoxic gas mixture (F_IO_2 = .05) than ventilated with high oxygen (F_IO_2 = 1.0). The exact mechanism(s) for differences is not clear.

T.J. Gregory *et al.* from the LSU Medical Center, New Orleans, Louisiana, compared changes in pressure flow characteristics of isolated blood-Krebs-Ringer perfused lungs of rats with mild or severe right ventricular hypertrophy, and control animals. Slopes and intercepts of the pressure-flow curves (estimated by linear regression analyses) increased in the monocrotoline-treated rats. The more severe the right ventricular hypertrophy, the greater were the changes in slope and intercept. The authors interpret these findings to indicate an increase in non-Starling components (slope) and Starling components (intercept) of the pressure flow curves. Changes in non-Starling components may be due to decreases in the vascular cross sectional area, while changes in the Starling components may be due to increased tone in a collapsible segment of the pulmonary vasculature.

The action of BW 755c, an antioxidant, which may inhibit both cyclooxygenase and lipoxygenase pathways, was tested on the hypoxic pressor response of isolated perfused (PSS -3% albumin blood solution) rat lungs. C. Marshall and B. Marshall, University of Pennsylvania, Philadelphia, found that with increasing doses of BW 755c (10 - 100 µM) in the perfusate, the pressor responses to hypoxia were diminished and almost totally abolished at the highest concentration (1000 µm).

These observations lend support to the contention that the pressor response to hypoxia may be due to 5-lipoxygenase products, since generally one observes an augmented pressor response when cyclooxygenase alone is inhibited. However, the role of leukotrienes in the pressor response to hypoxia has not been implicated in other species (Foster S, Garett RC and Thomas HM III, *Am Rev Resp Dis* **133**:A226, 1986; Leffler CW, Mitchell JA and Green RS, *Circ Res* **55**:780, 1984). This area of research needs further investigation.

D.J. Riley and his co-workers from the Department of Medicine, Rutgers Medical School, New Jersey, presented a series of four posters dealing with collagen synthesis and pulmonary hypertension. The first set of experimental data dealt with the effects of cis-4-hydroxy-L-proline (cHyp), an inhibitor of collagen production, on the development of pulmonary hypertension in rats exposed to 10% O_2 in N_2 for 3 weeks. Hypoxia increased right ventricular pressures (RVP) from 12 ±1.0 mmHg to 27 ±1 mmHg. However, cHyp partially inhibited this response (RVP = 20±2 mm Hg). Although hypoxia increased elastin, cHyp had no effect on this increment. On the other hand, cHyp prevented the increase in collagen levels in main pulmonary arteries due to an hypoxic episode. The authors conclude that collagen is the major connective tissue component contributing to pulmonary hypertension.

In the second presentation, this group suggested that synthesis of vascular collagen and elastin is regulated by gene transcription, as a result of elevated blood pressure. This conclusion is based on the fact that levels of mRNA for collagen and elastin were increased in pulmonary arteries following hypoxia, but not in aorta (which is not subjected to hypoxic hypertension).

A third set of experiments, carried out on chronically hypoxic rats (10 days), indicated that along with an increase in right ventricular pressure, vascular collagen increased early on (3 days after hypoxia) and tended to decrease after recovery (7 days). The increase in vascular collagen seems to be a function of increased synthesis and decreased degradation. The authors conclude that induction and regression of hypoxic pulmonary hypertension results in dynamic changes in vascular collagen metabolism.

In the last very interesting study described by this group, data were presented to indicate that mechanical tension, applied to pulmonary arteries *in vitro*, induced vascular collagen biosynthesis, which is probably regulated by gene transcription. Tissues stretched with a tension equal to 100 mmHg for 4 hr were found to have a marked increase in collagen synthesis (433 ±127 cpm/mg protein, 1hr) in contrast to controls (198 ±48 cpm/mg protein, 1hr). Levels of mRNA for Type 1 collagen, elastin and actin were increased by 54%, 179% and 140%, respectively, in the stretched tissue.

SIDNEY CASSIN   E. KENNETH WEIR

Clinical Pulmonary Hypertension

Clinical Pulmonary Hypertension: Introduction

Pulmonary hypertension is not a disease, *per se*, but rather a shared manifestation of a variety of illnesses ranging from the acute elevations in pulmonary artery pressure resulting from massive pulmonary thromboembolism to the gradual and subtle progression of disordered pulmonary hemodynamics in chronic respiratory disease. In some conditions, such as thromboembolism and chronic hypoxic lung disease, the factors producing pulmonary hypertension are known, while in others, such as Primary Pulmonary Hypertension, the etiology remains obscure. Although consistently effective therapeutic modalities for pulmonary hypertension are not yet available, the renewed interest in recent years in clinical disorders of the pulmonary circulation has led to important advances in our understanding of the pathophysiology of the human pulmonary circulation and to therapeutic approaches which have great promise.

Although invasive hemodynamic measurements remain necessary for confirmation of the diagnosis of pulmonary hypertension, new approaches have enabled investigators to utilize these measurements not only to establish the diagnosis but also to determine the potential of reversibility of pulmonary vascular disease. Aleksandrov and Kanjuh (1) reported that pulmonary wedge angiography in patients with congenital left-to-right shunts and pulmonary hypertension was useful in identifying patients who benefit from corrective surgery: In patients with a "dead tree", or obstructive pattern on angiography, there was a high (up to 40%) mortality from corrective surgery, suggesting that these patients do not benefit from this approach. Simonneau and his colleagues (2) reported that an infusion of prostaglandin I_2 (PGI_2), a potent pulmonary vasodilator, was useful in predicting pulmonary vascular reactivity: Four patients who had no response to PGI_2 also had no response to other, longer-acting and less titratable agents, while 10 patients who responded to PGI_2 manifested vasodilator responses to one or several of the other agents tested.

The Pulmonary Circulation
in Health and Disease

Clarification of mechanisms contributing to pulmonary vasoreactivity has led to new therapeutic approaches. Infants with congenital diaphragmatic hernia often die with intractable, acute pulmonary hypertension and severe derangements in gas exchange. Stolar *et al.* (3) reported their experience using venoarterial extracorporeal membrane oxygenation (ECMO) in seven infants. They found that five of these patients survived after 48-200 hours of ECMO with normal arterial blood gas measurements and no evidence of pulmonary hypertension. Their results suggest that, if such patients can be supported during the period of acute pulmonary vasoconstriction, the constrictor stimulus subsides and subsequent development may be normal. Treacher and his associates (4) found that the administration of verapamil, a calcium-channel blocking agent, to patients with pulmonary hypertension secondary to chronic obstructive airways disease resulted in a reduction in pulmonary artery pressure and vascular resistance without producing a deterioration in arterial oxygenation. Since pulmonary hypertension in the setting of chronic obstructive pulmonary disease is often progressive and its presence is a poor prognostic sign (5), the development of such therapeutic modalities may lead to more effective ways to both treat cor pulmonale and prevent its development.

LEWIS J. RUBIN

REFERENCES

1. Aleksandrov R, Kanjuh V. (1986) *J Crit Care* **1**:113.
2. Simonneau G, Herve P, Escourrou P, Baudouin C, Nebout T, Duroux P. (1986) *J Crit Care* **1**:117.
3. Stolar CJH, Dillon PW, Reyes C, Wung JT. (1986) *J Crit Care* **1**:118.
4. Treacher DF, Douglas A, Jones A, Bateman NT, Bradley RD, Cameron JR. (1986) *J Crit Care* **1**:119.
5. Weisse AP, Moschos CB, Frank MJ, Levinson GE, Cannilla JE and Regan TJ. (1975) *Am J Med* **58**:92.

Clinical Pulmonary Hypertension: An Overview

LEWIS J. RUBIN
Head, Pulmonary Division
Associate Professor of Medicine
University of Maryland
School of Medicine
Baltimore, Maryland 21201

I. INTRODUCTION

Elevations in pulmonary artery pressure can occur as a primary insult to the pulmonary circulation or as a consequence of a variety of cardiovascular respiratory diseases. In either case, the increased right ventricular afterload imposed by pulmonary hypertension results in right ventricular hypertrophy and, if sustained, right heart dilatation and failure. Although the true incidence of pulmonary hypertension is unknown — largely due to the invasive procedures required for confirming the diagnosis — it has been estimated that, next to coronary artery disease and hypertensive cardiovascular disease, pulmonary heart disease is the most common cardiac disorder beyond the fifth decade of life (1).

There has been great interest over the last several years in improving non-invasive diagnostic techniques and therapeutic approaches for pulmonary hypertension. Much of this work has followed a natural scientific progression from basic research to applied investigation. Although our understanding of the pathophysiology of the pulmonary circulation remains incomplete, substantial gains have been achieved in the approach to management of clinical pulmonary vascular disease.

II.   PULMONARY HYPERTENSION DUE TO
         CHRONIC OBSTRUCTIVE PULMONARY DISEASE

Chronic obstructive pulmonary disease (COPD) is one of the five leading causes of death in the United States, and the death rate from this condition continues to rise. The coexistence of pulmonary hypertension with COPD contributes substantially to both morbidity and mortality from this disorder (2).

The mechanisms responsible for the development of pulmonary hypertension in COPD are probably complex. Alveolar hypoxia is a major contributor to pulmonary vasoconstriction, and acidosis or hypercarbia potentiate hypoxic pulmonary vasoconstriction (3). Recently, mixed venous hypoxemia has been implicated as a stimulus for vasoconstriction, either by a direct effect on precapillary vessels or through its relationship with the alveolar gas milieu (4). Polycythemia, which results from chronic hypoxia as a compensation to maintain tissue oxygen delivery, may further compromise pulmonary blood flow by increasing the viscosity of blood (5). In patients with advanced disease a loss of cross-sectional vascular surface area due to destroyed lung parenchyma may also contribute to pulmonary hypertension. These, and other factors which remain unclarified, ultimately produce a remodeling of the pulmonary vascular bed.

Therapy of pulmonary hypertension in the setting of COPD is aimed primarily at improving intrapulmonary gas exchange and ameliorating the factors which are recognized to induce pulmonary vasoconstriction. Some bronchodilators, particularly theophylline and terbutaline, may have the additional beneficial effects of modest pulmonary vasodilation and augmentation of cardiac performance (6,7). Supplemental oxygen therapy used for at least 18 hours per day has been shown to improve survival nearly two-fold in hypoxemic COPD patients, although the pulmonary vasodilator effects of low oxygen therapy are variable and often incomplete (8). The entry criteria used by the Nocturnal Oxygen Therapy Trial (NOTT) are now widely accepted as the indication for the use of supplemental oxygen:

a) Stable arterial hypoxemia, i.e. arterial $PO_2 < 55$ torr breathing room air, repeated at least twice one week apart

or

b) $P_aO_2 < 59$ torr with either

1. P pulmonale on electrocardiogram
2. Hematocrit > 55 percent
3. Edema

The goal of oxygen therapy is to raise P_aO_2 to greater than 6O torr — a level which is associated with minimal hypoxic pulmonary vasoconstriction and at which hemoglobin is usually at least 9O% saturated with oxygen.

The development of pharmacologic agents which are potent vasodilators led to improved management of chronic left ventricular failure. By reducing left ventricular afterload, these drugs improve left ventricular output. A number of these drugs have also been demonstrated to exert pulmonary vasodilator effects in several animal models of acute and chronic pulmonary hypertension, and these studies have provided the rationale for clinical trials evaluating the effects of vasodilators in hypertensive pulmonary vascular disease.

Transmembrane calcium fluxes are important in the pulmonary vasoconstriction produced by alveolar hypoxia, and calcium channel blocking agents have been shown to reduce the pulmonary hypertension in several small series of COPD patients (9). Other agents, such as hydralazine, which may exert its cardiovascular effects by stimulating the vascular release of prostaglandin I_2, have been used successfully by some investigators, while others have reported conflicting results. While it seems clear that some vasodilator agents can improve pulmonary hemodynamics in some COPD patients, several questions must be answered before the potential role of this approach to therapy is clarified:
1) Which patients are most likely to have beneficial responses to therapy? Since it is clear that not all forms of pulmonary hypertension are characterized pathologically by medial hypertrophy, the correlate of vasoconstriction, it would be foolish to assume that all patients with pulmonary hypertension would respond to vasodilators. Alternatively, these agents may prove most useful as a preventive modality in patients at risk for developing pulmonary hypertension, since they have been shown to inhibit the pulmonary hypertension and remodeling which occurs in animals exposed to chronic hypoxia. 2) In responding patients, are the hemodynamic effects additive to those of supplemental oxygen? 3) What are the effects of vasodilators on exercise tolerance and "quality of life"? 4) What is the effect of vasodilator therapy on survival in COPD with pulmonary hypertension?

III.   PULMONARY THROMBOEMBOLIC DISEASE

Pulmonary thromboembolism causes approximately 50,000 deaths per year and contributes to an additional 150,000 deaths. The development of noninvasive diagnostic procedures has revolutionized the approach to patients suspected of having deep venous thrombosis and pulmonary embolism, and carefully performed studies have delineated their utility and limitations. Ventilation-perfusion lung scanning and impedence plethysmography are now available in most hospitals and are widely used in the initial approach to suspected thromboembolic disease. Radiolabelled fibrinogen and platelet studies have also been used with encouraging results. Computerized tomography and digital subtraction angiography have joined the ranks of noninvasive radiographic techniques which are being evaluated.

Therapy of pulmonary thromboembolism has largely been directed at preventing recurrence by using anticoagulants. The development of thrombolytic agents has given the clinician the ability to lyse clot, thereby clearing the pulmonary circulation of fresh thrombus. Although serious side effects of the currently available thrombolytic agents streptokinase and urokinase occur in approximately 7-10 percent of patients, those with extensive thrombosis of the venous system or massive embolism resulting in hemodynamic compromise may experience dramatic improvement with this form of therapy (10). The use of plasminogen activating factor (TPA) may prove to be as effective as conventional thrombolytic therapy but with a lower incidence of adverse effects.

Pulmonary thromboendarterectomy in patients with chronic, unresolved proximal thrombosis is a new therapeutic option for patients with this disorder (11). Although experience with this surgical procedure is limited, initial reports have shown hemodynamic and symptomatic improvement in a carefully selected population for whom there were no therapeutic alternatives several years ago.

A major emphasis has been placed on prevention of deep venous thrombosis in patients who are at risk. Low-dose heparin (5,000 units subcutaneously twice daily) in the peri-operative period or in patients who have other major risk factors has been shown to markedly reduce the incidence of thromboembolism. Adjusted-dose heparin (to achieve a partial thromboplastin time approximately 1 1/2 times control) has been shown to reduce the incidence of recurrence of thromboembolism to a level comparable to that achieved with warfarin, but is associated with a lower incidence of side effects (12). Inferior vena cava interruption with a filter inserted percutaneously via the internal jugular or femoral vein is an effective means of preventing recurrence of embolism in selected patients and is associated with a high degree of vascular patency and a low incidence of serious complications.

IV.   PRIMARY PULMONARY HYPERTENSION

Primary pulmonary hypertension is a rare condition which is characterized by extreme elevations in pulmonary artery pressure. The cause is unknown and death usually occurs within several years of diagnosis. For the clinician, this remains a frustrating disease since it typically affects young women; even the diagnostic studies, such as cardiac catheterization, are hazardous. Pathologically, six grades of vascular lesions have been identified, which may represent a continuum of progression, different disease processes, or both (13).

Not surprisingly, a variety of vasodilator agents have been used to treat this condition, with mixed results. Some patients manifest dramatic hemodynamic and symptomatic improvement, while others, presumably with "fixed" pulmonary vascular lesions, develop adverse reactions or even life-threating or fatal hypotension.

Infusions of potent, short-acting vasodilator compounds such as prostaglandin I_2 have been used to quantify the vasodilator potential in patients with primary pulmonary hypertension prior to administering drugs which are non-titratable and have a longer duration of action. The responses to PGI_2 have been shown to correlate with the subsequent responses to orally administered hydralazine and nifedipine. This method provides a safer, more measured approach to pharmacologic therapy of pulmonary hypertension.

Although thromboembolism is not the cause of primary pulmonary hypertension, it may be a life-threatening or fatal complication. A recent retrospective study suggested that patients with this disease who were treated with anticoagulants lived longer than those who were not (14).

Combined heart-lung transplantation has been performed successfully in a few patients with primary pulmonary hypertension (15). Limitations to this approach include the dearth of medical centers with active programs as well as the need for donors, the tenuous clinical status of potential candidates for transplant, the cost of the procedure, and the long-term complications of immunosuppressive therapy to prevent transplant rejection. Nevertheless, this approach should be considered when dealing with patients with primary pulmonary hypertension who are unresponsive to medical therapy and who are deteriorating clinically.

A major obstacle to developing strategies in the diagnosis and managment of primary pulmonary hypertension has been the infrequency with which it occurs. A National Institute of Health supported multi-center registry of patients with this disease has amassed clinical data on several hundred patients, and it is hoped that an analysis of this wealth of clinical information may provide important clues to the pathogenesis of this disease as well as provide guidelines for its diagnosis and management.

V.   THE FUTURE

Although major advances have been developed in recent years, the approach to clinical pulmonary hypertension remains only partially satisfactory. Newer imaging techniques, such as Doppler ultrasonography, radionuclide angiography, computerized tomography and magnetic resonance imaging are likely to be useful tools in the evaluation of disorders of the pulmonary circulation. Knowledge obtained from basic research on the responses of the pulmonary circulation to physiologic, pathophysiologic, and pharmacologic stimuli will be applied to the clinical laboratory, particularly as more selective agents are discovered. Techniques which have been used successfully in the treatment of other conditions, such as continuous delivery of medications like insulin, will be applied to administer medications into the pulmonary circulation. Prevention of disease will be addressed with greater accuracy, as the factors responsible for the development and progression of pulmonary vascular disease become clarified.

ACKNOWLEDGMENTS

The author appreciates the secretarial assistance provided by Ms. Diane Blueford.

REFERENCES

1. **Pulmonary Heart Disease.** (1984) (LJ Rubin, ed) Martinus Nijhoff Publishing:Boston.
2. Dodge R, Burrows B and Morrison D. (1984) *In* **Pulmonary Heart Disease.** (LJ Rubin, ed) Martinus Nijhoff Publishing:Boston.
3. Fishman AP. (1980) *Ann Rev Physiol* **42**:211.
4. Hyman AL, Higashida RT, Spannhake EW and Kadowitz PJ. (1981) *J Appl Physiol* **51**:1009.
5. Weisse AP, Moschos CB, Frank MJ, Levinson GE, Cannilla JE and Regan TJ. (1975) *Am J Med* **58**:92.
6. Parker JO, Kekar K and West RO. (1966) *Circulation* **33**:17.
7. Brent BN, Mahler DA and Berger HJ. (1982) *Am J Cardiol* **50**:313.
8. Nocturnal Oxygen Therapy Trial Group. (1980) *Ann Intern Med* **93**:391.
9. Simonneau G, Escourrau P, Duroux P and Lockhart A. (1981) *N Eng J Med* **304**:1582.
10. The Urokinase Pulmonary Embolism Trial. (1973) *Circulation* (suppl) **47**:II.
11. Moser KM, Spragg RG, Utley J and Dail, PO. (1983) *Ann Intern Med* **99**:299.
12. Hull R, Delmore T, Carter C, Hirsch J and Genton E. (1982) *N Eng J Med* **306**:189.
13. Hughes JD and Rubin LJ. (1986) *Medicine* **65**:56.
14. Fuster V, Steele PM, Edwards WD, Gersh BJ, McGrod MD and Fryer L. (1984) *Circulation* **70**:580.
15. Reitz BA, Wallwork JL, Hunt SA, Rennock JL, Billingham ME, Oyer PE, Stinson EB and Shumway NE. (1982) *N Eng J Med* **307**:557.

Epidemiologic and Clinical Characteristics of Primary Pulmonary Hypertension

STUART RICH
From the Section of Cardiology
Department of Medicine
University of Illinois College of
Medicine
Chicago, Illinois   60680

I.   INTRODUCTION

Primary pulmonary hypertension (PPH) is a term used for the entity of unexplained pulmonary hypertension in patients stricken with a clinical disease syndrome for which no obvious etiology can be determined. The relative rarity of this condition has created considerable difficulties in characterizing both the demographic and clinical manifestations of the disease. This review will attempt to clarify many of these uncertainties.

A patient is deemed to have pulmonary hypertension when the pressures within the pulmonary arterial bed exceed the upper limits of normal. The value for the upper limit of mean pulmonary artery pressure in adult males has been reported as 18 mmHg, and for systolic arterial pressure 25 mmHg (1). In addition, given that the pulmonary capillary wedge pressure can range between 1 and 12 mmHg, the calculated pulmonary vascular resistance (arrived at by dividing the pulmonary arterial pressure gradient by the cardiac index) should be less than 3.5 units (1).

Primary pulmonary hypertension is and likely will remain a diagnosis of exclusion. For that reason it is important for the physician to rule out all other secondary causes for the pulmonary hypertension. Several conditions have been

The Pulmonary Circulation
in Health and Disease

associated with pulmonary hypertension, some commonly and some far less common. For all practical purposes, the diagnosis of primary pulmonary hypertension should not be entertained if any of the following conditions coexist:

1. Chronic obstructive airways disease
2. Chronic interstitial lung disease
3. Elevated left heart filling pressures, secondary either to valvular or myocardial disease
4. A left-to-right shunt, either congenital or acquired
5. Pulmonary embolism, acute or chronic
6. Schistosomiasis (the most common cause of pulmonary hypertension world-wide)
7. Collagen vascular disease
8. Sickle cell anemia or a history of intravenous drug abuse, both of which have been associated with intravascular thrombus formation (2,3)

One cannot make the diagnosis of both primary and secondary pulmonary hypertension in the same patient. Since the pulmonary vascular response to increased downstream resistance can be highly variable (4), it may appear that the resulting pulmonary hypertension is out of proportion to an underlying disease process and therefore suggest a primary origin. However, it has been shown that if one alleviates the underlying condition (such as mitral valve replacement in a patient with mitral stenosis and severe pulmonary hypertension) the severity of a pulmonary hypertension will usually be reduced (5).

In order to confirm the presence of primary or unexplained pulmonary hypertension the physician must acquire extensive data on every patient, irrespective of whether the history or physical exam is suggestive of a secondary disorder. Particular attention should be placed on the childhood history as children may have an undetected left-to-right shunt in their early lives, only to develop Eisenmenger's syndrome later in life.

II.   EPIDEMIOLOGY OF PRIMARY PULMONARY HYPERTENSION

The general population incidence rate for primary pulmonary hypertension has not been established, but the incidence rates in patients undergoing right heart catheterization has been reported to be 1.1% (6). Although primary pulmonary hypertension is seen in the very young and elderly, it most frequently occurs between the ages of 15 and 35 years. Several small series seem to confirm a female to male predominance, with ratio ranging from 1.7 to 1 to as high as 4 to 1 (7-9; see Figure 1). Although its prevalence seems to be highest in the 3rd and

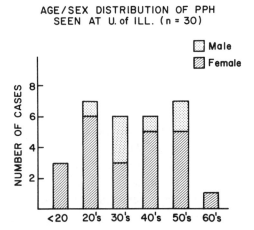

Figure 1. The distribution of age and sex of patients with PPH seen at the University of Illinois over the past two years is shown. There was a female to male predominance of 3.3:1. Note that men were often seen between the ages of 20 to 40, and that patients aged 50 and older were not uncommon.

4th decades, recent reports have documented the presentation of unexplained pulmonary hypertension in the elderly (10). Consequently one should not exclude the possibility of primary pulmonary hypertension in a patient who is either male or of greater age.

There have been no racial or geographic differences noted in the literature with regard to the prevalence of primary pulmonary hypertension, although there are two reports of geographic clustering. One was associated with the appetite suppressant drug aminorex (11), and the other is an unexplained epidemic which occurred in Sri Lanka between the years of 1968 and 1973 (12). Familial cases of primary pulmonary hypertension have been well documented. One recent review summarized the inheritance which was characterized by the infrequent expression of the gene within some families, and the widely different frequency of expression among other families (13). Fourteen separate families of primary pulmonary hypertension have already been reported in literature. The pattern has generally been one of autosomal dominance with a 2 to 1 female ratio, similar to the distribution of the disease in general. All of the other clinical manifestations of PPH in the families seem to be similar to those reported for non-familial primary pulmonary hypertension. The only distinction appears to be a somewhat shorter interval from the first symptom until the patient has the diagnosis made, which probably represents a heightened awareness of the patients to the symptoms due to their familial histories.

III.   CLINICAL FEATURES OF PRIMARY PULMONARY
        HYPERTENSION

The clinical symptoms of patients presenting with primary pulmonary hypertension vary: dyspnea, fatigue, chest pain, palpitations, leg edema, near syncope and syncope (14). Dyspnea is by far the most common symptom, although the pathophysiologic mechanism for it is not clear, since it cannot be explained purely on the basis of hypoxemia in most cases. Syncope has been related to fixed cardiac output with the inability to increase in response to increasing physical demands, and the leg edema as a manifestation of right ventricular failure. Chest pain is also unexplained, but has been suggested to represent right ventricular ischemia due to the marked pressure overload on the right ventricle. Stretching of the large pulmonary arteries has also been proposed as a potential etiology. Cyanosis, although not common, can be seen in patients in a peripheral pattern due to the low cardiac output they develop, or a central pattern from a right-to-left shunt across a patent foramen ovale. Clubbing, however, is distinctly rare in primary pulmonary hypertension and should alert the physician to seek out a secondary cause.

The physical findings of patients with primary pulmonary hypertension are typical of the patient with pulmonary hypertension of any cause. An increase in the pulmonic component of the second heart sound, and a right ventricular third and fourth heart sound are all frequently heard (15). The presence of these abnormalities may be associated with the severity of the disease. Tricuspid regurgitation and pulmonic insufficiency also commonly occur.

IV.   LABORATORY FINDINGS IN PATIENTS WITH
       PRIMARY PULMONARY HYPERTENSION

Because PPH is a diagnosis of exclusion, every patient in whom this diagnosis is entertained should undergo a thorough evaluation to exclude all possible secondary causes. The first step in the workup should be a quality standard PA and lateral chest x-ray. In primary pulmonary hypertension one would expect to see enlargement of the right descending pulmonary artery, and perhaps even bulging of the main pulmonary artery. In addition varying degrees of cardiomegaly and clear lung fields are the rule. However, it has been reported that clear lung fields on chest x-ray do not in and of themselves exclude interstitial lung disease as a secondary cause (16). The presence of wide spread interstitial infiltrates, hyperinflation or bullæ should alert the physician that secondary pulmonary hypertension exists.

The electrocardiogram of most patients with PPH will have evidence of right ventricular hypertrophy (RVH). One extensive review showed that, depending on the criteria used to make the diagnosis of RVH, its presence was noted in up to 98% of the cases (17). In addition, the changes on the electrocardiogram were able to reflect the prognosis of the patient, as those with greater alterations in R wave amplitude reflecting RVH seemed to have more severe disease and shorter survival (17). The absence of right axis deviation and features of RVH should be considered distinctly unusual and prompt the physician to pursue a secondary cause.

A lung scan is an imperative diagnostic test in any patient with unexplained pulmonary hypertension. The ventilation scan should be normal, but may also help identify the existence of obstructive lung disease if excessive air trapping is demonstrated, even in the patient without clinical symptoms. The perfusion scan is often abnormal in patients with various types of pulmonary vascular disease, but in PPH generally shows either completely normal distribution of the labelled albumin, or diffuse patchy abnormalities in a non-segmental distribution that is not consistent with pulmonary embolic disease (18; Figure 2). Chronic thromboembolic pulmonary hypertension may closely mimic PPH, especially by the absence of a history consistent with acute pulmonary embolism (19). It is quite important, however, to distinguish the two entities since the ultimate therapy may have an enormous impact on the natural history of the patient. When the lung scan is at all suggestive of thromboembolic disease we strongly advocate performing a pulmonary angiogram. Although it has been widely held that this is a very morbid procedure in the face of pulmonary hypertension, it has been our experience that the risk of this procedure may be overstated. The literature reports that mortality due to pulmonary angiography in a patient with pulmonary hypertension is related to right ventricular end-diastolic pressure (namely the failing right ventricle), rather than the level of pulmonary artery pressure (20). In such cases we opt for a selective injection of the pulmonary vascular bed based on the distribution of tracer by the lung scan, thus delivering a smaller volume load to the heart. In addition, it has been our experience that the hypotensive episodes following pulmonary angiography may be vagally mediated, and therefore we administer intravenous atropine to any patient with pulmonary hypertension undergoing pulmonary angiography at the first suggestion of either a relative bradycardia (slowing of the resting heart rate ten beats/minute or more) or any reduction in systemic blood pressure (which we

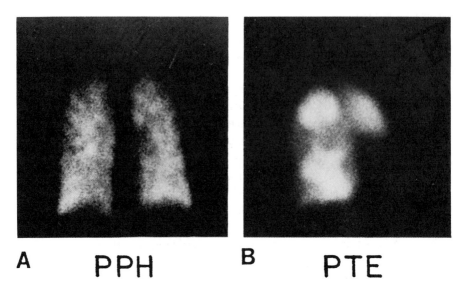

A   PPH   B   PTE

Figure 2. The lung scans of two patients with pulmonary hypertension are shown. The one on the left (A) has PPH and a diffuse patchy pattern that is nonsegmental in nature and not suggestive of pulmonary emboli. The scan on the right (B) is from a patient who had chronic persistent proximal pulmonary emboli. The segmental nature of the defects is apparent. Neither patient had a history of acute dyspnea or any clinical findings of deep vein thrombosis.

monitor continuously). By following this strategy, we have not had a single adverse reaction to pulmonary angiography in our series.

Pulmonary function tests need to be performed in order to evaluate the presence of underlying obstructive or restrictive lung disease. Although both obstructive and restrictive changes in pulmonary function testing have been reported in patients with PPH, these findings may be related to the small size of the series and a somewhat selected population (21, 22). Pulmonary function tests in patients with PPH should be normal, although arterial hypoxemia on room air and a reduction in diffusing capacity to carbon monoxide seem to be the rule (8,21,23; Figure 3). In the patient in whom central hypoventilation or sleep apnea is a consideration, a full sleep apnea workup should be entertained. Although pulmonary hypertension is not commonly associated with sleep apnea it has definitely been reported to be a consequence, and is a much more treatable condition (24).

The echocardiogram may be a very useful diagnostic tool in patients with pulmonary hypertension. It helps the clinician evaluate left ventricular dysfunction, mitral valve disease or any impairment to blood inflow of the left ventricle. In the patient with primary pulmonary hypertension it will typically show a large right ventricle, small left ventricle, and paradoxical motion of the intraventricular septum (25). Tricuspid regurgitation and pulmonic insufficiency are also common secondary findings in any patient with pulmonary hypertension.

Upon evaluating the ventricular septum in the parasternal short axis view, it has been shown that as the pulmonary hypertension worsens, not only does the paradoxical septal motion increase, but the curve of the ventricular septum loses its normal concave shape (with respect to the left ventricle) and becomes increasingly convex (26, 27; Figure 4). Although the sensitivity of this abnormality with respect to screening for pulmonary hypertension has not been tested, in our experience we have been able to detect subtle abnormalities in ventricular septal motion in patients with minimal elevations in pulmonary pressure. In addition, we have noted restoration of the normal septal architecture in patients with pulmonary hypertension who have responded to drug treatment in concert with the reversal in the level of their pulmonary artery pressures.

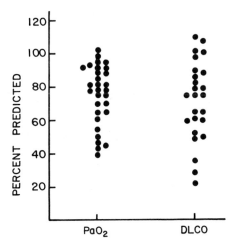

Figure 3. Values for systemic arterial blood gas on room air (P_aO_2) and diffusing capacity (D_LCO) are plotted for 30 patients with PPH evaluated at the University of Illinois and shown as the percent of predicted normal value based on age, sex and height from previously published norms. Arterial hypoxemia and low diffusing capacities were more the rule rather than the exception.

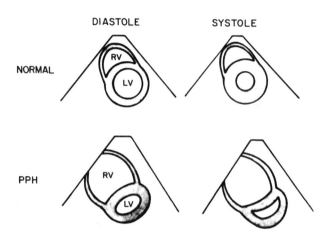

*Figure 4. Graphic representations of the left and right ventricles as seen
in the short axis view on 2-D echo are illustrated for normal and PPH patients.
Normally the LV assumes a circular shape, both in diastole and in systole. In
PPH the septum becomes progressively flattened and may actually reverse its
curvature in systole. The curvature of the septum in systole has been correlated
with the severity of the pulmonary hypertension.*

    The diagnosis of primary pulmonary hypertension can finally be made
with certainty only with a cardiac catheterization. Again, amplifying the
statements made earlier, the catheterization study should not be performed just to
document the level of pulmonary pressure, but also should be used to help exclude
any other secondary causes for pulmonary hypertension that might have gone
undetected. For that reason, we always perform some method of excluding an
underlying left-to-right shunt (preferably a hydrogen curve), as well as assess left
ventricular filling pressure either by direct measurement of the left ventricle, or the
recording of a pulmonary capillary wedge pressure whose reliability has been
confirmed by ability to withdraw arterial blood through the wedged catheter, along
with an adequate wave form.

    In the patient with primary pulmonary hypertension, one will typically
find severe elevations in pulmonary artery pressure (with pulmonary artery mean
pressures commonly in excess of 60 mmHg) with an associated low-normal or
reduced cardiac index (28). The pulmonary capillary wedge pressure by definition
should be normal, and the right atrial pressure will reflect right ventricular function
in the course of the disease. Published series on patients who present both early

and late with PPH have recorded similar levels of pulmonary hypertension, suggesting that the pulmonary artery pressures may rise fairly rapidly in the clinical course of the disease (29).

V.   PREDICTORS OF PROGNOSIS

From the literature it has been suggested that median survival in primary pulmonary hypertension is approximately $2^1/2$ years from the time of diagnosis (30). The prognosis does not appear to be uniformly dismal in all patients, however. It has been established that patients may have the disease for several years, and even spontaneous regression has been reported (31). For that reason it is important to characterize the underlying hemodynamics if, for no other reason, than to be able to better direct interventions in future PPH patients. Studies on survival have shown that the right atrial pressure and stroke volume index predict prognosis (29). Since these two parameters reflect underlying right ventricular function, this is really no surprise. In addition, survival has also been related to arterial blood gas saturation with oxygen, which also is a manifestation of underlying cardiopulmonary function (17).

It is not the purpose of this review to discuss the effectiveness of the vasodilator drug intervention in these patients. However, we have shown that the acute response to vasodilator challenge at least appears to separate out those with poor prognosis from those whose prognosis is somewhat better (32). The ability to lower pulmonary vascular resistance with acute vasodilator challenge has been interpreted as indicating some functional reserve capacity within the pulmonary arterial bed which would allow the patient to adjust themselves to day-to-day activity changes. Patients who are unable to alter their cardiac outputs and drop their calculated pulmonary resistances with challenge of any vasodilator appear to be in a more advanced stage of their disease. It has not been shown, however, that chronic therapy of patients with vasodilator drugs in a group that does have favorable acute responses alters their clinical courses or survival (32).

REFERENCES

1.   Grossman W. (1980) **Cardiac Catheterization and Angiography.** Lea and Febiger:Philadelphia, 2nd edition.
2.   Collins FS and Orringer EP. (1982) *Am J Med* 73:814.
3.   Hook RJ, Bailey GL, Daroca PH, Brazda F, Johnson FB and Klein RC. (1980) *Chest* 77:277.
4.   Dexter L. (1979) *Arch Int Med* 139:922.

5. Zener JC, Hancock EW, Shumway NE and Harrison DC. (1972) *Am J Cardiol* **30**:820.

6. Storstein O, Efskind L, Muller C, Rokseth R and Sanders S. (1966) *Acta Med Scand* **79**:197.

7. Wagenvoort CA and Wagenvoort N. (1970)*Circulation* **42**:1163.

8. Walcott G, Burchell HB and Brown AL. (1970) *Am J Med* **49**:70.

9. Watanabe S and Ogata T. (1976) *Jap Heart J* **40**:603.

10. Phipps B, Wang B, Chang CHJ and Dunn M. (1983) *Chest* **84**:899.

11. Kay JM, Smith P and Heath D. (1971) *Thorax* **26**:262.

12. Wagenvoort CA and Wagenvoort N. (1977) **Pathology of Pulmonary Hypertension.** John Wiley and Sons:New York.

13. Lloyd JE, Primm RK and Newman JH. (1984) *Amer Rev Respir Dis* **129**:194.

14. Hughes JD and Rubin LJ. (1986) *Medicine* **65**:65.

15. Weir EK. (1984) *In* **Pulmonary Hypertension** (EK Weir and JT Reeves, eds) Futura:Mount Kisco.

16. Elper GR, McLoud TC, Gaensler EA, Mikus JP and Carrington CB. (1978) *N Engl J Med* **298**:934.

17. Kanemoto N. (1980) *Eur J Cardiol* **12**:181.

18. Wilson AG, Harris CN, Lavender JP and Oakley CM. (1973) *Br Heart J* **35**:917.

19. Moser KM, Spragg RG, Utley J and Daily PO. (1983) *Ann Intern Med* **99**:299.

20. Mills SR, Jackson DC, Older RA, Heaston DK and Moore AV. (1980) *Radiology* **136**:295.

21. Horn M, Ries A, Neveu C and Moser KM. (1983) *Amer Rev Resp Dis* **128**:163.

22. Fernandez-Bonetti P, Lupi-Herrera E, Martinez-Guerra ML, Barrios R, Seoanne M and Sandoval J. (1983)*Chest* **83**:732.

23. Gazetopoulos N, Salonikides N and Davies H. (1974) *Br Heart J* **36**:19.

24. Podszus T, Bauer W, Mayer J, Penzel T and Peter JH. (1986) *Am J Cardiol* **33**:438.

25. Goodman DJ, Harrison DC and Popp RL. (1974) *Am J Cardiol* **33**:438.

26. Tanaka H, Tei C, Nakao S, Tahara M, Sakurai S, Kashima T and Kahehisa T. (1980) *Circulation* **62**:588.

27. King ME, Braun H, Goldblatt *et al.* (1983)*Circulation* **68**:68.

28. Kanemoto N and Sasamoto H. =(1979) *Jap Heart J* **20**:395.

29. Rich S and Levy PS. (1984) *Am J Med* **76**:573.

30. Fuster V, Giuliana ER, Brandenbury RO *et al.* (1981) *Am J Cardiol* **47**:422.

31.   Fujii A, Rabinovitch M and Matthews EC. (1981) *Br Heart J* **46**:574.
32.   Rich S, Brundage BH and Levy PS. (1985) *Circulation* **71**:1191.

Diagnosis and Long-Term Management of Venous Thromboembolism

RUSSELL D. HULL
Chief of Medicine,
Chedoke Division
Chedoke-McMaster Hospitals
Hamilton, Ontario, Canada

GARY E. RASKOB
Clinical Trial Specialist
Department of Medicine
McMaster University
Hamilton, Ontario, Canada

I.   INTRODUCTION

Recent clinical trials have produced substantial advances in the diagnosis and long-term treatment of venous thromboembolism [venous thrombosis (VT) and/or pulmonary embolism (PE)]. The purpose of this article is to provide an overview of the diagnosis and long-term treatment of venous thromboembolism, and to review the recent advances in these two aspects of management.

II.   DIAGNOSIS OF VENOUS THROMBOEMBOLISM

It is now widely recognized that the clinical diagnosis of PE is highly non-specific (1-8). Multiple studies indicate that more than half of all patients with clinically suspected PE do not have this diagnosis confirmed by objective testing (1-8). Similarly, it is widely documented that the clinical diagnosis of VT is also highly non-specific (9-16). Patients with relatively minor symptoms and signs may have extensive VT, and patients with florid symptoms, suggesting extensive deep vein thrombosis (DVT), frequently are shown to be free of this disorder by objective testing.

Despite the overwhelming evidence for the non-specificity of the clinical diagnosis of both VT and PE, many patients still have management decisions made on clinical grounds alone. The reasons for this include lack of experience with objective testing, the perceived inconvenience to both doctors and patients, the expense of investigation, and the possible morbidity caused by objective testing. All of these perceived disadvantages are outweighed by the advantages of investigating all patients. The cost of investigation is substantially less than the cost of unnecessary hospital admission or prolongation of hospital stay, and of unnecessary anticoagulant therapy in patients who have an incorrect diagnosis made (17). The inconvenience of investigation is also minimal compared with the inconvenience of unnecessary hospitalization and treatment. Although there is some morbidity associated with the use of the invasive procedures, venography and pulmonary angiography, there is virtually none associated with the use of non-invasive testing. Noninvasive testing avoids the need for venography in most of patients with clinically suspected VT (14-16,18), and offers a replacement for pulmonary angiography in many patients with clinically suspected PE (8). Furthermore, the morbidity from unnecessary anticoagulant therapy and inappropriate hospitalization exceeds that caused by pulmonary angiography and venography, and these tests should be used when other approaches are unavailable or inconclusive.

A.   The Diagnostic Reference Standards for Venous Thromboembolism

1.   Pulmonary Angiography

Pulmonary angiography is the accepted diagnostic reference standard for PE (19,20). A diagnosis of PE is made if there is a constant intraluminal filling defect seen on multiple films, or if sharp cut-offs can be seen in vessels greater than 2.5 mm in diameter, which are constant in multiple films (21). Other abnormalities, such as oligemia, vessel pruning, and loss of filling of small vessels, are non-specific and may result from a variety of pulmonary disorders (*e.g.* pneumonia, atelectasis, emphysema, etc). Loss of filling may also occur for technical reasons but this artifact can often be avoided by careful attention to technique with repeated injection of small volumes of dye (*e.g.*, 20 cc).

Selective pulmonary angiography (22,23) is a safe technique in the absence of severe chronic pulmonary hypertension or severe cardiac or respiratory decompensation (7,8,24). Although the risk of pulmonary angiography has been substantially reduced in recent years by the use of the selective technique, its invasive nature and the associated risks contraindicate its use in a significant number of very ill patients whose clinical course has been complicated by suspected PE. In our experience, approximately 20% of patients with clinically suspected PE and abnormal perfusion lung scan findings cannot undergo pulmonary angiography because of the severity of their primary illness (7,8).

Clinically significant complications including tachyarrythmias, endocardial or myocardial injury, cardiac perforation, cardiac arrest, and hypersensitivity reactions to contrast medium occur in up to 3-4% of patients undergoing selective pulmonary angiography (24). Patients with a history of allergy to radiopaque dye should not have pulmonary angiography performed.

2. Venography

Venography is the accepted diagnostic reference standard for VT (13,18,25,26). The presence of a constant intraluminal filling defect, which is seen on multiple films, is considered diagnostic of acute VT (13,18,25,26). Other less reliable criteria include (i) nonfilling of a segment of the deep venous system with abrupt termination of the column of contrast medium at a constant site below the segment and reappearance of the contrast medium at a constant site above the segment, and (ii) nonfilling of the deep venous system above the knee, despite adequate venographic technique. These latter two venographic abnormalities may be caused by incomplete mixing of contrast medium with blood, by external compression of a vein, or by injecting the contrast medium too far proximally in the foot.

Venography is a difficult technique to perform well and requires considerable experience to execute adequately and interpret accurately. Misinterpreting an inadequate venogram (usually in the direction of a falsely positive diagnosis) is becoming an important problem with the increasing use of venography in centres without a special interest or expertise in this technique. Radiologists and clinicians must be sensitive to the technical pitfalls of venography, and either repeat the venogram when the result is inadequate or base management decisions on the results of non-invasive testing.

Venography is an invasive procedure that produces significant foot or calf pain in some patients (27). The procedure may also be complicated by superficial phlebitis and even DVT in a small percentage (1-2%) of patients who have normal venograms (13,27). Other less common complications of venography include hypersensitivity reactions to the radiopaque dye, and local skin and tissue necrosis due to extravasation of contrast at the site of injection (27).

TABLE I. The essential design features for studies evaluating the efficacy of diagnostic test.

---

1. Evaluation in a consecutive series of patients, all of whom undergo both the diagnostic test and the reference test in order to determine the four indices of efficacy: sensitivity, specificity, positive predictive value, and negative predictive value.

2. Evaluation of the diagnostic test in a broad spectrum of patients with and without the disease in question. Failure to include a broad spectrum of patients may results in a falsely high estimate of efficacy.

3. Avoidance of diagnostic suspicion bias by interpreting the results of the diagnostic test and reference test independently and without knowledge of the results of each other or of the patient's clinical findings.

4. Long-term clinical follow-up to determine the safety of withholding treatment in patients with a negative test result.

B. Methodologic Criteria for the Evaluation of Less-Invasive Diagnostic Approaches for Suspected Venous Thromboembolism

Due to the pitfalls and limitations of pulmonary angiography and venography, extensive efforts have been made to replace these invasive techniques with less invasive diagnostic tests. The early studies (28,29) with less invasive tests for PE (serum enzymes and bilirubin, and arterial blood gases) were inadequately designed and the diagnostic recommendations drawn from these studies were spurious. A falsely high specificity for the diagnosis of PE was attributed to perfusion lung scanning, which was subsequently refuted by multiple studies (1,3-8). The uncritical clinical acceptance of a diagnostic test for PE or VT has serious implications, because it may result in inappropriate and potentially dangerous management.

The major reason for the early inappropriate application of the above diagnostic tests for PE was a premature clinical acceptance of diagnostic efficacy based on studies that failed to include the essential design features (30) required to adequately assess the efficacy of a diagnostic test. These essential design features are summarized in Table I. The efficacy of a diagnostic test lies in its ability to indicate the presence or absence of disease. Efficacy is measured by four indices: sensitivity (proportion of positive test results among patients with the disease), specificity (proportion of negative test results among patients without the disease), positive predictive value (the likelihood that the patient with positive test results will have the disease), and negative predictive value (the likelihood that patients with negative test results will not have the disease).

To adequately determine the efficacy of a diagnostic test, it is essential that the test be evaluated prospectively in a broad spectrum of patients suspected to have the disease of interest (both with and without the disease), all of whom undergo testing with a diagnostic reference test (30). In this way, it is possible to identify disorders that produce falsely positive and falsely negative results, and to determine the clinical utility of the test in various patient subgroups. Failure to evaluate the test in a broad spectrum of patients may result in falsely high indices of efficacy (30), particularly when applied to certain subgroups. Bias can be avoided by evaluating consecutive patients, and by assessing the test results blindly, without knowledge of the reference test (or other diagnostic tests), or the patient's condition (30).

The final step in the process of evaluating a new diagnostic test is to confirm the clinical validity of a negative test result. Clinical validity should be determined by long-term follow up in consecutive patients in whom treatment has been withheld on the basis of negative test results.

C. Less Invasive Diagnostic Approaches for Clinically Suspected Pulmonary Embolism

1. Summary

Measurements of serum enzymes and bilirubin, and arterial blood gases, are both insensitive and non-specific (1,28,29), and should not be used for diagnostic purposes in patients with suspected PE.

The radiologic abnormalities associated with PE are non-specific and occur in many other pulmonary disorders. In addition, patients with PE may have a normal chest x-ray at presentation (1,3-8). The chest x-ray is helpful, however, in demonstrating other causes for the patient's condition (*e.g.* pneumothorax) and is important in interpreting the lung scan findings.

The ECG is frequently normal in patients with suspected PE, and the classical findings reported to be associated with PE (right axis shift, and S1, Q2, T3 pattern) are non-specific and occur uncommonly (29). The ECG may be useful for differentiating between PE and myocardial infarction.

Perfusion lung scanning plays a pivotal role in the diagnostic work-up of patients with suspected PE. A normal perfusion scan excludes the diagnosis of clinically important PE; however, an abnormal perfusion scan is highly non-specific (1,3-8).

Ventilation imaging was introduced into clinical practice for the diagnosis of PE to improve the specificity of an abnormal perfusion scan by differentiating embolic occlusion of the pulmonary vasculature from perfusion defects occurring secondary to a primary disorder of ventilation (31,32). The basic premise that perfusion defects which ventilate normally (ventilation-perfusion mismatch) are due to PE, whereas matching ventilation-perfusion abnormalities are due to other conditions, was not supported by early studies in experimental animals (33,34), and has recently been shown to be incorrect based on the finding of prospective clinical trials (7,8)(see below; Diagnostic Value of Ventilation Lung Scanning).

Ventilation scanning is only helpful if the perfusion defect is segmental (or larger) and associated with ventilation mismatch (*i.e.*, a high probability scan); in these patients, anticoagulant therapy can usually be commenced without further investigation. The remaining ventilation-perfusion scan patterns do not have sufficiently high or low predictive value to either rule in or rule out PE (7,8), and further investigations are required.

2.   Diagnostic Value of Ventilation Lung Scanning

The published data (4-6,31,32,35) supporting the clinical application of ventilation-perfusion lung scanning were, until recently, taken largely from retrospective studies, or from non-consecutive prospective patient series, none of which satisfied the essential study design criteria outlined in Table I. The initial studies (31,32), which included only small numbers of patients, reported a falsely high degree of efficacy for ventilation-perfusion lung scanning.

Attempts were made to improve the specificity of ventilation-perfusion lung scanning by classifying the perfusion defects according to size, number, and the presence of matched or mismatched ventilation defects (4-6,35). Multiple large defects with normal ventilation were associated with a very high probability (>90%) of PE, while other lung scan patterns were reported to be associated with a low frequency (<10%) of PE, leading to the concept of "low-probability" patterns. Recently, the concept that a "low-probability" lung scan pattern could be used to rule out PE has been shown to be incorrect (7,8; see below).

The results of our recent prospective study (7,8) have provided new data concerning the predictive value of the individual ventilation-perfusion lung scan patterns, and provide the basis for a practical approach to the diagnosis of PE outlined later in this article. In this study, a consecutive series of patients with clinically suspected PE and an abnormal perfusion lung scan were entered prospectively in a protocol requiring ventilation-perfusion lung scanning, pulmonary angiography and objective testing for VT in all patients (unless these tests were contraindicated because of concurrent life-threatening cardiac or respiratory illness).

TABLE II: Frequency of pulmonary embolism (PE) associated with the individual ventilation-perfusion scan patterns*.

Ventilation-perfusion scan pattern	Frequency of PE
One or more segmental or greater defects	
Mismatch	51/59 (86%)
Match	10/28 (36%)
One or more subsegmental defects	
Mismatch	16/40 (40%)
Match	6/24 (25%)
Indeterminate	5/24 (21%)

* From Hull *et al.* (8).

The results of ventilation-perfusion lung scanning, therefore, did not influence the decision to perform pulmonary angiography, thus avoiding "work-up" bias that would have occurred if pulmonary angiography was done selectively on the basis of the lung scan findings. Bias due to diagnostic suspicion (in which knowledge of one test finding may influence interpretation of another) was avoided by interpreting all of the test findings independently and without knowledge of each other or the patient's clinical findings.

The frequency of PE by pulmonary angiography associated with the individual ventilation-perfusion scan patterns is shown in Table II (8). Patients with large perfusion defects (one or more segmental or greater defects) and ventilation mismatch have a high probability (86%) of pulmonary embolism; this observation is consistent with the findings previously reported in the literature (4-6,35). Our results differ, however, from previous findings in patients with a ventilation-perfusion match, and in those with subsegmental perfusion defects. In these latter two groups, the frequency of PE ranged from 25 to 40% (Table II) and is not sufficiently low to rule out PE. Contrary to current clinical practice, these findings indicate that the strategy of using a "low probability" lung scan pattern to rule against PE is incorrect and should be abandoned. The use of an improved method of ventilation scanning (Tc-99m aerosol ventilation imaging)(36), which provided excellent ventilation imaging did not improve the specificity of the ventilation-perfusion lung scan abnormalities (8). The observed frequencies of PE in patients with "low probability" lung scan patterns, (segmental or greater defects with ventilation match, or subsegmental defects) indicate that it is inappropriate to

with ventilation match, or subsegmental defects) indicate that it is inappropriate to withhold anticoagulant therapy solely on the basis of a "low probability" lung scan, and further objective testing is required to establish or refute the diagnosis of venous thromboembolism.

3.   The Association Between Deep Venous Thrombosis and Pulmonary Embolism: The Role of Objective Testing for Venous Thrombosis in Patients with Suspected Pulmonary Embolism

The detection of VT in patients with clinically suspected PE is clinically very useful since in most cases, the treatment of DVT and PE is the same. Thus, detection of DVT provides an indication for therapy and may circumvent the need for pulmonary angiography, a distinct advantage because objective testing for DVT is less invasive, less complex, and more readily available.

Both impedance plethysmography (IP) and venography have now been formally evaluated prospectively in patients with suspected PE and abnormal perfusion lung scans (7,8). IP has the potential advantage that it is non-invasive and free of morbidity, and can easily be performed in the emergency room or

TABLE III: Frequency of proximal-vein thrombosis detected by impedance plethysmography associated with the individual ventilation-perfusion scan patterns*

Ventilation-perfusion scan pattern	Frequency of proximal vein thrombosis
One or more segmental or greater defects	
Mismatch	29/59 (49%)
Match	7/28 (25%)
One or more subsegmental defects	
Mismatch	6/40 (15%)
Match	4/24 (17%)
Indeterminate	5/24 (21%)

* From Hull et al. (8).

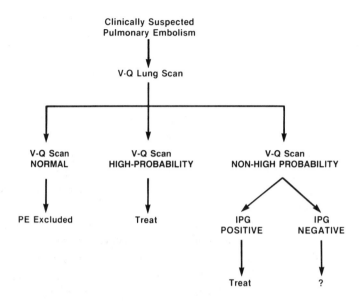

Figure 1. Practical diagnostic approach for clinically suspected pulmonary embolism. V-Q = Ventilation-Perfusion; IPG = Impedance Plethysmography.

doctor's office, and is readily repeatable. IP was positive in approximately 45% of patients with PE by pulmonary angiography (8). Others have reported a higher frequency (37).

The results of IP were also compared with the venographic findings in these patients with clinically suspected PE (7). Almost 90% of the proximal-vein thrombi shown by venography were detected by IP (even though most of the thrombi were asymptomatic), and a positive IP result was highly predictive of venous thromboembolism (a positive predictive value of greater than 95%)(7).

A gradient was noted for the frequency of proximal vein thrombosis detected by IP among patients with a range of ventilation-perfusion defects (Table III)(7,8), and this frequency differed sharply from that found in patients with normal lung scans (<1%) (7). Thus, patients presenting with clinically suspected PE and abnormal findings by perfusion lung scanning, including those scan patterns that have been traditionally regarded as "low probability", have a substantial frequency of extensive deep-vein thrombosis. This observation has important management implications because recent randomized clinical trials (38-

40) have shown that failure to treat proximal-vein thrombosis is associated with a high risk (47%) of recurrent venous thromboembolism.

4.   A Practical Diagnostic Strategy for Clinically
         Suspected Pulmonary Embolism

A diagnostic algorithm for the management of clinically suspected PE is shown in Figure 1. Following a history and physical examination, electrocardiogram, and chest x-ray, all patients should undergo perfusion lung scanning. A normal perfusion lung scan excludes clinically important PE. In our recent study (7), approximately 40% of patients with suspected PE had a normal perfusion lung scan.

If the perfusion lung scan demonstrates one or more segmental (or greater) perfusion defects, ventilation lung scanning should be performed because the probability of PE is markedly increased if a mismatch is found (positive predictive value 86%), providing an end point for commencing anticoagulant therapy in the majority of these patients. For the remaining ventilation-perfusion scan patterns, the predictive values (Table II) are neither sufficiently high nor low to confirm or exclude the presence of PE, and further testing is required.

Alternative approaches are available which would reduce the need for pulmonary angiography in patients with abnormal but non-high probability ventilation-perfusion lung scans. In these patients, venography or IP could be performed as the initial step of the diagnostic work up. If objective testing confirms the presence of DVT, anticoagulant therapy can be commenced without the further procedure of pulmonary angiography. If venography is negative, further testing is required, because a negative venogram occurs in up to 30% of patients with PE by angiography (7), and therefore, does not exclude a diagnosis of PE.

The correct approach to patients with non-high probability lung scan patterns who have a negative result by IP (or venography) at presentation (and, therefore, either don't have VT or have calf vein thrombosis) remains to be adequately defined (Figure 1). One approach would be to perform pulmonary angiography in all of these patients to detect the 15-50% of patients who have PE. An alternative and more practical strategy which we are currently exploring in patients with good cardiorespiratory reserve, non-high probability lung scans, and negative IP at presentation, is to use surveillance with serial IP testing to detect recurrent or extending VT. The rationale of this approach is based on the premise that clinically significant recurrent PE is very unlikely in patients who do not have proximal vein thrombosis (14-16,41), and that serial IP testing can be used to detect extending deep-vein thrombosis.(14-16). Serial IP has been used successfully to detect clinically important VT in patients with clinically suspected

DVT who are negative at presentation (14-16) and therefore, holds promise in patients with suspected PE who are stable clinically. This approach is likely to be more successful than venography alone because, in patients negative by venography at presentation, the putative thrombus may have embolized completely but, in the absence of further testing, could reoccur undetected and lead to serious recurrent PE. Furthermore, because of its invasive nature, venography cannot be readily repeated.

If anticoagulant therapy is started on the basis of documented DVT, the patient's respiratory illness should be closely monitored to detect a non-embolic disorder that may be present. The objective confirmation of DVT provides an indication for anticoagulant therapy but does not necessarily establish a diagnosis of PE because VT may have occurred in association with another primary respiratory illness. By closely monitoring the patient's respiratory status, other diseases such as pneumonia, which initially may not have been an obvious component of the diagnosis, can be detected and managed appropriately. If the cause of the respiratory disorder remains uncertain, pulmonary angiography will distinguish between PE and other respiratory problems.

D.   Non-Invasive Approaches for the Diagnosis of VT

1.   Summary

Several noninvasive techniques for the diagnosis of VT have been introduced recently, but only three have been extensively evaluated: IP (43-51), Doppler ultrasonography (52-55), and ^{125}I-fibrinogen leg scanning (56-59). On applying the essential study design criteria (Table I) to clinical trials evaluating non-invasive testing for VT, only two approaches have been evaluated by studies meeting all of the essential criteria: these approaches are combined IP and ^{125}I-fibrinogen leg scanning (15,60,61), and more recently, the approach of IP alone performed serially (14-16).

Until recently, the insensitivity of IP for detecting isolated calf-vein thrombosis was a potential limitation to its clinical application. This limitation can be overcome for practical clinical purposes, either by adding ^{125}I-fibrinogen leg scanning (which is highly sensitive to calf vein thrombosis) to IP (15,60,61) or by performing serial IP (14-16). The combined approach of IP and leg scanning can replace venography in most patients with clinically suspected VT (60,61). However, serial IP alone has now replaced this combined approach as the preferred diagnostic approach in patients with their first episode of suspected VT (14-16). Serial IP is effective, and limits the need for venography to less than 5% of asymptomatic patients. Venography may be required in the occasional patient who has a clinical condition known to produce falsely positive results by IP (for example, congestive cardiac failure, or severe peripheral vascular disease). Leg scanning combined with IP remains a useful approach in selected patients with clinically suspected acute recurrent VT (62).

It is currently uncertain if serial Doppler ultrasonography, or other non-invasive tests (*e.g.* strain gauge plethysmography) performed serially, can be used in place of IP, because these alternatives have not been evaluated by clinical trials incorporating long-term follow up to validate the safety of withholding therapy in patients with negative findings by serial testing.

2.   The Non-Invasive Approach of Serial IP Alone

Multiple studies (43-51) have evaluated the sensitivity and specificity of occlusive cuff IP for proximal vein thrombosis in patients with clinically suspected VT (Table IV). The cumulative sensitivity and specificity are 95% and 96% respectively. Thus, in symptomatic patients, a positive result by IP is highly specific for acute proximal vein thrombosis, and can be used as a basis for commencing therapy. A negative IP result at presentation essentially excludes thepresence of obstructive proximal-vein thrombosis, but does not exclude the presence of isolated calf-vein thrombosis; in these patients, serial IP is required.

TABLE IV: Sensitivity and specificity of occlusive impedance plethysmography (IPG) for proximal-vein thrombosis in patients with symptomatic venous thrombosis

Investigator	Sensitivity*		Specificity†	
Hull et al., 1976[45]	93%	(124/133)	97%	(386/397)
Hull et al., 1977[60]	98%	(59/60)	95%	(108/114)
Toy and Schrier, 1978[47]	94%	(15/16)	100%	(9/9)
Flanigan et al., 1978[48]	96%	(52/54)	95%	(93/98)
Hull et al., 1978[46]	92%	(155/169)	96%	(305/317)
Gross and Burney, 1979[49]	100%	(9/9)	94%	(32/34)
Cooperman et al., 1979[50]	87%	(20/23)	96%	(72/75)
Wheeler and Anderson, 1980[14]	98%	(88/90)	92%	(191/209)
Hull et al., 1981[61]	95%	(74/78)	98%	(157/160)
Peters et al., 1982[51]	92%	(36/39)	93%	(115/124)

* Proportion of patients with positive venograms who have a positive IPG.
† Proportion of patients with normal venograms who have a normal IPG.

The use of repeated IP evaluations is based on the premise, now confirmed by clinical observation (14-16), that calf-vein thrombi are only clinically important when they extend into the proximal veins, at which point detection with IP is possible. Since extension occurs only in a minority of patients with calf-vein thrombosis (approximately 20%), by detecting only those patients who extend, treatment is confined to those patients who are most likely to benefit.

The approach of serial IP alone, initally reported by Wheeler based on a large retrospective study (14), has now been evaluated by two large prospective clinical trials (15,16). Based on the data provided by these two studies, the following conclusions can be made:

a) A positive result by IP (in the absence of conditions known to produce false positive results) in a patient with clinically suspected DVT is highly predictive of acute proximal vein thrombosis (positive predictive value greater than 90%);

b) It is safe to withhold therapy in patients with clinically suspected DVT who remain negative by serial IP over a 10 day period;

c) IP has a high clinical utility, as it was successfully performed in 98% of the more than 1400 patients studied.

3.   A Practical Non-Invasive Diagnostic Approach for
      Clinically Suspected Venous Thrombosis

A practical non-invasive diagnostic approach to clinically suspected VT is shown in Figure 2. If IP is positive in the absence of clinical conditions which are known to produce false-positive results, the diagnosis of VT is established and the patient is treated accordingly. A positive result in the presence of conditions known to produce false-positive results (*e.g.* congestive cardiac failure), should be confirmed by venography. If the result of the initial IP evaluation is negative, anticoagulant therapy is withheld, and IP is repeated the following day, and again on day three, day five to seven, and on day ten. If IP becomes positive during this time, a diagnosis of VT is made and anticoagulant therapy is commenced.

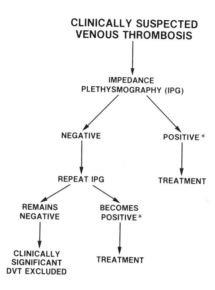

*Figure 2. Practical non-invasive approach for the diagnosis of clinically suspected deep-vein thrombosis using serial impedance plethysmography. * In the absence of clinical conditions known to produce false-positive results (e.g., congestive cardiac failure).*

III.   LONG-TERM MANAGEMENT OF VENOUS THROMBOEMBOLISM

A.   Summary

Heparin followed by long-term anticoagulant therapy remains the treatment of choice in most patients with acute venous thromboembolism. Oral anticoagulant therapy for three months, overlapped with intravenous heparin for four to five days prior to cessation of heparin therapy, is the standard long-term anticoagulant approach (38-40,63). Adjusted dose subcutaneous heparin is an effective and safe alternative to warfarin sodium for the long-term treatment of venous thromboembolism (39); it is the long-term regimen of choice in pregnant patients, and in patients returning to geographically remote areas lacking facilities for anticoagulant monitoring. Inferior vena caval interruption, using a transvenously-inserted filter, is the management of choice in patients in whom anticoagulant therapy is contraindicated, and in the very rare patient in whom anticoagulant therapy is ineffective.

Recent data indicate that failure to follow the initial course of heparin with adequate long-term therapy exposes patients with proximal vein thrombosis (VT involving the popliteal or more proximal veins) to a 40 to 50% risk of recurrent venous thromboembolism (38); this risk is markedly reduced to less than 2% by long-term anticoagulant therapy with warfarin sodium (38-40).

B. Oral Anticoagulant Therapy

Oral anticoagulants (*e.g.* warfarin sodium) antagonize the effect of Vitamin K by inhibiting its effect on the hepatic synthesis of factors II, VII, IX, and X, resulting in the synthesis of biologically inactive forms of these coagulation proteins (63). The anticoagulant effect of the Vitamin K antagonists is delayed until the normal clotting factors are cleared from the circulation, and the peak inhibitory effect on the synthesis of biologically active Vitamin K-dependent clotting factors only takes place 36 to 72 hours after drug administration. Oral anticoagulants also inhibit the synthesis of protein C, a proenzyme activated by thrombin to form activated protein C (63). Activated protein C inhibits activated factor V and activated factor VIII and is a potentially important anticoagulant.

The laboratory test most commonly used to measure the effect of oral anticoagulants is the one-stage prothrombin time (PT), which is sensitive to reduced activity of factors II, VII and X, but is insensitive to reduced activity of factor IX. The optimal therapeutic range for oral anticoagulant therapy monitored using the prothrombin time has been controversial because, until recently, it had not been adequately evaluated in clinical trials (64). Further confusion about the appropriate therapeutic range was created by the fact that different tissue thromboplastins used for measuring the prothombin time vary considerably in their sensitivity to the Vitamin K dependent clotting factors,and in response to oral anticoagulants. In North America, the thromboplastin reagents are usually obtained from rabbit brain tissue, whereas in the United Kingdom and parts of Europe, the thromboplastin is obtained from human brain (64). The rabbit brain thromboplastins which are commercially available in North America (*e.g.* Simplastin, Dade-C, etc.) are generally less sensitive to reductions in the Vitamin K dependent coagulation factors than is standardized human brain thromboplastin (40,64). A prothrombin time ratio of 1.5 to 2.0 times control using a rabbit brain thromboplastin is equivalent to a ratio of 4.0 to 6.0 times control using human brain thromboplastin. Conversely, a prothrombin time ratio using human brain thromboplastin of 2.0 to 3.0 times control is equivalent to a prothrombin time ratio of approximately 1.25 to 1.5 times control using rabbit brain thromboplastin (40,64).

The traditionally recommended therapeutic range in North America for patients with venous thromboembolism (*i.e.* a prothrombin time ratio of 1.5 to 2.0 times control using rabbit brain thromboplastin), although effective, is associated with a high risk of bleeding (20%)(38-40). A recent randomized trial (40) indicates that patients with venous thromboembolism can now be treated with a low risk (4%) of bleeding, without loss of effectiveness for preventing recurrent venous thromboembolism, by adjusting the dose of warfarin sodium to achieve a less intense anticoagulant effect (1.25 to 1.5 times control using a rabbit brain thromboplastin).

In order to promote standardization of the prothrombin time for monitoring anticoagulant therapy, the World Health Organization (WHO) has developed an international reference thromboplastin from human brain, and has recommended that the prothrombin time ratio be expressed according to a uniform system known as the International Normalized Ratio (INR)(64). The INR is the prothrombin time ratio obtained by testing a given plasma sample using the WHO reference thromboplastin. For practical clinical purposes, the INR for a particular plasma sample is equivalent to the prothrombin time ratio obtained using a human brain thromboplastin known as the Manchester Comparative Reagent (MCR), which is widely used in the United Kingdom (64). In patients with venous thromboembolism, the recommended less intense therapeutic range of 1.25 to 1.5 times control using a rabbit brain thromboplastin corresponds to an INR of 2.0 to 3.0 (40,64).

1.   Protocol for Oral Anticoagulant Therapy Using Warfarin Sodium

Warfarin sodium is administered in an initial dose of 10 mg per day for the first two days, and the daily dose is then adjusted according to the prothrombin time. Heparin therapy is discontinued on the fourth or fifth day following the initiation of warfarin therapy, provided the prothrombin time is prolonged into the therapeutic range (see above).

A four to five day overlap period of heparin and warfarin therapy is important. Experimental evidence indicates that the maximal antithrombotic effect of oral anticoagulant therapy is delayed for as long as five days (63), even though the anticoagulant effect, reflected by an increase in the prothrombin time (due mainly to a reduction in factor VII), may be evident within two to three days. Factor VII and Protein C (a naturally occurring anticoagulant) have similar short half-lives; therefore, in the early stage of warfarin administration, the levels of functionally active factor VII and protein C fall while the levels of functionally active factors II, IX and X remain relatively normal. Consequently, in the early stages of warfarin therapy, the anticoagulant effect of low-functional factor VII is counteracted by the potentially thrombogenic effect of low levels of functional protein C, while the levels of other Vitamin K dependent coagulation proteins are relatively normal (63). After 72 to 96 hours, the levels of functional factors II, IX and X fall and the optimal anticoagulant activity of warfarin therapy is expressed. For these reasons, it is important to overlap oral anticoagulant therapy with heparin therapy for four to five days even though the prothrombin time may be prolonged into the therapeutic range after two to three days.

Once the patient's condition is stable, the prothrombin time is monitored weekly throughout the course of oral anticoagulant therapy. However, if there are factors which may produce an unpredictible response to warfarin (*e.g.*, concominent drug therapy), the prothrombin time is monitored more frequently to minimize the risk of complications due to poor anticoagulant control.

Oral anticoagulant therapy is continued for three months in patients with their first episode of proximal-vein thrombosis or PE. A longer course of therapy is indicated in patients in whom there is a continuing risk factor for venous thromboembolism. In patients with a continuing risk factor that is potentially reversible, oral anticoagulant therapy should be continued until the risk factor is reversed. Oral anticoagulant therapy should be continued indefinitely in patients with an irreversible risk factor (for example, antithrombin III deficiency or protein C deficiency). In patients with objectively documented recurrent VT, discontinuation of oral anticoagulant therapy at three months is associated with a 20% risk of recurrent venous thromboembolism during the following year (62); in these patients, oral anticoagulant therapy should be continued for at least one year.

2.   Adverse Effects of Oral Anticoagulants

The major side effect of oral anticoagulant therapy is bleeding. Bleeding during well-controlled oral anticoagulant therapy is usually due to surgery or other forms of trauma, or to local lesions such as peptic ulcer or carcinoma (38-40). Spontaneous bleeding may occur if warfarin sodium is given in an excessive dose resulting in marked prolongation of the prothrombin time; this bleeding may be severe and even life-threatening. The risk of bleeding can be substantially reduced in patients with VT by maintaining the prothrombin time (using rabbit brain thromboplastin) at approximately 1.25 times control (INR 2.0 to 3.0), without loss of effectiveness for preventing recurrent venous thromboembolism (40).

Non-hemorrhagic side effects of coumarin anticoagulants are uncommon and the coumarins (*e.g.* warfarin sodium) are the oral anticoagulants of choice. The non-hemorrhagic side effects occur more frequently with the indanedione derivatives, and include skin necrosis, dermatitis, and a syndrome of painful blue toes. Hypersensitivity reactions have been reported to occur in 1 to 3% of patients receiving indanedione derivatives, and include rash, fever, hepatitis, leukopenia, renal failure, and diarrhea; these side effects are sometimes fatal. The indanedione derivatives also produce red discoloration of the urine in many patients which is sometimes confused with hematuria.

Oral anticoagulants cross the placenta and may cause fetal malformations when used during pregnancy. Two specific fetopathic syndromes as a result of oral anticoagulant administration during pregnancy are now well-recognized. Administration of oral anticoagulants during a critical period (the sixth to ninth week of gestation) may induce the syndrome of "warfarin embryopathy" in the fetus (a syndrome which includes a variety of skeletal abnormalities ranging from stippled epiphyses to frank skeletal hypoplasia). A second specific fetopathic syndrome of oral anticoagulant administration during the second or third trimester of pregnancy has been reported, characterized by multiple central nervous system abnormalities, such as abnormalities of the ventricular system (the Dandy-Walker malformation), dorsal midline dysplasia, optic atrophy, and agenesis of the corpus

TABLE V: Drug interactions with oral anticoagulants

Increase anticoagulant effect	Decrease anticoagulant effect
Allopurinol	Barbiturates
Anabolic steroids	Cholestyramine
Chloramphenicol	Dichloralphenazone
Clofibrate	Diuretics
Co-trimoxazole (trimethoprim & sulphamethoxazole)	Estrogens
Dextrothyroxine	Glutethimide
Disulfiram	Griseofulvin
Mefanamic acid	Heptabarbitone
Neomycin	Phenytoin
Nortriptyline	Rifampicin
Oxphenbutazone	
Phenylbutazone	
Phenyramidol	
Quinidine	
Salicylate	
Sulphaphenazole	
Sulphafurazole	
Sulphinpyrazone	

callosum. Thus, exposure to oral anticoagulants during the first trimester results in the risk of warfarin embryopathy, whereas, exposure in the second and/or third trimesters appears to independently predispose to the development of central nervous system abnormalities. Therefore, oral anticoagulants are contraindicated at any time during pregnancy, and should not be used in women planning a pregnancy.

3.   Factors that Interact with the Effect of Oral Anticoagulants

A large number of drugs interact with oral anticoagulants and may produce either a prolongation or reduction in the anticoagulant effect (Table V). Special care should be taken to adjust the dose of oral anticoagulant therapy during the time that other drugs are being taken to minimize the risk of complications due to inadequate anticoagulant control.

Increased sensitivity to oral anticoagulants occurs in vitamin K deficiency, impaired liver function, and thyrotoxicosis due to more rapid metabolism of the vitamin K-dependent clotting factors.

C.   Adjusted Subcutaneous Heparin Therapy

Adjusted dose subcutaneous heparin therapy is the long-term regimen of choice in pregnant patients, and in patients who return to geographically remote areas in whom long-term anticoagulant monitoring is impractical. The starting dose of long-term subcutaneous heparin is determined from the patient's initial intravenous heparin dose requirements; a starting subcutaneous dose equivalent to one-third of the patient's 24 hour intravenous heparin dose is administered every 12 hours. For example, if the patient required 30,000 units/24 hours of continuous intravenous heparin to maintain the APTT above 1.5 times the control value, the starting dose of long-term subcutaneous heparin would be 10,000 units every 12 hours. The subcutaneous dose is adjusted during the first three days of long-term therapy to maintain the mid-interval APTT (determined six hours after injection) at 1.5 times the control value (39). Following this initial adjustment, the dose is fixed and further anticoagulant monitoring is not required. A recent randomized clinical trial (39) indicates that this approach is effective for preventing recurrent venous thromboembolism and is associated with a low-risk (2%) of bleeding complications.

Long-term subcutaneous heparin has the potential disadvantage of inducing osteoporosis if administered for longer than three months. If treatment with adjusted dose subcutaneous heparin for longer than three months is necessary, these patients should be evaluated at regular intervals with an objective technique for measuring bone density.

D.   Inferior Vena Caval Interruption

Inferior vena caval interruption should be used in the following circumstances:

a) The patient with acute VT and an absolute contraindication to anticoagulant therapy;
b) The rare patient with massive PE who survives, but in whom recurrent embolism may be fatal;
c) The very rare patient who suffers from objectively documented recurrent VT during adequate anticoagulant therapy.

Inferior vena caval interruption has the potential of increasing the risk of long-term sequelæ (*e.g.*, a more severe post-phlebitic syndrome), and it may be ineffective for preventing late embolic recurrence due to the development of collaterals which bypass the inferior vena caval interruption. The frequency of these late complications can be reduced by using the Greenfield filter (a transvenously-inserted filter), which is associated with a very low frequency of loss of patency. The Greenfield filter does not require concomitant anticoagulant therapy to maintain patency, and because the hemodynamic disturbances are less, the sequelæ of venous outflow obstruction are minimized.

REFERENCES

1.   Urokinase pulmonary embolism trial: A national co-operative study. (1973) *Circulation* **47**(Supp II):1.
2.   Bell WR, Simon TL and Demets DL. (1977) *Am J Med* **62**:355.
3.   Bell WR and Simon TL. (1976) *Am Heart J* **92**:700.
4.   Alderson PO, Rujanavech N, Secker-Walker RH and McKnight RC. (1976) *Radiology* **120**:633.
5.   Biello DR, Mattar AG, McKnight RC *et al.* (1979) *Am J Radiol* **133**:1033.
6.   McNeil BJ. (1980) *J Nucl Med* **21**:319.
7.   Hull R, Hirsh J, Carter C, *et al.* (1983) *Ann Intern Med* **98**:891.
8.   Hull R, Hirsh J, Carter C *et al.* (1985) *Chest* **88**:819.
9.   Haeger K. (1969) *Angiology* **20**:219.
10. Kakkar VV, Howe CT, Flanc C *et al.* (1969) *Lancet* **2**:230.

11. McLachlin J, Richards T and Paterson JC. (1962) *Arch Surg* **85**:738.

12. Nicolaides AN, Kakkar VV, Field ES *et al.* (1971) *Br J Radiol* **44**:653.

13. Hull R, Hirsh J, Sackett DL *et al.* (1981) *Circulation* **64**:622.

14. Wheeler HB and Anderson FA, Jr. (1982) *In* **Non-Invasive Diagnostic Techniques in Vascular Disease.** (EF Bernstein, ed) CV Mosby:St. Louis, 2nd ed.

15. Hull R, Hirsh J, Carter CJ *et al.* (1985) *Ann Intern Med* **102**:21.

16. Huisman MV, Buller HR, Ten Cate JW and Vreeken J. (1986) *N Engl J Med* **314**:823.

17. Hull T, Hirsh J, Sackett DS *et al.* (1981) *N Engl J Med* **304**:1561.

18. Salzman EW. (1986) *N Engl J Med* **314**:847.

19. Robin ED. (1977) *Ann Intern Med* **87**:775.

20. Dalen JE. (1974) *In* **Cardiac Catheterization and Angiography.** (W Grossman, ed) Lea and Febiger:Philadelphia, 2nd edition.

21. Bookstein JJ and Silver TM. (1974) *Radiology* **110**:25.

22. Bookstein JJ. (1969) *Radiology* **93**:1007.

23. Grollman JH, Gyepes MT and Helmer E. (1970) *Radiology* **96**:202.

24. Mills SR, Jackson DC, Older RA, Heaston DK and Moore AV. (1980) *Radiology* **136**:295.

25. Rabinov K and Paulin S. (1972) *Arch Surg* **104**:134.

26. Lea Thomas M. (1972) *Arch Surg* **104**:145.

27. Bettman MA and Paulin S. (1977) *Radiology* **122**:101.

28. Wacker WE, Rosenthal M, Snodgrass PJ and Amader E. (1961) *JAMA* **178**:8.

29. Szucs MM, Brooks HL, Grossman W *et al.* (1971) *Ann Intern Med* **74**:161.

30. Ransohoff DF and Feinstein AR. (1978) *N Engl J Med* **299**:926.

31. Denardo G, Goodwin DA, Ravasini R *et al.* (1974) *N Engl J Med* **282**:1334.

32. Williams O, Lyall J, Vernon M *et al.* (1974) *Br Med J* **1**:600.

33. Austin JM and Sagel SS. (1972) *Invest Radiol* **7**:135.

34. Robinson AE, Puckett CL, Green JD *et al.* (1973) *Radiology* **109**:283.

35. Cheely R, McCartney WH, Perry JR *et al.* (1981) *Am J Med* **70**:17.

36. Alderson PO, Biello Dr, Gottschalk A *et al.* (1984) *Radiology* **153**:515.

37. Sasahara AA, Sharma GVRK and Parisi AF. (1979) *Am J Cardiol* **43**:1214.

38. Hull R, Delmore T, Genton E *et al.* (1979) *N Engl J Med* **301**:855.

39. Hull R, Delmore T, Carter C *et al.* (1982) *N Engl J Med* **306**:189.

40. Hull R, Hirsh J, Carter C, *et al.* (1982) *N Engl J Med* **307**:1676.

41. Moser KM and Lemoine JR. (1981) *Ann Intern Med* **94**:439.

42. Wheeler HR, Pearson D, O'Connell D *et al.* (1972) *Arch Surg* **104**:164.

43. Wheeler HB, O'Donnell JA, Anderson FA *et al.* (1975) *Angiology* **26**:199.

44. Johnston KW, Kakkar VV, Spindler JJ *et al.* (1974) *Am J Surg* **127**:349.

45. Hull R, van Aken WG, Hirsh J *et al.* (1976) *Circulation* **53**:696.

46. Hull R, Hirsh J, Powers P *et al.* (1978) *Circulation* **58**:898.

47. Toy PT and Schrier SL. (1978)*West J Med* **129**:89.

48. Flanigan DP, Goodreau JJ, Burnham SJ *et al.* (1978) *Lancet* **2**:331.

49. Gross WE and Burney RE. (1979) *J Am Coll Emerg Phys* **8**:110.

50. Cooperman M, Martin EW Jr, Satiani B *et al.* (1979) *Am J Surg* **137**:252.

51. Peters SH, Jonker JJ, de Boer AD *et al.* (1982) *Thromb Hemost* **48**:397.

52. Evans DS. (1971) *Ann R Coll Surg Engl* **49**:225.

53. Homes MCCG. (1973) *Med J Aust* **1**:427.

54. Sigel B, Felix WR, Popky GL *et al.* (1972) *Arch Surg* **104**:174.

55. Strandness DE and Sumner DS. (1972) *Arch Surg* **104**:180.

56. Browse NL. (1972) *Arch Surg* **104**:160.

57. Flanc C, Kakkar VV and Clark MB. (1968) *Br J Surg* **55**:742.

58. Kakkar VV. (1972) *Arch Surg* **104**:152.

59. Kakkar VV. (1977) *Semin Nucl Med* **7**:229.

60. Hull R, Hirsh J, Sackett DL *et al.* (1977) *N Engl J Med* **296**:1497.

61. Hull R, Hirsh J, Sackett DL *et al.* (1981) *Ann Intern Med* **94**:12.

62. Hull R, Carter C, Jay R *et al.* (1983) *Circulation* **67**(4):901.

63. Wessler S and Gitel SN. (1984) *N Engl J Med* **311**:645.

64. Hirsh J, Deykin D and Poller L. (1986) *Chest* **89**(Feb suppl):11S.

Management of Chronic Unresolved Large Vessel Thromboembolism

KENNETH M. MOSER
PAT O. DAILY
KIRK L. PETERSON
From the Departments of Medicine and
Surgery,
University of California, San Diego,
School of Medicine,
San Diego, California 92103

I. INTRODUCTION

Pulmonary hypertension due to chronic thromboembolic obstruction of the major (main, lobar, segmental) pulmonary arteries has been, in the past, chiefly an autopsy diagnosis. Patients with persistent, unexplained dyspnea on exertion and right ventricular failure were found, at autopsy, to have organized, endothelialized thromboembolic residuæ obstructing major pulmonary arteries. They were reported as interesting medical curiosities (1-3).

Advances in diagnostic and cardiac surgical technics, and our understanding of the pathophysiology of thromboembolism, have changed the status of this disorder. Demonstration that surgical thromboendarterectomy is both feasible and associated with substantial hemodynamic improvement has changed the prognosis of these patients (4-7).

We report here 42 patients with this disorder who have undergone thromboendarterectomy at the UCSD and San Diego VA Medical Centers between July, 1970, and December, 1985.

The Pulmonary Circulation
in Health and Disease

TABLE I. Characteristics of the 42 patients being reported.

Case	Age	Sex	Date of surgery	Duration of symptoms[1]	PAP	PCW	CO	PVR	NYHA
1	68	M	7/70	16.0	56	5	3.7	1208	4
2	37	M	2/75	0.5	42	8	3.9	864	3
3	31	M	7/76	2.0	43	9	3.6	756	3
* 4	65	M	9/76	3.0	52	15	4.6	698	4
5	31	M	5/78	8.0	41	5	5.2	554	3
6	55	F	4/79	2.0	49	12	3.81	767	4
7	24	M	1/80	1.0	45	4	5.8	565	3
8	42	M	2/81	1.5	50	4	3.1	1184	4
9	68	F	8/80	4.0	58	8	4.08	1018	4
10	42	M	2/81	1.5	27	5	3.9	451	3
11	61	M	4/81	3.0	65	8	2.44	1869	4
12	60	M	5/81	4.0	58	8	3.8	1116	4
* 13	21	F	6/81	3.0	38	9	4.17	556	4
14	39	M	6/81	16.0	66	6	4.2	1142	4
15	26	F	9/81	0.8	62	10	3.1	1600	4
16	70	M	5/83	3.0	40	10	3.1	800	4
* 17	56	F	10/83	8.0	70	10	2.2	1891	4
18	38	M	3/84	8.0	44	11	5.15	512	3
* 19	70	M	3/84	2.0	50	10	3.2	1020	4
20	35	M	3/84	5.0	48	13	3.52	800	4
* 21	67	M	3/84	2.0	60	8	4.6	698	4
22	38	M	5/84	1.5	65	9	2.41	1856	4
23	64	M	8/84	6.0	43	12	3.5	708	4
24	40	M	9/84	24.0	60	8	4.05	1024	4
25	54	M	10/84	0.4	35	8	3.2	675	4
26	20	M	10/84	2.0	47	9	3.1	984	4
27	24	M	11/84	1.0	38	12	2.4	867	3
28	54	M	1/85	4.0	52	8	4.0	900	3
29	43	M	2/85	4.0	45	2	5.98	590	4
* 30	41	M	2/85	1.0	48	5	3.6	952	4
31	56	F	3/85	1.0	50	6	4.4	1000	3
32	39	M	4/85	6.0	55	7	4.4	891	4
33	69	F	6/85	2.0	46	8	4.4	691	4
34	28	M	6/85	2.0	45	12	3.2	825	4
35	51	M	6/85	1.5	33	8	3.12	640	3
* 36	37	M	7/85	7.0	65	9	3.24	971	4
37	36	M	8/85	5.0	45	12	4.6	600	4
38	73	M	10/85	2.5	45	12	4.7	560	3
39	38	F	11/85	8.0	48	10	3.7	816	4
40	40	M	11/85	2.5	42	11	4.6	540	3
41	38	M	11/85	0.8	50	9	4.1	800	4
42	24	M	12/85	6.0	45	6	4.22	739	3

[1]Duration of symptoms = duration before surgery (in years)
PAP = mean pulmonary artery pressure in mmHg
PCW = pulmonary capillary (wedge) pressure in mmHg
C.O. = cardiac output in liters/minute
PVR = calculated resistance in dynes/sec-cm^5
NYHA = cardiac class, New York Heart Association criteria
* died post-operatively

II.   FREQUENCY

The frequency of this disorder is unknown. It is estimated that some 500,000 patients/year in the United States experience embolism, of whom 450,000 survive. Among these survivors, prior reports indicate that significant residual embolic obstruction is rare (8-10). However, such data are derived from patient groups in which the diagnosis of acute embolism was made and therapy given. Many patients in our series were neither diagnosed nor operated upon during their acute embolic episode(s).

In 1983, we reported results in the first fifteen patients operated upon during the period 1970 - 1982, a rate of approximately 1.3 patients/year (5). Between 1983 and late 1985, an additional 27 patients have been operated, or approximately 9 patients/year. This experience suggests that recognition is increasing.

Thus, the condition is uncommon, but not as rare as previously believed. What might be a reasonable estimate of its frequency? If, among the 450,000 survivors of pulmonary embolism each year, 1% have massive embolism which fails to resolve, some 4500/year exist; if the estimate is a more likely 0.1%, (1/1000), then there are 450 instances per year. Whatever the estimate, it seems evident that a number of such patients are being carried under alternative diagnoses. This frequency is not likely to change significantly with use of new therapies (e.g., thrombolytic agents) because, as noted, many of these patients escape diagnosis and, therefore, therapy.

III.   DIAGNOSIS

Quite characteristically, the diagnosis of chromic thromboembolic major vessel pulmonary hypertension (C T-E PH) has been long delayed. The duration of symptoms (dyspnea on exertion and others) before surgery averaged 4.4 years (range 0.4 - 26 years) (Table I). The reasons for this delay have been multiple.

First, many patients have not had an obvious history of venous thromboembolism. Second, PH, like all forms of PH, presents in a subtle fashion. There are many other causes for its primary early symptoms (dyspnea on exertion and easy fatigue), and the physical findings of PH are easy to overlook. The dominant symptoms are dyspnea on exertion and fatigue. Other common symptoms include near-syncope on exertion and anginal pain. Physical findings depend upon the severity and duration of PH. The only physical finding with any specificity is the presence of "thrombus stenosis" murmurs, so-called because they are generated by flow through partial stenoses of the pulmonary arteries due to organized thrombus (4). These murmurs are like those heard in congenital

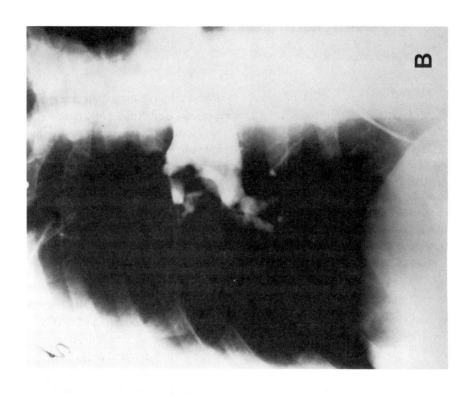

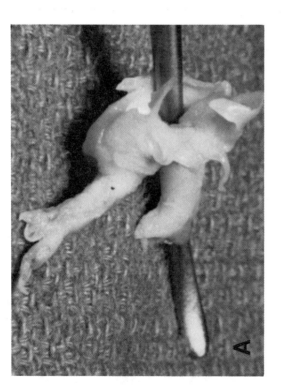

Figure 1.

A. Chronic thrombotic material removed from right upper lobe. Probe goes through narrow, stenotic channel. Loud murmur was present over this area.

B. Angiogram showing the stenotic area in right upper lobe (and obstruction elsewhere).

pulmonary artery stenosis. Perhaps their most important characteristic is that they are heard outside of the normal cardiac "listening areas." Location is determined by location of the stenotic area(s). Correlation with sites of anatomic stenosis has been excellent (Fig. 1). We have heard one or more such murmurs in 33% of operated patients.

Chest X-ray is often unremarkable, but may offer clues (Fig. 2). The central pulmonary arteries may be enlarged symmetrically (as in PPH); but more commonly, there is vascular *asymmetry* in C T-E PH, due to asymmetry in the distribution of obstruction and/or the fact that despite severe PH, organized thrombus prevents artery distension. The electrocardiographic findings are non-specific and there are no characteristic hematologic abnormalities. Pulmonary spirometric tests, usually normal, may be misleading by disclosing a restrictive

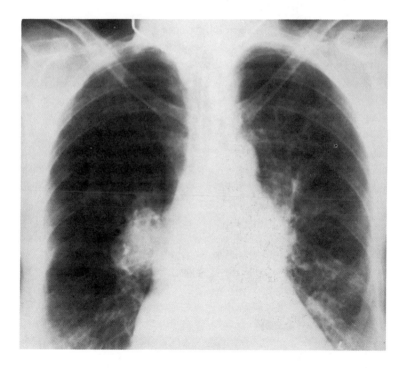

Figure 2. Striking chest X-ray in patient who proved to have thrombus totally occluding distal right main PA and several arteries on left. Note differences in vessel size and uneven flow distribution.

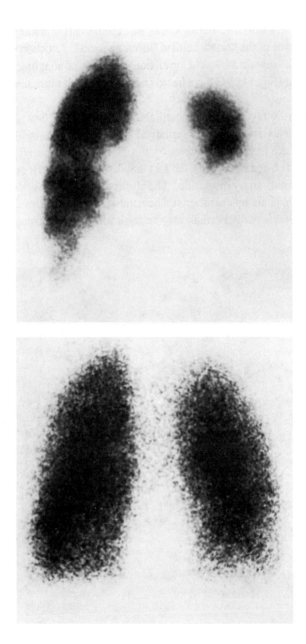

Figure 3. Perfusion scan (top) showing multiple, bilateral segmental defects which are "mismatched" by ventilation scan (bottom).

defect. Lung biopsies from several such patients have not disclosed interstitial fibrosis. Others have reported instances of unexplained restriction in patients with PPH (13). Therefore, C T-E PH should not be abandoned as a diagnosis when spirometric tests disclose restriction. Of particular importance are our findings regarding the diffusing capacity for carbon monoxide, a test described by some as a sensitive indicator of pulmonary vascular disease (14). That has not been the case with C T-E PH (13). The single breath D_{co} has been normal in 12/42 (29%) patients and only modestly reduced in many others. Thus, a normal or slightly reduced D_{co} does not exclude severe C T-E PH.

Arterial blood gas analysis has often provided the first unequivocal evidence of physiologic abnormality in these patients. Resting arterial hypoxemia (with normo- or hypo-capnia) is very common. All patients had either resting hypoxemia or a decline in P_aO_2 with exercise.

Lung scanning has proven an invaluable diagnostic tool. We have found that all patients with C T-E PH have one or more segmental or larger perfusion defects which, on ventilation scanning, are normally ventilated (15,16). These findings contrast sharply with those in PPH, in which we have found no patients with a segmental or larger defect that is "mismatched" on ventilation scan (Fig. 3). Thus, the perfusion scan has been extremely useful not only in alerting physicians to the diagnosis but also in distinguishing T-E PH from PPH.

Unfortunately, other types of pulmonary hypertension also may present with large perfusion defects, including fibrosing mediastinitis (17), pulmonary artery agenesis (18), congenital branch stenosis, tumors primary in (or compressing) large pulmonary arteries, and some instances of COPD.

Therefore, perfusion scans, while of great value, cannot be the final diagnostic step. Right heart catheterization and pulmonary angiography are the minimal additional requirements. Right heart catheterization cannot make the diagnosis of C T-E PH. However, it is central to establishing the severity of PH and excluding competing diagnoses such as left atrial or ventricular disease, pulmonary venous obstruction and intracardiac shunts. Pulmonary angiography is usually the definitive diagnostic step. Observing special precautions (to be discussed subsequently), we have found the procedure to be safe. Most often, pulmonary angiography establishes the diagnosis. However, in some patients the angiograph is equivocal in terms of thrombus location; in these, we now undertake direct visualization with a specially-designed fiberoptic angioscope (19).

IV.   NATURAL HISTORY

Our experience with chronic T-E PH has established some features of its natural history; but others remain to be defined.

Virtually all patients have shown symptomatic deterioration over months to years prior to surgery. One explanation for such deterioration would be multiple embolic recurrences. However, there is evidence that this is rarely the case. Among patients in whom serial scans and/or pulmonary angiograms have been available, there has been evidence of change in less than 5%. Furthermore, a number of patients have clearly progressed after non-occlusive interruption of the inferior vena cava (although this is, of course, not an absolute form of protection). Finally, the organized thromboemboli removed are always well-organized (with occasional evidence of more recent proximal thrombus extension).

Thus, while some patients have had recurrence or extension, the usual course appears to have been one major embolic event which fails to resolve. Among patients in whom that initial event was recognized, there is usually a history of acute symptoms followed by substantial symptomatic recovery. In our view this apparent recovery is in part due to thrombus organization and in part due to compensation via right ventricular dilatation and hypertrophy. Virtually all patients who reported such "recovery" still noted persistent dyspnea on exertion; and among those with follow-up scans, there was nominal scan improvement.

The explanation for progressive deterioration appears to lie in two events. First, the extreme exaggeration of PH (and, often, hypoxemia) which they demonstrate during exertion. Since these patients rarely limit exertion (indeed, some purposely exercise to "get in shape"), perhaps episodic right ventricular ischemia occurs, leading to progressive RV dysfunction. A second event, which we believe occurs in all patients, is development of progressive pulmonary arterial hypertensive changes in the smaller pulmonary arteries in the non-obstructed lung zones. Such changes, documented in more than 15 patients by lung biopsy, exaggerate the degree of PH and right ventricular afterload.

V.   SELECTION CRITERIA AND EVALUATION SEQUENCE:

Some 15 years ago, we established criteria for offering patients surgical thromboendarterectomy. We should emphasize that these criteria were not designed to select the "optimal" patients; i.e., those in whom the best outcomes might have been anticipated. Rather, they were designed to screen out: (1) patients who could safely be followed rather than operated; (2) patients in whom operation was contraindicated on the basis of thrombus location or associated disease.

These criteria include: (1) a calculated pulmonary vascular resistance above 300 dynes/sec-cm^5; (2) chronic thrombus located within the main, lobar and/or segmental pulmonary arteries; (3) absence of significant coexisting disease; (4) an informed decision on the part of the patient that surgical intervention is desired.

As already noted, patients are not excluded on the basis of the severity of hemodynamic compromise. Indeed, most patients have been seriously disabled, with 29 in NYHA Class IV and 13 in Class III preoperatively (Table I). Further, we have, on a number of occasions, violated criterion (3) and agreed to operate on patients with significant, coexisting disease, after extensive discussion of the increased risks involved. As to thrombus location, thrombi located in main or lobar arteries have consistently been associated with an ability to restore vessel patency at surgery. However, if all obstructions appear to begin at or beyond the segmental level, their successful removal is questionable. One concern at the onset of the series was that proximal thrombi might extend so far distally that endarterectomy would be impossible. We have found, however, that virtually all thrombi which present in main or lobar vessels are of modest length and usually extend only one "branch order" beyond their proximal origin. Some have suggested that bronchial arteriography might be useful in this context (6). We have not found it helpful. Table I summarizes the pre-operative features of the 42 patients. The average pulmonary artery pressure was 48.9 ($\pm$ 9.3); the average cardiac output, 3.86 ($\pm$ 0.84); and the average PVR, 897 ($\pm$ 352).

The evaluation sequence upon which we base surgical selection has evolved over a period of years. The procedures include, in addition to a detailed history and physical, a complete blood count, platelet count, prothrombin time and partial thromboplastin time, measurement of Anti-thrombin III, Protein C, Protein S, Factor X, a comprehensive admission chemistry panel, blood typing and cross-matching, electrocardiogram, chest x-ray, pulmonary spirometric tests, D_{co}, rest and exercise (if possible) arterial blood gas studies, 2-D echocardiogram-Doppler, perfusion and ventilation lung scans and impedance plethysmography (IPG).

The IPG is an important element of the evaluation not only in documenting a potential embolic source but also in deciding whether and when insertion of an IVC filter should be undertaken. In this series, IPGs were done unless a recent venogram was available. Of the 22 patients with a history compatible with prior DVT, 18 had either a positive IPG or venogram or both. More instructive, however, was the finding that, of the 20 patients with no history of DVT, the IPG or recent venogram or both were positive in 10 (50%).

With these data in hand, the remainder of the diagnostic sequence is planned. Right heart catheterization is the next procedure performed. If catheterization discloses significant pulmonary hypertension (PVR > 300

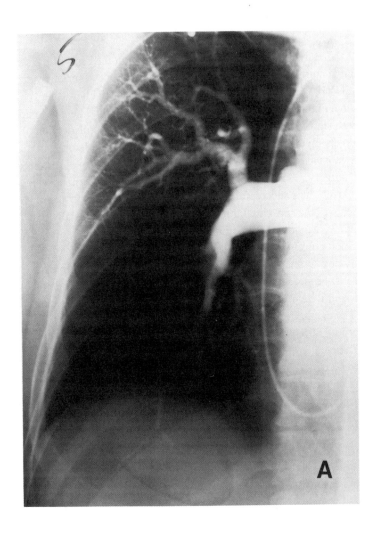

Figure 4. Angiogram of right (A) and left (B) pulmonary arterial tree demonstrating extensive chronic thrombotic obstruction.

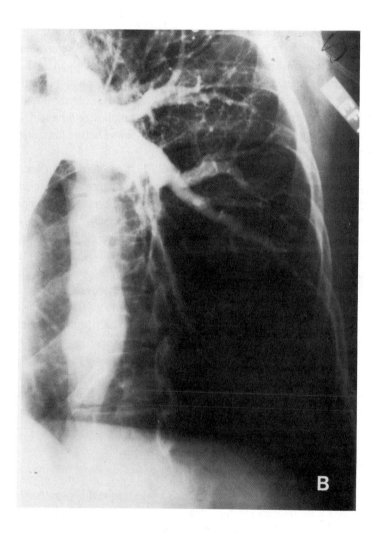

Figure 4B.

dynes/sec-cm[5]) and no alternative diagnosis is suggested, pulmonary angiography is performed. Special precautions are observed to limit risk and obtain images that allow accurate thrombus localization (20). These precautions include catheter insertion through arm or neck veins, unless a normal venogram or IPG is available; interruption of heparin therapy only the evening before and morning of the procedure; administration of supplementary oxygen throughout; and the use of non-ionic contrast media. There are rarely more than two contrast injections done: one into the right main PA; one into the left. Large, cut films are obtained (Fig. 4). The field of view is carefully pre-positioned to emphasize the main, lobar and segmental arteries. The films are processed and reviewed before the catheter is moved.

Angiographic interpretation in C T-E PH is much more difficult than in acute embolism. Such difficulty reflects the variable patterns of organization and recanalization encountered. Our interpretive skills have evolved by comparing, in each patient, angiographic findings with findings at surgery.

If, even after angiography, question persists regarding diagnosis or thrombus location, angioscopy is performed (19). Finally, it is now routine to perform coronary angiography in all patients above 35, or with special coronary disease risk factors at any age, or with angina. In addition, left heart catheterization may be needed if competing diagnoses (e.g., fibrosing mediastinitis) are entertained (17). CAT scanning may be performed if fibrosing mediastinitis is considered. MRI is currently under evaluation.

With all of the data available, the patient and relatives/friends meet with the physician team and discuss the potential of surgical intervention, and its timing. If indicated, insertion of an IVC filter is performed and a date set for thromboendarterectomy.

VI.   SURGICAL APPROACH

Perhaps the most important aspects of the surgical approach are: (1) the recognition that pulmonary thromboendarterectomy bears no resemblance to acute embolectomy; and (2) that the procedure should not be undertaken, even by the most skilled of cardiovascular surgeons, without witnessing the procedure and discussing it in depth with those who have performed it repetitively. Pulmonary thromboendarterectomy is time-consuming, difficult and tedious. If mortality is to be avoided and a good surgical result obtained, all technical details must be optimized. Our approach has evolved over a period of years (4, 5, 7, 21, 22), and in patients who have presented a variety of challenges anatomically and functionally.

The median sternotomy approach should be used. Thoracotomy, in our view, should not be done. Luxuriant bronchial collaterals are associated with severe bleeding risks; violation of the pleural space makes intra- and post-operative management extremely difficult. Adequate exposure to the entire proximal pulmonary arterial tree is provided via median sternotomy.

A bloodless field is essential to optimal endarterectomy. To achieve this, cardiopulmonary bypass, hypothermia and cardioplegia are needed. It is vital to recognize that no "embolus" is present. Rather, organized, endothelialized fibrotic masses, incorporated into the arterial walls, are encountered (Fig. 5).

It has become routine to explore the atrial septum and close atrial septal openings, if present. If very severe tricuspid insufficiency is present, tricuspid annuloplasty also has been done (four cases).

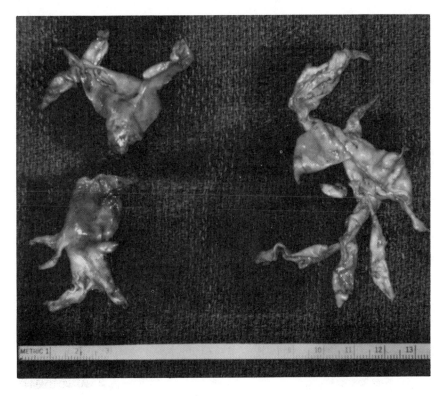

Figure 5. Extensive, organized material removed from right and left lungs at thromboendarterectomy. Meticulous dissection in a bloodless field was essential.

All patients are placed on mechanical compressive devices of the lower extremities during and after surgery.

If the patient has coronary artery disease requiring bypass, this is done in concert with the thromboendarterectomy.

VII.   POST-OPERATIVE CONSIDERATIONS

These patients experience all of the complications common to other forms of open heart surgery. In addition, they may develop certain special complications. One of these is bilateral hypothermic injury of the phrenic nerves. This was encountered in seven patients in the series; two expired and all had prolonged, difficult courses post-operatively. All patients who survived have

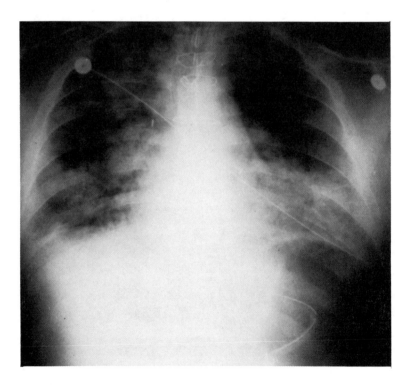

Figure 6. Reperfusion pulmonary edema. Chest X-ray at 48 hours after surgery. Edema is limited to those zones supplies by vessels from which chronic obstructions were removed.

recovered full diaphragmatic function, at three to eight months post-operatively. A special insulating device between the heart and pericardium have eliminated this complication (22) in the 20 patients operated since late 1984.

The most consistent complication encountered post-operatively is what we have called reperfusion pulmonary edema (RPE) (Fig. 6). This unusual form of pulmonary edema is limited to those lung regions supplied by pulmonary arteries which have been opened at thrombo-endarterectomy (23). It usually appears within 24 hours of surgery but, in some patients, has been delayed until 72 hours. A detailed analysis has shown that neither the time of onset nor the duration of RPE relate to such factors as pre-operative or post-operative pulmonary arterial, wedge or left atrial pressures, patient age, or pre-operative duration of symptoms (23). Its basis remains unknown.

RPE is a major post-operative problem because it induces significant and persistent post-operative hypoxemia, necessitating prolonged mechanical ventilation and use of increased F_IO_2. All patients receive DVT prophylaxis by mechanical compression of the lower extremities during and after surgery. If there is no contraindication, heparin is initiated at 24-36 hours post-operatively (5000 units subcutaneously every eight hours).

A variety of psychiatric aberrations (including euphoria, paranoia, depression, hallucinations) are common in the post-operative period. Their genesis is under investigation.

VIII.   EARLY FOLLOW-UP APPROACH

All patients, except one, have demonstrated substantial hemodynamic improvement in the immediate post-operative period (Table II). The patient with no PVR decline was the only one in whom no significant thrombus could be removed. The PVR is a better monitor of the immediate results of thromboendarterectomy than the pulmonary arterial pressure because it is characteristic for the cardiac output to increase sharply in the post-operative period. Thus, the pulmonary arterial pressure may underestimate the decrement in resistance achieved.

The immediate post-operative pulmonary hemodynamics do not, however, necessarily reflect longer-term results. The use of positive pressure ventilation and the presence of RPE often maintain PAP and PVR above levels observed subsequently. Furthermore, the anatomic pulmonary vascular changes previously described appear to resolve slowly so that maximum hemodynamic improvement often occurs only after 6-9 months.

TABLE II. Hemodynamic values before surgery (pre) and during first several days after surgery.

PAm		PCW		CO		PVR[1]	
Pre	Post	Pre	Post	Pre	Post	Pre	Post
48	2.96	9	11	3.86	5.67	897	278
(±9.3)	(±8.3)	(±3)	(±3)	(±0.84)	(±1.08)	(±352)	(±135)

[1]PAm = pulmonary arterial mean pressure in mmHg; PCW = wedge (or left atrial) pressure in mmHg; CO = cardiac output in l/min; PVR = pulmonary vascular resistance in dynes/sec/cm^5.

IX.   DEATHS

Among the 42 patients operated to date, seven deaths have occurred in the post-operative period, placing mortality at 16.6%. These deaths occurred from less than 24 hours to 126 days after surgery (Table III). Analysis of those patients who died disclosed that all were in NYHA Class IV, had severe pulmonary hemodynamic compromise and most had a significant coexisting disorder. All patients, save one, had a successful thromboendarterectomy with a marked, immediate decline in pulmonary vascular resistance post-operatively.

Some comment on the specific circumstances surrounding each mortality is warranted because these experiences have conditioned modifications in evaluation, surgical approach and/or post-operative management.

Two patients died of acute myocardial infarction. One was 65 years old, developed infarction on the 17th post-operative day when he was fully ambulatory. He died of unrelenting left ventricular failure two days later. Autopsy disclosed a large left ventricular infarct and patent pulmonary arteries. The second patient was 37 years old, had been markedly obese in the past, had undergone gastric stapling 20 months before, but still was obese. A coronary angiogram done elsewhere eight months before, and reviewed by us, was normal. An echocardiogram at our institution disclosed normal LV function. The day following surgery, he suddenly developed hypotension, marked reduction of cardiac output, elevation of left atrial pressure, and EKG evidence of myocardial infarction. He expired four days after surgery. Autopsy disclosed a severe, discrete stenosis of the LAD coronary artery and extensive left ventricular infarction.

Experience with these two patients led to our policy of obtaining coronary angiography in all patients 35 years or older, with angina or special risk factors for CAD.

TABLE III. Seven patients have died in the post-operative period, one after transfer to another hospital. See text for details.

Case #	Age	NYHA	Time Post-Op (days)	Cause
4	65	4	19	Myocardial Infarct (LV)
13	21	4	55	ARDS
17	56	4	<1	Myocardial Infarct (RV)
19	70	4	126	Diaphragmatic paresis; multiple complications
21	67	4	45	Diaphragmatic paresis; multiple complications
30	41	4	<1	No thrombus removed
36	37	4	4	Myocardial Infarct (LV)

A severely disabled 56 year old woman, with prolonged RV failure and hypoxemia, developed significant RPE six hours after chest closure. Despite ventilator support, marked arterial hypoxemia (P_aO_2 40-50) developed. A decline in cardiac output ensued and EKG evidence of RV ischemia appeared. She expired some hours thereafter. Autopsy disclosed extensive ischemic changes throughout the very hypertrophied RV.

A 21 year old female developed marked RPE immediately following thrombo-endarterectomy. The RPE involved all lobes, thrombi having been removed from all lobar arteries. This cleared slowly over three weeks. However, two days after mechanical ventilation was discontinued, ARDS developed and mechanical ventilation was resumed. She expired on the 55th post-operative day. Autopsy disclosed only severe ARDS.

One patient, admitted in prolonged, severe RV failure had, on angiography and angioscopy, multiple segmental and subsegmental obstructions. After extensive discussion with the patient regarding these highly unfavorable findings, surgery was undertaken at his request. At surgery, only one segmental occlusion in the left lower lobe could be alleviated. After chest closure, the patient's cardiac output could not be sustained and he expired six hours after surgery.

The remaining two post-operative deaths were occasioned by a complex of post-operative complications. Both developed bilateral diaphragmatic paresis and marked RPE post-operatively. Both required prolonged mechanical ventilation. One died on the 45th post-operative day; the other, after transport to another

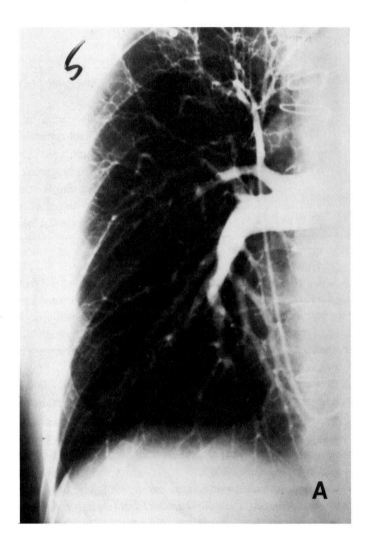

Figure 7. Follow-up angiogram of right (A) and left (B) pulmonary vessels at 9 months after thromboendarterectomy. Same patient as in Figure 4.

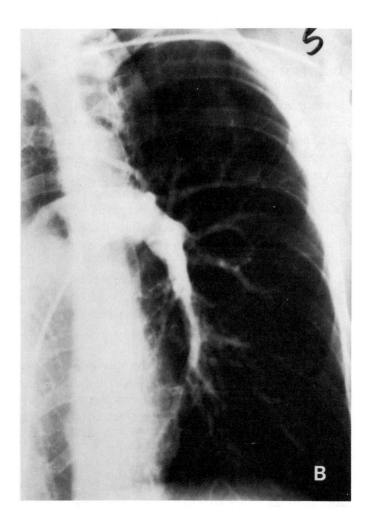

Figure 7B.

hospital, 126 days after surgery. The combination of diaphragmatic paresis and RPE mandated sustained mechanical ventilation, the complications of which are well-recognized.

X.   LONGTERM FOLLOW-UP

Patients referred for this procedure have come from many locales. While all are requested to return at 6-12 months after surgery, this has not been achieved in all patients. Therefore, follow-up data is a composite of information obtained by telephone-mail contact with the patient and the patient's physician, as well as by evaluation at UCSD.

The average duration of follow-up among survivors has been 28 months, with a range of seven months to 16 years. [The last patient included here in the series was operated in 12/85]. Follow-up has disclosed that symptomatic and physiologic improvement appear to continue for 9-12 months following surgery. In part, this reflects recovery from a major procedure. However, two other events also occur. One is the resolution of the post-operative hypoxemia. Of the 35 survivors, 29 demonstrated continued hypoxemia (P_aO_2 < 60 torr at rest or during exercise) at discharge and left the hospital on nasal oxygen. All patients have been able to discontinue use of supplementary oxygen at six weeks to four months post-discharge.

Another important feature is the long-term behavior of pulmonary hemodynamics. As noted in Table IV, there is a further decline in PAm and PVR at follow-up. This decline reflects, we believe, the resolution of both RPE and pulmonary arterial hypertensive changes. Results of follow-up angiograms have paralleled the hemodynamic data (Fig. 7).

TABLE IV. Serial pulmonary vascular resistance values in 17 patients in whom repeat cardiac catheterization was done four months to one year after theomboendarterectomy.

PVR Pre-operative	PVR Early (first 3 days postop)	PVR Late (4 mos-1 yr postop)
985	302	229
(±414)	(±138)	(±129)

TABLE V. NYHA classification of survivors before surgery and at time of last follow-up.

	Pre-op	Post-op
Class IV	22	0
Class III	13	1
Class II	0	18
Class I	0	16

There have been no embolic recurrences during the follow-up period, although two patients have had recurrent DVT. Twenty-six of the 35 survivors have had inferior vena caval interruption before or during admission, and all have been on long-term anticoagulant protection.

Perhaps most important has been the change in functional class after surgery (Table V). Of the 22 survivors in Class IV before surgery, one was in Class III, twelve in Class II and nine in Class I when last seen. Of the 13 in Class III, pre-op, five were in Class II and eight in Class I when last seen. In many instances, patients with prolonged, near-total disability have returned to normal activity.

REFERENCES

1.   Carroll D. (1950) *Am J Med* **9**:175.
2.   Ring A and Bakke JR. (1956) *Ann Intern Med* **43**:781.
3.   Ball KP, Goodman JF and Harrison CV. (1956)*Circulation* **14**:766.
4.   Moser KM, Houk VN, Jones RC *et al.* (1965) *Circulation* **32**:377.
5.   Moser KM, Spragg RG, Utley J and Daily P. (1983) *Ann Intern Med* **99**:299.
6.   Sabiston DC, Wolfe WG, Oldham HM *et al.* (1977) *Ann Surg* **185**:699.
7.   Daily PO, Johnson GG, Simmons CJ and Moser KM. (1980) *J Thor Cardiovasc Surg* **79**:523.
8.   Dalen JE, Banas JS, Brooks HL *et al.* (1969) *N Eng J Med* **280**:1194.
9.   Paraskos JA, Adelstein SJ, Smith RE *et al.* (1973) *N Eng J Med* **289**:55.
10. Hall RJC, Sutton AC and Kerr IH. (1977) *Brit Heart J* **39**:1128.
11. Horn M, Ries A, Neveu C and Moser K. (1983)*Amer Rev Resp Dis* **128**:163.

12.   Ryan KL, Fedullo PE, Clausen J and Moser KM. (1986) *Amer Rev Resp Dis* **133**:222.
13.   Goldring R. Personal Communication.
14.   Nadel JA, Gold WM and Burgess JH. (1968) *Am J Med* **44**:16.
15.   Moser KM, Fedullo PF, Shure D *et al.* (1986)*Amer Rev Resp Dis* **133**:A221.
16.   Fishmann AJ, Moser KM and Fedullo PF. (1983)*Chest* **84**:679.
17.   Berry D, Peterson K and Moser KM. (1986)*Chest* **89**:296.
18.   Bluck MC and Moser KM. (1970) *Circulation* **41**:859.
19.   Shure D, Gregoratos G and Moser KM. (1985) *Ann Intern Med* **103**:844.
20.   Peterson K, Moser KM, Nicod P *et al.* (submitted for publication).
21.   Utley JR, Spragg RG, Long WB *et al.* (1982) *Surgery* **92**:1096.
22.   Daily PO, Moser KM, Dembnitsky W. *et al.* (In press) *J Thor and Cardiovasc Surg* .
23.   Levinson RM, Shure D and Moser KM. (In press) *Amer Rev Resp Dis* .

Exogenous Influences on the Initiation and Course of Pulmonary Hypertension

DR. JOHANNES MLCZOCH
Oberarzt der Kardiol. Univ. Klinik
Garnisongasse 13
A-1090 Vienna, Austria

I.   INTRODUCTION

The first example that an exogenous stimulus can induce pulmonary hypertension was the finding that alveolar hypoxia leads to hypoxic pulmonary vasoconstriction. The possibility that other exogenous influences such as drugs and diet could also affect the pulmonary circulation is of increasing interest. However, the facts are still few and most of the thoughts on pathophysiology are still speculative.

In coronary heart disease the demonstration of spontaneous coronary vasospasm has opened a new understanding of many events. In the pulmonary circulation, the role of vasospasm is still yet to be defined, although in pulmonary hypertension spontaneous changes in pulmonary artery pressure and pulmonary vascular resistance are surprisingly frequent (1).

We do not know if the pulmonary vascular bed is subject to continuous active vasodilatation. If this is the case, pulmonary vasoconstriction might occur because of a reduction of dilatation. On the other hand, active vasoconstriction also occurs, and can be elicited in many different ways. In principle, there are two basic means by which an exogenous stimulus can enter to provoke vasoconstriction:

1. by inhalation
2. by ingestion.

The following presentation will focus on the second possibility.

An ingested substance might affect the pulmonary circulation by several means. The substance might either be toxic, or break down into toxic metabolites or be toxic to the pulmonary vessels because of incomplete detoxification in the liver. Another possibility is the activation of different systems within the circulation; for example, the complement system, coagulation system or specific blood cells. In this situation, however, the question arises, why the lung is more or less the only target organ. General activation of any system should produce changes not restricted to the pulmonary vascular bed. The epidemic increase in pulmonary hypertension related to the intake of the anorectic substance aminorex showed rather clearly, that not every person who took aminorex developed pulmonary hypertension, and therefore a predisposition has to be present. This individual predisposition could be temporary, perhaps associated with metabolic changes like acidosis induced by fasting, or permanent, like a latent endothelial cell dysfunction or other unidentified genetic determinant.

The next important question in the case of a dietary-induced pulmonary hypertension is whether the withdrawal or lack of ingestion stops the process responsible for the development of pulmonary hypertension. A trigger effect might lead to a self-perpetuating process, with pulmonary hypertension regardless of whether the exposure continues or not. Under these circumstances, once the damage is initiated, the pulmonary circulation remains damaged even if an improvement of resting pressures is achieved.

II.   POSSIBLE MECHANISMS LEADING TO PULMONARY HYPERTENSION

A.   Alveolar Hypoxia

Alveolar hypoxia leads to pulmonary vasoconstriction. This well known and often discussed phenomenon seems *quoad vitam* a local reflex mechanism to prevent perfusion of underventilated pulmonary segments. The underlying mechanism is not yet identified and I am not going into details, because this has already been discussed extensively by McMurtry *et al.*

B.   Pulmonary Vasospasm

Pulmonary vasoconstriction can occur without alveolar hypoxia. In patients with pulmonary hypertension, prolonged measurements of pulmonary artery pressure and pulmonary vascular resistance show a surprisingly variable hemodynamic pattern, suggesting intermittent vasoconstriction (1). The reasons for this vasoconstriction are not clear, and although many vasoactive substances have been identified in different animal experiments, their role in man is still not certain. It also seems that different receptors might be stimulated by one substance at the same time, thus leading either to vasoconstriction or vasodilatation or possibly no hemodynamic change. This has been shown for serotonin, where serotonin infusion into the human pulmonary circulation does not change the pulmonary pressures (2), whereas isolated pulmonary artery strips do contract with serotonin (3).

Spontaneous vasomotion in the normal pulmonary vascular bed has not yet been demonstrated. Patients with known vasoconstriction in other vascular beds have been investigated to look for pulmonary vasoconstriction after peripheral stimulation. Patients with Raynaud's disease and scleroderma did not show any changes in pulmonary hemodynamics (4). Recently, in our department patients with Prinzmetal angina have been exposed to a cold pressor test, and an increase in pulmonary vascular resistance has been demonstrated which could be prevented by Nifedipine (5).

C.   Endothelial Dysfunction or Damage

Normal endothelial cell function may be important for the low pressure system in the pulmonary vasculature. Toxic substances or metabolites could induce endothelial damage leading to activation of circulating cells. In the mouse, dietary-induced endothelial damage has been found in the systemic vasculature after ingestion of a high cholesterol diet (6). No direct changes have so far been reported in the pulmonary endothelium.

D.   Activation of Circulating Cells

Circulating cells could either be activated by damaged endothelium or by endogenous influences. Extracorporeally circulating blood reperfused into isolated perfused lungs resulted in the elevation of pulmonary vascular resistance. This increase could be prevented by removal of leukocytes, or leukocytes and platelets, from the blood used as perfusate (7). The second interesting finding was that the primary site of pulmonary reactivity has to be in the precapillary bed. Perfusion with leukocyte- and platelet-poor blood did not change the baseline pulmonary vascular resistance, suggesting the key role for either one or both cells.

It also has been shown that leukocyte-aggregation in the lung injures pulmonary endothelium (8). Such changes could also be elicited by infusion of complement-activated plasma (9). Increased platelet deposition in the lung has been reported after intravenous injection of oleic acid (10). However, it is not clear from these experiments if the lung injury after oleic acid is mediated by platelets or if the platelet deposition is the result of lung injury.

Thrombocytopenia also occured in two-thirds of the patients with acute lung injury due to acute respiratory failure (11). Platelet lifespan was reduced and the turnover rate increased. Platelet sequestration was demonstrated in the lung, liver and spleen.

Again, it is not possible to say whether platelets cause or exacerbate acute lung disease. In patients with sudden death, platelet aggregates in the small pulmonary arteries have been found, and this was the main postmortem finding in these patients (12).

It also has been hypothesized that abnormal intrapulmonary platelet production might be a possible cause of vascular and lung disease (13).

E.   Blood Coagulation Changes

The question whether altered blood coagulation can lead to vascular changes resulting in pulmonary hypertension has not been answered. In Indian soldiers developing pulmonary hypertension at high altitude, an increase in platelet adhesiveness, platelet factor III, factor V and factor VIII was found, whereas all soldiers had an increase in fibrin activity and plasma fibrinogen (14). In these patients, however pulmonary pressures were not measured, so no direct correlation was possible and these findings might be nonspecific. Too many systems might interfere, and the role of the fibrinolytic system and especially of inhibitors has not yet been investigated.

The finding that the fibrinolytic activity did not increase after venous occlusion in patients with pulmonary hypertension (15) could be interpretated as evidence for endothelial dysfunction. This dysfunction could provide the predisposition needed for the development of pulmonary hypertension. In all these thoughts and speculations there remains one unsolved problem: are these vascular changes restricted to the pulmonary circulation, and if so,why?

III.   THE AMINOREX STORY

The evidence that anorectic substances like Aminorex can definitely be involved in the initiation of pulmonary vascular changes is in my opinion overwhelming. This is based on a clear-cut epidemiological relationship between the intake of Aminorex and the development of pulmonary hypertension (16). The evidence is not so clear regarding the number of tablets taken. In addition, the incidence of pulmonary hypertension without a history of anorectic drug intake also increased at that time in the three countries involved. Early lung biopsies showed endothelial proliferation with luminal obstruction (17). Postmortem findings showed histologically the typical picture of plexiform pulmonary arteriopathy, a finding of long-standing pulmonary hypertension, which is also found in cardiac shunt disorders with pulmonary hypertension (18).

Follow up studies showed an unpredictable course, even after withdrawal of the possible initiating agent (19, 10, 21). In some patients pulmonary hypertension was progressive, while in others normalisation was almost achieved, at least at rest. As a group, the patients with the lower pulmonary artery pressures at the time of diagnosis had a better prognosis than those with high pulmonary pressures (19). However, long-term survival was also possible with very high pulmonary pressures at the time of diagnosis. The initial high mortality decreased and long term follow up revealed a survival rate of about 45%, 10 years after the diagnosis was established (19). It seems, therefore, that Aminorex had some influence on the initiation but may not have been relevant for the long-term course of the pulmonary hypertension.

It makes the identification of the pathophysiological mechanism very difficult if we assume that the initiation of pulmonary hypertension was only possible because of the coincidental presence of some events like predisposition and activation of certain mechanisms. If, for example, the activating mechanism was not identified, or looked for, at the time of the diagnosis, it would no longer be possible to repeat this specific starting mechanism. The hypothesis that platelets might be the activating factor, leading to endothelial reaction followed by pulmonary hypertension (22), cannot be evaluated after Aminorex is withdrawn or even during Aminorex medication, if activation could have occurred only over a short time through coincidence of some additional factors. These factors could act like a trigger mechanism, with self-perpetuation. It was therefore not surprising that measures of platelet function like platelet aggregation (22), platelet factor IV and the levels of β thromboglobulin (23) were not different from normal controls. Platelet survival time was shortened and thromboxane B levels were increased (24), but we do not know if pulmonary hypertension itself changes these parameters. An interesting finding in these patients was that fibrinolytic activity was impaired in about 2/3 of patients showing no increase in fibrinolytic activity after venous occlusion (15). This could be interpreted as a marker of endothelial dysfunction. However, again it would be difficult to explain why a generalized endothelial dysfunction leads only to pulmonary vascular changes.

IV.   THE TOXIC OIL SYNDROME

In 1981 another epidemic occurred, this time in Spain, with development of a multisystemic disease. Over 20,000 patients have been officially reported as suffering from the so-called Toxic Oil Syndrome after consumption of a toxic cooking oil (25). Lopez Sendon reported at the last European Congress of Cardiology in 1984 (26) that in the second phase of the disease pulmonary hypertension became increasingly common. In addition to pulmonary hypertension, scleroderma-like skin lesions and alterations resembling systemic sclerosis have also been observed. Histological specimens taken from different organs showed endothelial lesions with swelling, cytoplasmatic vacuolation and necrosis of endothelial cells. Later, endothelial proliferation with lumen obstruction and, in advanced stages, obliterative fibrosis of the intima were the main histological findings.

As in the Aminorex cases the possible initiating agent — the toxic oil — was only the starting mechanism, and the disease progressed later on. The toxic component has not been identified and the way by which changes developed is unclear. The presence of pulmonary hypertension was more frequent in women and some familial incidence was present.

The initial atypical pneumonia was followed by a symptom-free interval. Then the patients presented with right heart failure and evidence of pulmonary hypertension. Pulmonary capillary wedge pressure was found to be normal, with an increase in pulmonary vascular resistance unrelated to hypoxia. At this stage of the disease, platelet abnormalities were found in nearly all patients studied. Platelet factor IV and β thromboglobulin were abnormally increased, compared to normal values in patients with toxic oil syndrome without pulmonary hypertension. As in the Aminorex story, endothelial lesions and platelet abnormalities may be responsible for the pulmonary hypertension either alone or in combination with other factors.

V.   DRUG AND DIETARY INDUCED PULMONARY HYPERTENSION

No substances have so far been identified which cause reproducible pulmonary vasoconstriction or pulmonary hypertension after oral intake. However, there are possible connections between some groups of substances and the finding of pulmonary hypertension. The question remains in all of them whether the intake and the pulmonary hypertension are coincidental findings or cause-effect related. At least in some cases the documentation is in favour of the latter, as for example in two cases of pulmonary hypertension after the intake of fenfluramine (27). Other anorectic substances have also been noted in the history of patients with pulmonary hypertension. None of these were withdrawn from the market like Aminorex, and no new cases of pulmonary hypertension have been reported in this regard.

Oral contraceptive drugs have been implicated in the development of pulmonary hypertension (28). It remains, however, unclear whether oral contraceptives might affect the pulmonary vasculature directly or only indirectly via thromboembolic disease. Taking into account the number of oral contraceptive drugs taken, the incidence of pulmonary hypertension is evidently rare in these individuals, thus making a direct link between drug intake and the development of pulmonary hypertension very unlikely.

The axis gut-liver-lung has been discussed, especially in view of the finding that pulmonary hypertension is found in patients with liver cirrhosis. If the escape of an otherwise metabolized agent is the missing link for the pulmonary vascular changes, no such substance has been identified. Individual susceptibility is again out of question, since only a few patients with severe liver disease develop pulmonary hypertension (29).

No examples of dietary-induced pulmonary hypertension are available in man. Only experimental pulmonary hypertension after feeding *Crotalaria spectabilis* or similar plants are well documented (30), and endothelial damage seems to be the starting point for the pulmonary vascular changes (31).

VI.   SUMMARY

Various forms of exogenously induced pulmonary hypertension might all be initiated by the same initial mechanism. This mechanism acts either alone or in combination with one or more predisposing factors. Which comes first - vasoconstriction or endothelial damage? Besides all these open questions, the main question for me is, if endothelial interaction with, for example, platelets or other circulated cells, is the starting process, why is it restricted only to the pulmonary vascular bed? Is the predisposing factor restricted to the lung?

In our present understanding only the initiation seems possible. There are no indicators that the course of pulmonary hypertension can be altered by exogenous factors, other than hypoxia, or that pulmonary hypertension might be reversible if these influences are withdrawn.

A prolonged maintenance of pulmonary hypertension by exogenous means only seems unlikely because pulmonary vascular changes probably occur as a result of the pulmonary hypertension. However, the finding that vasodilators like prostacyclin reduce the pulmonary vascular resistance in patients with longstanding pulmonary hypertension showed that, at least to some degree, potentially reversible vasoconstriction is present (32). Until we know more, the words of Fishman are still valid: "The prospects are tantalizing, but further speculation would at this point simply be an exercise in fantasy (29)."

REFERENCES

1. Rich ST, D'Alonzo GE, Dantzker DR, and Levy PS. (1985) *Am J Cardiol* **55**:159.
2. Grover RF, Olson SK and Blount SG. (1958) *Clin Res* **6**:62.
3. Gillis CN and Pitt BR. (1982)*Ann Rev Physiol* **44**:269.
4. Shuck JW, Oetgen WJ and Tesar JT. (1985) *Amer J Med* **78**:221.
5. Stefenelli T. (submitted).
6. Davenport WD and Ball CR. (1981)*Atherosclerosis* **40**:145.
7. Van Zandwijk N, Lenssen FTJ, Van der Meer J, Wagenvoort CA and Groen AS. (1979)*Europ Surg Res* **11**:301.
8. Malik AB, Johnson A and Blumenstock FA. (1983)*Gen Pharmac* **14**:200.
9. Hohn DC, Meyers AJ, Gherini ST, Beckmann A, Markison RE and Churg AM. (1980) *Surgery* **88**:48.
10. Spragg RG, Abraham JL and Loomis W.H. (1982) *Amer Rev Respir Dis* **126**:553.
11. Schneider RC, Zapol WM and Carvalho AC. (1980) *Amer Rev Respir Dis* **122**:445.
12. Birkle H. (1974) *Science* **185**:1062.
13. Martin JF, Slater DN and Trowbridge EA. (1983) *Lancet* **i**:793.
14. Singh I and Chohan IS. (1972) *Brit Heart J* **34**:611.
15. Fuchs J, Mlczoch J, Niessner H and Lechner L. (1981) *Europ Heart J* **2**(suppl A):169.
16. Gurtner HP. (1985) *Schweiz med Wschr* **115**:782.
17. Obiditsch-Mayer I. (1969) Wien Z Inn Med., **50**:486.
18. Wagenvoort CA and Wagenvoort N. (1977) **Pathology of Pulmonary Hypertension.** John Wiley & Sons:New York.
19. Mlczoch J, Probst P, Szeless St and Kaindl F. (1980) *Cor Vasa* **22**(4):251.
20. Voss H, Feigel H and Bücking J. (1983)*Z Kardiol* **72**:215.
21. Turina J, Wirz P and Krayenbühl HP. (1977)*Schweiz med Wschr* **49**:107.
22. Mlczoch J. (1980) *Acta Med Austriaca* **Suppl 9**:1.
23. Mlczoch J, Schernthaner G, Mühlhauser I, Silberbauer K. (1981) *Z Kardiol* **70**:837.
24. Mlczoch J, Sinzinger H. (1983)*Europ Heart J* **4**(suppl. E):30.
25. Garcia-Dorado D, Miller D, Garcia EJ, Delcan JL, Maroto E and Chaitman BR. (1983) *J Am Coll Cardiol* **1**(5):1216.
26. Lopez Sendon J. (1984) Lecture Europ Congr of Cardiol Düsseldorf.

27. Douglas JG, Munro JF, Kitchin AH, Mdir AL and Proudfoot AT. (1981) *Brit Med J* **283**:881.

28. Kleiger RE, Boxer M, Ingham RE and Harrison DC. (1976) *Chest* **69**:143.

29. Fishman AP. (1974) *Circulation Research* **35**:657.

30. Heath D and Smith P. (1977) *Medical Clinics of North America* **61**:1279.

31. Sugita Takash, Hyers TM, Dauber IM, Wagner WW, McMurtry IF and Reeves JT. (1983) *J Appl Physiol* **54**:371.

Index